COVID-19 Critical and Intensive Care Medicine Essentials

Denise Battaglini • Paolo Pelosi
Editors

COVID-19 Critical and Intensive Care Medicine Essentials

Springer

Editors
Denise Battaglini
Anesthesia and Critical Care Unit
Ospedale San Martino
Genova, Italy

Paolo Pelosi
Anesthesia and Critical Care
Ospedale San Martino
Genoa, Italy

ISBN 978-3-030-94991-4 ISBN 978-3-030-94992-1 (eBook)
https://doi.org/10.1007/978-3-030-94992-1

This Springer imprint is published by the registered company Springer Nature Switzerland AG
The registered company address is: Gewerbestrasse 11, 6330 Cham, Switzerland

Contents

About the Editors

Denise Battaglini is Consultant in Intensive Care and research assistant at San Martino Policlinico Hospital, Genoa, Italy. Dr. Battaglini is attending a PhD in Translational Medicine at the University of Barcelona, Spain. She attended two research fellowships in pneumonia and respiratory physiotherapy at the University of Barcelona, Spain, and in neurological and pulmonary critical care at Federal University of Rio de Janeiro, Brazil. Further, Dr. Denise Battaglini is serving representative roles for the Italian Society of Anaesthesia, Analgesia, Reanimation, and Intensive Care (SIAARTI) and European Society of Intensive Care Medicine (ESICM). She was former national representative of young Anaesthesiologists and Intensivists in SIAARTI and member of national representatives of the European Society of Anaesthesiology (ESA). She is involved in several research projects regarding critical care management of patients with COVID-19, pulmonary diseases, and neurocritical care. Her actual research interests include pulmonary critical care, neurointensive care, and translational medicine.

Paolo Pelosi is the Director of Anaesthesia and Intensive Care as well as Regional Poison Control Center at San Martino Policlinico Hospital, IRCCS for Oncology and Neurosciences, Genoa, Italy. Prof. Pelosi is also the Director of the Specialty School in Anesthesiology, Reanimation, Critical Care and Pain Medicine at the University of Genoa, Italy. He was former president of the European Society of Anaesthesiology (ESA), former president of

Italian College of Professors in Anesthesiology and Critical Care (CPAR), and the president elect of the Italian Society of Anaesthesia, Analgesia, Reanimation, and Intensive Care (SIAARTI). Prof. Pelosi was a Fellow of the European Respiratory Society (FERS) and Fellow of the European Society of Anaesthesiology and Intensive Care (FESAIC). He published more than 750 original papers.

Part I

Fundamentals of COVID-19

1 Essential Multiorgan Pathophysiology of COVID-19

Denise Battaglini and Paolo Pelosi

1.1 Introduction

In late December 2019, an outbreak caused by severe acute respiratory syndrome coronavirus 2 (SARS-CoV-2) started from the city of Wuhan, China and rapidly spread worldwide. Despite global efforts to contain the pandemic, as halfway through the year 2021, the pandemic is still far from being over [1]. Typical manifestations of coronavirus disease-2019 (COVID-19) include mild-to-moderate "flu-like" symptoms, although more severe manifestations have been reported [2]. The pathophysiology of COVID-19 is complex, and its clinical spectrum might not be limited to local pneumonia, but rather may represent a multisystem

D. Battaglini (✉)
Anesthesia and Intensive Care, San Martino Policlinico Hospital, IRCCS for Oncology and Neuroscience, Genoa, Italy

Department of Medicine, University of Barcelona, Barcelona, Spain

P. Pelosi
Anesthesia and Intensive Care, San Martino Policlinico Hospital, IRCCS for Oncology and Neuroscience, Genoa, Italy

Department of Surgical Sciences and Integrated Diagnostics, University of Genoa, Genoa, Italy

D. Battaglini, P. Pelosi (eds.), *COVID-19 Critical and Intensive Care Medicine Essentials*, https://doi.org/10.1007/978-3-030-94992-1_1

illness with potential for severe acute respiratory distress syndrome (ARDS) and multiorgan impairment [3].

In this context, the aim of the present handbook is to provide an overview of possible multisystemic manifestations and therapeutic strategies, in order to guide the clinician to deal with COVID-19 critical illness and to prevent potential systemic consequences.

1.2 Structure of SARS-CoV-2 Host Cell Infection and Systemic Replication

The SARS-CoV-2 is an enveloped single-stranded ribonucleic acid (RNA) virus belonging to the β-coronavirus genus. The 70% of SARS-CoV-2 viral genome is composed of two open-reading frames with several conserved nonstructural protein sequences [4]. Two polypeptides are encoded between these open reading frames, and processed by viral proteases to produce nonstructural proteins, which are involved in replication and suppression of host innate immune defenses [4]. The SARS-CoV-2 is composed of four main structural proteins: the spike (S), envelope (E), membrane glycoproteins (M), and the nucleocapsid protein (N). The nucleocapsid protein N is a phosphorylated protein that directly binds to viral RNA. The E glycoprotein is an integral membrane structure that is involved in the maturation and pathogenesis of coronaviruses, while the M glycoprotein plays a key role in viral assembly and delineates the shape of the viral envelope. The S glycoprotein is a transmembrane structure present in the surface of the virus and composed by two functionally distinct subunits (S1 and S2) that are cleaved by the cell proteases of the host. The S1 subunit (N-terminal), which contains the receptor-binding motif [5], is released during the fusion process and changes the conformation of the S2 subunit (composed by fusion peptide, heptad repeat 1 and 2, and the transmembrane domains) [4, 5]. Upon anchoring the S proteins, SARS-CoV-2 recognizes ACE2, that is a component of the renin–angiotensin–aldosterone system (RAAS), and binds to its receptor, therefore fusing its membrane and activating entry-proteases (including TMPRSS2) and cathepsins B and L [5, 6] for entry into host cells. Once entering the cells, SARS-CoV-2 reduces surface tissue expression of ACE2 and inhibits the RNA expression. ACE2 is expressed in several cells that are infected by SARS-CoV-2 via several mechanisms: (1) direct pathological damage induced by the virus, (2) dysregulation of immune response, (3) ACE2 downregulation and dysregulation of the RAAS system, (4) direct endothelial cell damage, and (5) fibrosis [4].

All these mechanisms are responsible of the activation of the host immune response to viruses. Notably, the coronavirus S protein is responsible of conformational changes and membrane fusion processes that make this mechanism a target of innate and adaptive immune responses [5]. Following entry into host cells, SARS-CoV-2 replicates at the site of infection. The open reading frames 1a and 1b produces two polyproteins (pp1a and pp1b) that in turn release 16 nonstructural proteins that are implied in proteolytic processing, RNA synthesis, RNA proofreading, and RNA modification [5]. At this point in the host, neutrophils are rapidly recruited to the site of infection, while innate cells recognize viral replication and secrete cytokines. In turn, viral antigens are recognized by antigen-presenting cells and carried to the local lymph nodes, thus activating T helper cell response, that is also responsible of recalling B cells to secrete antibodies [7]. The activation of a systemic immune response is therefore predictable, with possible disease progression and multisystem illness with involvement of different organs and potential for multisystemic complications [8], Fig. 1.1.

1.3 Respiratory System

The lung is the primarily affected organ and initial reservoir of SARS-CoV-2 because of its large surface area and highly vascularization, thus allowing for systemic dissemination. SARS-CoV-2 enters via ACE2 that are expressed in various cell types and the respiratory tract (mucosal membranes, alveolar epithelial cells, nasal surface) [4]. Upon SARS-CoV-2 respiratory infection several symptoms have been recognized, varying from mild

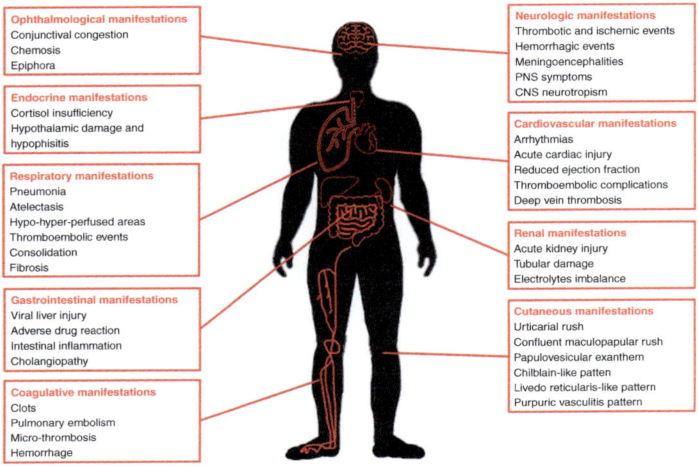

Fig. 1.1 Multisystem COVID-19 critical illness. Typical multiorgan manifestations of COVID-19. *CNS* central nervous system, *PNS* peripheral nervous system

illness characterized by fever, dry cough and tiredness to acute respiratory distress syndrome (ARDS) as the worst. Distinct phenotypes have been identified at computed tomography (CT) scan as possible different stages of the same disease [9, 10]. Gattinoni et al. [11] and Robba et al. [12] proposed the existence of 2 (H and L) or 3 phenotypes (1, 2, and 3), respectively. The phenotype L/1, which is characterized by low compliance, with impaired distribution of lung perfusion and shunting and focal hypo/overperfused ground-glass opacities; the phenotype 2, which is a transitional phase between the 1 and 3, and the phenotype H/3, which is characterized by inhomogeneously distributed atelectasis, patchy ARDS-like pattern. Finally, as proposed by Tonetti et al. [13] the phenotype F could be an evolution of mechanical stretch of lung epithelial cells with pathological fibro-proliferations. The identification of phenotypes represents a key strategy to individualize mechanical ventilation in patients with COVID-19. We described regional aeration and perfusion distribution in nonintubated and intubated patients with COVID-19 [14]. Phenotype/L1 is characterized by hypoxia mainly due to increased low/*V*/*Q* areas, less true shunt, with high *V*/*Q* and dead space, thus better responding to higher noninvasive respiratory support and higher inspiratory oxygen fractions. Noninvasive respiratory support should be cautiously used, especially in patients who do not improve within hours due to the potential occurrence of patients self-inflicted lung injury [15, 16]. Phenotype H/3 is characterized by hypoxia mainly due to increased true shunt, maintaining high *V*/*Q* and dead space, better to early intubation (within 2 days from hypoxia), moderate levels of positive end-expiratory pressure (PEEP), and prone position. In general, patients with COVID-19 requiring mechanical ventilation present relatively low recruitability and poor response to recruitment [17, 18].

1.4 Cardiovascular System

Cardiac injury during SARS-CoV-2 infection is very common, ranging from 7.2 to 22% in the intensive care unit (ICU) [19, 20]. Patients affected by cardiac injury reported older age, more cardiovascular comorbidities such as hypertension, higher leukocyte count, and pro-inflammatory response than patients without cardiovascular symptoms [19, 20]. Cardiac dysfunction in COVID-19 may present with acute cardiac injury, reduced ejection fraction, increased levels of troponins, heart attack, deep venous thrombosis, and thromboembolic complications. Moreover, patients with cardiovascular dysfunction are more likely to exhibit systemic complications, including electrolyte disbalance, coagulation disorders, and kidney injury, with a higher fatality rate. This suggests that patients should be strictly monitored for cardiac complications including bedside assessments of cardiac function, and the use of electrocardiogram, standard cardiac biomarkers like brain natriuretic peptide (BNP) and troponins that have shown prognostic values in the prevention of COVID-19 cardiovascular dysfunction [21]. Indeed, cardiac troponins were associated with higher mortality in elderly COVID-19 patients, although serial troponin testing did not add additional prognostic information [22].

1.5 Coagulation Disorders

SARS-CoV-2 binding to ACE2 receptors on the endothelial cells surface may lead to the activation of the coagulation and pro-inflammatory cascades due to the exposure of tissue factor and collagen to blood and release of von Willebrand factor (vWF) [23]. Platelets are exposed and recruited by adenosine monophosphate and vWF, followed by activation, aggregation, and plug formation. After activating the intrinsic and extrinsic pathways, and the common coagulation pathway, fibrin strands and stable fibrin clots are formed [23]. Coagulation derangements are associated with pro-inflammatory mechanisms and a high incidence of thromboembolic and hemorrhagic events. The clinical course of coagulation derangements may be dominated by thrombosis, bleeding, or both, with a high rate of pulmonary embolism and vasculitis [23]. Screening tests for coagulation disorders are highly recommended, including clinical evaluation, cardiac biomarkers, D-dimer, platelet count, fibrinogen, international normalized ratio (INR) or prothrombin, activated prothrombin time (aPTT) to monitor daily and associated with bedside ultrasound tests [23].

1.6 Kidney Injury

As for the direct action of SARS-CoV-2 on RAAS, the homeostasis of blood pressure and water–salt balance may be altered [24]. Renin acts by cleaving angiotensinogen and producing angiotensin I (Ang I) that is transformed to angiotensin II (Ang II). Ang II binds to two receptors (AT 1 and 2) that are implicated in several biological functions like vasoconstriction, blood pressure control, promotion of oxidative stress, and cell apoptosis. After SARS-CoV-2 binding to ACE2, the external domain of ACE2 is cleaved and the internal domain is internalized with downregulation and increased Ang II levels, that may lead to an increased pro-inflammatory storm [24]. Based on autopsy results, kidney damage resulted in proximal tubular injury, erythrocyte aggregation, and obstruction of peritubular capillary loops, interstitial edema, inflammatory infiltrates [24]. The glomerular involvement was limited mainly to patients with previous comorbidities such as diabetic nephropathy or hypertension. As for clinical manifestations, several patients reported hypocalcemia, hypokalemia, and hyponatremia, and in more severe cases acute renal failure, often requiring continuous renal replacement therapy [24]. Therefore, a daily evaluation of blood urea nitrogen, creatinine clearance, electrolyte status, and fluid balance in ICU COVID-19 patients should be pursued [4, 24].

1.7 Gastrointestinal System

ACE2 is also present in the luminal surface of intestinal epithelial cells, being responsible of amino acid uptake; it can be also found on cholangiocytes being responsible of possible virus-induced cytotoxicity [4]. Gastrointestinal symptoms are among the most common manifestations of SARS-CoV-2 infection following respiratory symptoms. Abdominal pain, nausea, diarrhea, and vomiting can be manifestations of direct gastrointestinal invasion. Also, altered liver function has been observed in several COVID-19 patients with altered bilirubin levels, aspartate aminotransferase and alanine aminotransferase, and γ-glutamyl transferase [4]. For this reason, the complete panel of tests of liver function should be periodically monitored as well as dietetic recommendations should be pursued [25]. Moreover, attention should be paid to gut microbiota dysbiosis in order to individualize nutritional treatment and systemic therapies. When poorly considered, this condition may lead to more vulnerability and an inappropriate response to critical circumstances [25].

1.8 Nervous System

Neurological manifestations of COVID-19 are more frequent than expected. Several mechanisms have been proposed for SARS-CoV-2 neurologic derangement, including (1) viral neurotropism,

(2) hyperinflammation and hypercoagulation, and (3) brain–lung crosstalk [16]. SARS-CoV-2 may pass through neurons of the olfactory bulb, causing virus spread across the blood–brain barrier and binding to endothelial cells. However, given the low proportion of patients with positive cerebrospinal fluid, this mechanism of action has been almost abandoned [16]. Rather, the theories of pro-inflammatory and pro-coagulative disorders and of brain–lung cross talk have proved to be more suitable for the underlying neurological conditions caused by SARS-CoV-2. Indeed, around 2.2% of COVID-19 patients experienced stroke [26], and especially those who undergo extracorporeal membrane oxygenation support that is a known risk factor of possible altered coagulative status. In a recent meta-analysis, the pooled prevalence of ischemic stroke was 2.8% in patients admitted to ICU [27], while the incidence of delirium was as much as 24.3% [28]. Besides, many other clinical neurological manifestations are possible during COVID-19 and a strategy including multimodal neuromonitoring at bedside should be highly recommended for monitoring neurologic function daily especially in patients who are paralyzed and mechanically ventilated and cannot be awaked for clinical reasons [29].

1.9 Other Manifestations

Cutaneous manifestations of COVID-19 have been distinguished in six main clinical patterns, including (1) urticarial rush, (2) confluent morbilliform maculopapular erythematous rush, (3) papulovesicular exanthem, (4) chilblain-like pattern, (5) livedo reticularis-like pattern, and (6) purpuric vasculitis pattern [30].

Again, endocrinological manifestations has been reported in several COVID-19 patients, these included molecular mimics to the host adrenocorticotropic hormone (ACTH), or direct infection with degeneration and necrosis of the adrenal gland, and ACE2 expression on the hypothalamic and pituitary tissues with direct damage and possible hypophysitis [31].

Finally, ophthalmological complications included conjunctival congestion, chemosis, or epiphora, and the ocular via has also been proposed as a possible transmission route of infection [31].

1.10 Conclusions

Although SARS-CoV-2 presents primarily with lower respiratory tract symptoms, increasing evidence suggests multiorgan involvement in patients who have been infected. The systemic involvement is guided mainly by the viral binding to ACE2 receptors that are located in several tissues. The more the organ involvement, the more the patient morbidity and mortality. A strategy comprising daily clinical and laboratory evaluation of patients at higher risk of systemic disease should be strictly recommended.

References

1. Wouters OJ, Shadlen KC, Salcher-Konrad M, et al. Challenges in ensuring global access to COVID-19 vaccines: production, affordability, allocation, and deployment. Lancet. 2021;397(10278):1023–34. https://doi.org/10.1016/S0140-6736(21)00306-8.
2. Nalbandian A, Sehgal K, Gupta A, et al. Post-acute COVID-19 syndrome. Nat Med. 2021;27(4):601–15. https://doi.org/10.1038/s41591-021-01283-z.
3. Robba C, Battaglini D, Pelosi P, Rocco PRM. Multiple organ dysfunction in SARS-CoV-2: MODS-CoV-2. Expert Rev Respir Med. 2020;14(9):865–8. https://doi.org/10.1080/17476348.2020.1778470.
4. Lopes-Pacheco M, Silva PL, Cruz FF, et al. Pathogenesis of multiple organ injury in COVID-19 and potential therapeutic strategies. Front Physiol. 2021;12:593223. https://doi.org/10.3389/fphys.2021.593223.
5. V'kovski P, Kratzel A, Steiner S, Stalder H, Thiel V. Coronavirus biology and replication: implications for SARS-CoV-2. Nat Rev Microbiol. 2021;19(3):155–70. https://doi.org/10.1038/s41579-020-00468-6.
6. Shang J, Wan Y, Luo C, et al. Cell entry mechanisms of SARS-CoV-2. Proc Natl Acad Sci. 2020;117(21):11727–34. https://doi.org/10.1073/pnas.2003138117.
7. Rouse BT, Sehrawat S. Immunity and immunopathology to viruses: what decides the outcome? Nat Rev Immunol. 2010;10(7):514–26. https://doi.org/10.1038/nri2802.

8. Hamming I, Timens W, Bulthuis M, Lely A, Navis G, van Goor H. Tissue distribution of ACE2 protein, the functional receptor for SARS coronavirus. A first step in understanding SARS pathogenesis. J Pathol. 2004;203(2):631–7. https://doi.org/10.1002/path.1570.
9. Orlandi D, Battaglini D, Robba C, et al. COVID-19 phenotypes, lung ultrasound, chest computed tomography, and clinical features in critically ill mechanically ventilated patients. Ultrasound Med Biol. 2021;47(12):3323–32. https://doi.org/10.1016/j.ultrasmedbio.2021.07.014.
10. Pelosi P, Ball L, Barbas CSV, et al. Personalized mechanical ventilation in acute respiratory distress syndrome. Crit Care. 2021;25(1):250. https://doi.org/10.1186/s13054-021-03686-3.
11. Gattinoni L, Chiumello D, Caironi P, et al. COVID-19 pneumonia: different respiratory treatments for different phenotypes? Intensive Care Med. 2020;46(6):1099–102. https://doi.org/10.1007/s00134-020-06033-2.
12. Robba C, Battaglini D, Ball L, et al. Distinct phenotypes require distinct respiratory management strategies in severe COVID-19. Respir Physiol Neurobiol. 2020;279:103455.
13. Tonelli R, Marchioni A, Tabbì L, et al. Spontaneous breathing and evolving phenotypes of lung damage in patients with COVID-19: review of current evidence and forecast of a new scenario. J Clin Med. 2021;10(5):975. https://doi.org/10.3390/jcm10050975.
14. Ball L, Robba C, Herrmann J, et al. Lung distribution of gas and blood volume in critically ill COVID-19 patients: a quantitative dual-energy computed tomography study. Crit Care. 2021;25(1):214. https://doi.org/10.1186/s13054-021-03610-9.
15. Battaglini D, Robba C, Ball L, et al. Noninvasive respiratory support and patient self-inflicted lung injury in COVID-19: a narrative review. Br J Anaesth. 2021;127(3):353–64. https://doi.org/10.1016/j.bja.2021.05.024.
16. Battaglini D, Brunetti I, Anania P, et al. Neurological manifestations of severe SARS-CoV-2 infection: potential mechanisms and implications of individualized mechanical ventilation settings. Front Neurol. 2020;11:845. https://doi.org/10.3389/fneur.2020.00845.
17. Ball L, Robba C, Maiello L, et al. Computed tomography assessment of PEEP-induced alveolar recruitment in patients with severe COVID-19 pneumonia. Crit Care. 2021;25(1):81. https://doi.org/10.1186/s13054-021-03477-w.
18. Robba C, Ball L, Battaglini D, et al. Early effects of ventilatory rescue therapies on systemic and cerebral oxygenation in mechanically ventilated COVID-19 patients with acute respiratory distress syndrome: a prospective observational study. Crit Care. 2021;25(1):111. https://doi.org/10.1186/s13054-021-03537-1.
19. Wang D, Hu B, Hu C, et al. Clinical characteristics of 138 hospitalized patients with 2019 novel Coronavirus-infected pneumonia in Wuhan, China. JAMA. 2020;323(11):1061. https://doi.org/10.1001/jama.2020.1585.

20. Shi S, Qin M, Shen B, et al. Association of cardiac injury with mortality in hospitalized patients with COVID-19 in Wuhan, China. JAMA Cardiol. 2020;5(7):802. https://doi.org/10.1001/jamacardio.2020.0950.
21. Li J-W, Han T-W, Woodward M, et al. The impact of 2019 novel coronavirus on heart injury: a systematic review and meta-analysis. Prog Cardiovasc Dis. 2020;63(4):518–24. https://doi.org/10.1016/j.pcad.2020.04.008.
22. De Marzo V, Di Biagio A, Della Bona R, et al. Prevalence and prognostic value of cardiac troponin in elderly patients hospitalized for COVID-19. J Geriatr Cardiol. 2021;18(5):338–45. https://doi.org/10.11909/j.issn.1671-5411.2021.05.004.
23. Robba C, Battaglini D, Ball L, et al. Coagulative disorders in critically ill COVID-19 patients with acute distress respiratory syndrome: a critical review. J Clin Med. 2021;10(1):140. https://doi.org/10.3390/jcm10010140.
24. Wang M, Xiong H, Chen H, Li Q, Ruan XZ. Renal injury by SARS-CoV-2 infection: a systematic review. Kidney Dis. 2020;16:1–11. https://doi.org/10.1159/000512683.
25. Battaglini D, Robba C, Fedele A, et al. The role of dysbiosis in critically ill patients with COVID-19 and acute respiratory distress syndrome. Front Med. 2021;8:671714. https://doi.org/10.3389/fmed.2021.671714.
26. Cho S-M, Premraj L, Fanning J, et al. Ischemic and hemorrhagic stroke among critically ill patients with Coronavirus disease 2019 Critical Care Consortium Study. Crit Care Med. 2021;49(12):e1223. https://doi.org/10.1097/CCM.0000000000005209.
27. Huth SF, Cho S-M, Robba C, et al. Neurological manifestations of Coronavirus disease 2019: a comprehensive review and meta-analysis of the first 6 months of pandemic reporting. Front Neurol. 2021;12:664599. https://doi.org/10.3389/fneur.2021.664599.
28. Shao S-C, Lai C-C, Chen Y-H, Chen Y-C, Hung M-J, Liao S-C. Prevalence, incidence and mortality of delirium in patients with COVID-19: a systematic review and meta-analysis. Age Ageing. 2021;50(5):1445–53. https://doi.org/10.1093/ageing/afab103.
29. Battaglini D, Santori G, Chandraptham K, et al. Neurological complications and noninvasive multimodal neuromonitoring in critically ill mechanically ventilated COVID-19 patients. Front Neurol. 2020;11:602114. https://doi.org/10.3389/fneur.2020.602114.
30. Genovese G, Moltrasio C, Berti E, Marzano AV. Skin manifestations associated with COVID-19: current knowledge and future perspectives. Dermatology. 2021;237(1):1–12. https://doi.org/10.1159/000512932.
31. Gavriatopoulou M, Korompoki E, Fotiou D, et al. Organ-specific manifestations of COVID-19 infection. Clin Exp Med. 2020;20(4):493–506. https://doi.org/10.1007/s10238-020-00648-x.

Part II

Pneumological Critical Care of COVID-19

2 Clinical Presentation and Phenotypes in COVID-19

Roberto Boccafogli, Chiara Robba, and Lorenzo Ball

2.1 Introduction

Since the beginning of the COVID-19 pandemic, clinicians have highlighted the existence of different clinical presentations of the disease [1, 2]. The presence of a broad spectrum of respiratory compromise has been initially interpreted as the manifestation of different clinical phenotypes, with peculiar pathophysiological aspects translating into different requirements of respiratory support. The exceptional circumstances under which early research was performed resulted in several hypotheses based on pathophysiological reasoning, observation of case series, and autoptic

R. Boccafogli
Department of Surgical Sciences and Integrated Diagnostics (DISC), University of Genoa, Genoa, Italy

C. Robba · L. Ball (✉)
Department of Surgical Sciences and Integrated Diagnostics (DISC), University of Genoa, Genoa, Italy

Anesthesia and Intensive Care, Ospedale Policlinico San Martino, IRCCS per l'Oncologia e le Neuroscienze, Genoa, Italy
e-mail: lorenzo.ball@unige.it

D. Battaglini, P. Pelosi (eds.), *COVID-19 Critical and Intensive Care Medicine Essentials*, https://doi.org/10.1007/978-3-030-94992-1_2

studies. Based on the available evidence, COVID-19 phenotypes should be interpreted as different radiological and clinical patterns explained by an evolving spectrum of manifestations depending on the interaction of direct viral action, host inflammatory response, patient comorbidities and physical status, and the time elapsed from the onset of symptoms [3, 4].

This chapter discusses the classification of COVID-19 phenotypes based on imaging and respiratory mechanics parameters, also in relation with the differences and similarities with the acute respiratory distress syndrome (ARDS) from causes other than COVID-19.

2.2 Definition of Phenotypes

The first report [1] identified two extreme conditions, "non-ARDS COVID-19" or "type L" phenotype and "ARDS type" or "type H." The letters L and H refer to the respiratory system elastance, which is Low in the L Type and High in the H type. Another research group [2] proposed a numbered classification ranging from 1, corresponding to the L Type to 3, corresponding to the H type. According to this classification, phenotype 2 represents a commonly seen mixed pattern where different lung regions present radiographic characteristics of both phenotypes 1/L and 3/H. A later report [5] hypothesized the existence of a late phenotype with predominantly fibrotic characteristics, named Type F phenotype. Figures 2.1 and 2.2 illustrate the most relevant characteristics of the phenotypes discussed in this chapter.

2.2.1 Phenotype L (or Phenotype 1)

Phenotype L/1 is the earliest stage of COVID-19 pneumonia. While most patients with mild respiratory failure presenting with this early clinical manifestation will recover either spontaneously or with the implementation of antiviral and immunomodulatory

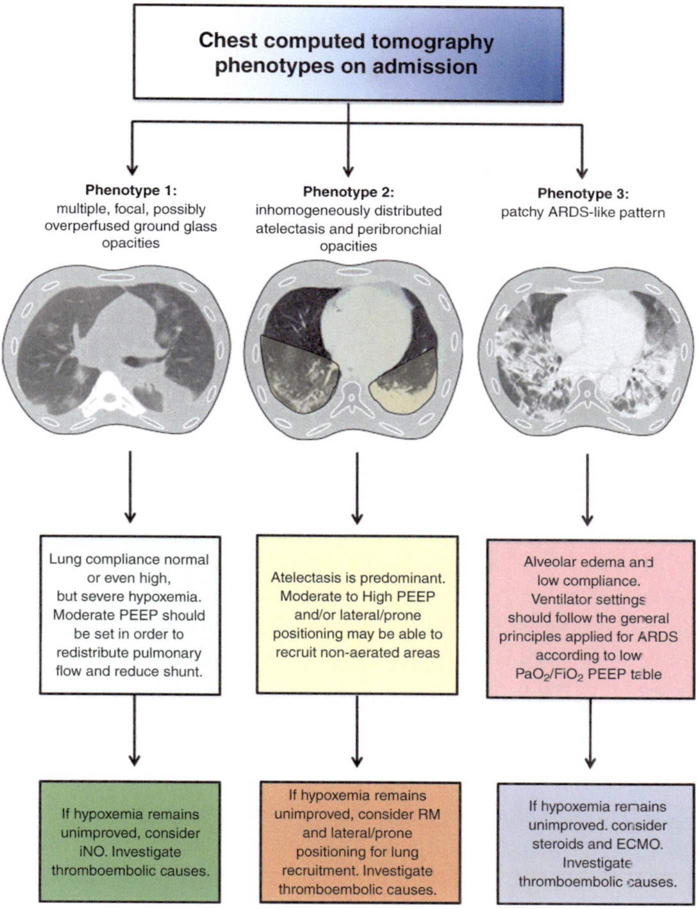

Fig. 2.1 Phenotypes 1, 2 and 3. Phenotype 1 and 3 correspond 3 to phenotype L and H according to Gattinoni [1], respectively. (Reproduced with permission from [2]). This illustration was published before the results of the RECOVERY trial, the indications for steroid therapy was thereafter extended to all COVID-19 patients requiring oxygen administration or higher degree of respiratory support

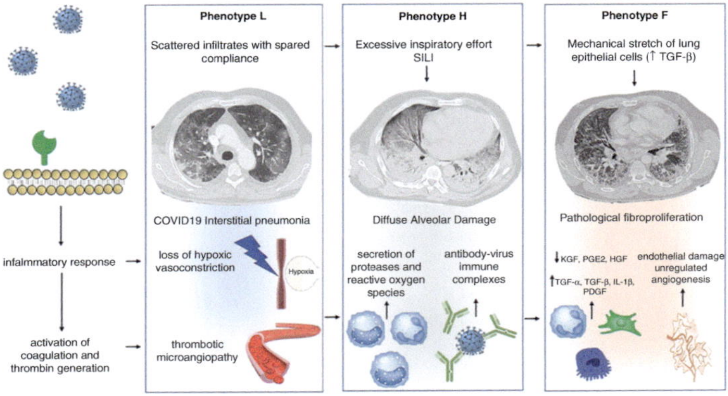

Fig. 2.2 Phenotypes L, H, and F according to the definitions of Gattinoni [1] and Tonelli [5]. (Reproduced from [5] under the Creative Commons Attribution CC BY license (https://creativecommons.org/licenses/by/4.0/))

therapy, in a certain proportion of patients this pattern could evolve to more advanced involvement of the respiratory function, typical of other phenotypes. This phase, or phenotype, of the disease has peculiar features that might deserve attention for the clinician. Computed tomography (CT) findings do not show atelectasis, but rather focal or diffuse ground-glass opacities, primarily located below the visceral pleura and along lung scissures [6]. The lung weight might be normal or only slightly increased [1, 7], suggesting the predominance of ground-glass over edema. As the main determinant of lung elastic properties is loss of aeration and lung collapse, these CT findings are reflected by preserved or low (i.e., only mildly increased) respiratory system elastance. Despite the small extension of atelectasis and nonaerated regions, which are the main determinants of gas exchange in conventional ARDS, these patients might have moderate-to-severe hypoxemia. This could be explained by an impairment of hypoxic vasoconstriction: ground-glass regions receive proportionally more perfusion than ventilation, resulting in low ventilation to perfusion (VA/Q) ratio contributing to venous admixture and hypoxemia [1]. Therefore, this stage of the disease is characterized by marked decoupling of oxygenation impairment from respiratory mechanics compromise. The physiologic response to hypoxemia is increased tidal volume and minute ventilation [8], but since these patients have near normal compliance, the inspiratory effort might only be marginally increased. As dyspnea is importantly affected by respiratory drive and the need of increasing the inspiratory effort, some of these patients can present with severe hypoxemia without dyspnea, a phenomenon that has been referred to as "happy hypoxemia" [9]. These mechanisms were observed during the first pandemic surge and subsequently subject to extensive investigation. Several physiological studies confirmed the presence of large areas of low VA/*Q* especially in earlier stages of the disease [10, 11] and an inspiratory effort lower than that of patients with acute respiratory failure from other causes [12].

The respiratory management of patients in this stage remains controversial, especially when conventional oxygen therapy fails in maintaining adequate oxygenation. High-flow nasal oxygen have been widely used in these patients for their ability to deliver a high fraction of inspired oxygen throughout the respiratory cycle [13]. Positive-pressure respiratory support, either delivered as continuous positive airway pressure (CPAP) or bilevel noninvasive ventilation (NIV) has also been extensively used. However, in the context of low extension of atelectasis, improvement of oxygenation might be explained by redistribution of blood flow rather than recruitment, and transpulmonary pressures might be increased compared to spontaneous breathing [12]. While prompt intubation had been proposed at the beginning of the pandemic, its risk–benefit profile has been questioned in the earliest stages of the disease [14].

While understanding the pathophysiological mechanisms underlying phenotype L/1 is crucial for a thorough comprehension of COVID-19, it must be stressed that most patients admitted to the hospital present with later evolutive phases of the disease, as detailed in the following paragraphs.

2.2.2 Phenotype 2

Phenotype 1/L might persist, resolve, or worsen. Mechanisms of worsening include host inflammatory response [3], increased alveolar capillary membrane permeability, and the exposure of lungs to negative intrathoracic pressures due to increased respiratory drive [2]. Patients with phenotype 2 present CT findings including ground-glass opacities overlapping with regions of atelectasis, especially in the dorsal regions (Fig. 2.2). Increased respiratory drive, applied to lungs with worsening elastance, might promote patient self-inflicted lung injury (P-SILI) [15]. Since both CPAP and NIV could potentially increase transpulmonary pressures, noninvasive respiratory support, while of sure value in improving oxygenation, might contribute to worsening of lung injury [12]. Patients receiving noninvasive support should be monitored for sign of increased respiratory drive and tachypnea and intubation should not be delayed when necessary. The gold standard for assessment of respiratory effort remains the measurement of esophageal pressure, which is underused [16], requires expertise and poses challenges in spontaneously breathing patients related to the need of positioning an esophageal balloon. Therefore, adequate monitoring of patients receiving noninvasive respiratory support might be challenging, especially when intensive care resources are overwhelmed during the pandemic surges.

2.2.3 Phenotype H (or Phenotype 3)

The most advanced acute phase of COVID-19 pneumonia is represented by phenotype H/3. As illustrated in Fig. 2.1, this phenotype is characterized at the CT scan by a typical patchy ARDS-like pattern, with large areas of ground glass overlapping to relevant amounts of atelectasis, further increased as compared to phenotype 2. Nonaerated lung tissue is predominantly located in the dorsal and caudal regions [7], as occurs in ARDS from causes other than COVID-19. When this ARDS-like pattern is established, respiratory system compliance is often low as in conventional ARDS [17]. However, when compared to historical cohorts of ARDS patients, intubated COVID-19 patients have a slightly higher respiratory system compliance [18]. Moreover, a matched-control study comparing patients with COVID-19 with ARDS patients with similar compliance, COVID-19 patients had more severe hypoxia [19]. This could be explained by the coexistence of ground glass regions characterized by high VA/Q with nonaerated regions with right-to-left true shunt, as suggested by the findings of a recent study based on dual-energy computed tomography, a technique able to study the distribution of lung aeration and perfusion in vivo [11]. Lung weight in phenotype 3 is markedly increased, similarly to conventional ARDS [1, 7]. In these patients, higher positive end-expiratory pressure (PEEP) could improve the respiratory function recruiting nonaerated regions. However, studies reported a high variability in response to PEEP in terms of recruitment [7, 10, 20] and a tendency toward worsening of respiratory system compliance and partial tension of carbon dioxide ($PaCO_2$) at higher PEEP [7, 20]. This advanced phase of the disease is also characterized by severe pulmonary coagulopathy, with a high incidence of pulmonary embolism and microthrombosis, a finding that constitutes the pathophysiological rationale for using higher doses of antithrombotic drugs, with dosing higher than those used for routine thromboprophylaxis in critically ill patients [21]. Also accounting for these peculiar aspects of COVID-19 related ARDS, most of these patients were managed with protective ventilation strategies derived from conventional ARDS protocols [17].

2.2.4 Phenotype F

Patients receiving prolonged mechanical ventilation for severe COVID-19 pneumonia often develop signs of radiological lung fibrosis [5]. Figure 2.2 illustrates the potential mechanisms underlying the transition from phenotype L/1 to H/3 and finally to a fibrotic phenotype F. These patients are at high risk of developing established fibrosis, a potentially irreversible condition. Of notice, a study in postmortem lung biopsies found that radiological pseudofibrotic findings are not necessarily associated with increased collagen deposition, a hallmark of histological fibrosis, suggesting that CT finding might overestimate the severity of fibrotic progression [22]. This could explain why most survivors still improve their respiratory function over time after discharge from the intensive care unit.

2.3 Clinical Message and Conclusions

COVID-19 pneumonia is characterized by a time-dependent evolution and peculiar pathophysiological aspects that have important clinical implications. Further research is necessary to better clarify the optimal pharmacological treatment and respiratory support in these patients.

Financial Support and Sponsorship None.

References

1. Gattinoni L, Chiumello D, Caironi P, Busana M, Romitti F, Brazzi L, Camporota L. COVID-19 pneumonia: different respiratory treatments for different phenotypes? Intensive Care Med. 2020;46(6):1099–102. https://doi.org/10.1007/s00134-020-06033-2.
2. Robba C, Battaglini D, Ball L, Patroniti N, Loconte M, Brunetti I, Vena A, Giacobbe DR, Bassetti M, Rocco PRM, et al. Distinct phenotypes require distinct respiratory management strategies in severe COVID-19. Respir Physiol Neurobiol. 2020;279:103455.
3. Gandhi RT, Lynch JB, del Rio C. Mild or moderate Covid-19. N Engl J Med. 2020;383:1757–66.
4. Berlin DA, Gulick RM, Martinez FJ. Severe Covid-19. N Engl J Med. 2020;383:2451–60.
5. Tonelli R, Marchioni A, Tabbì L, Fantini R, Busani S, Castaniere I, Andrisani D, Gozzi F, Bruzzi G, Manicardi L, et al. Spontaneous breathing and evolving phenotypes of lung damage in patients with COVID-19: review of current evidence and forecast of a new scenario. J Clin Med. 2021;10:975.
6. Inui S, Fujikawa A, Jitsu M, Kunishima N, Watanabe S, Suzuki Y, Umeda S, Uwabe Y. Chest CT findings in cases from the cruise ship "Diamond Princess" with Coronavirus Disease 2019 (COVID-19). Radiol Cardiothorac Imaging. 2020;2:e200110.
7. Ball L, Robba C, Maiello L, Herrmann J, Gerard SE, Xin Y, Battaglini D, Brunetti I, Minetti G, Seitun S, et al. Computed tomography assessment of PEEP-induced alveolar recruitment in patients with severe COVID-19 pneumonia. Crit Care. 2021;25:81.
8. Vaporidi K, Akoumianaki E, Telias I, Goligher EC, Brochard L, Georgopoulos D. Respiratory drive in critically ill patients. Pathophysiology and clinical implications. Am J Respir Crit Care Med. 2020;201:20–32.

9. Dhont S, Derom E, Van Braeckel E, Depuydt P, Lambrecht BN. The pathophysiology of "happy" hypoxemia in COVID-19. Respir Res. 2020;21:198.
10. Mauri T, Spinelli E, Scotti E, Colussi G, Basile MC, Crotti S, Tubiolo D, Tagliabue P, Zanella A, Grasselli G, et al. Potential for lung recruitment and ventilation–perfusion mismatch in patients with the acute respiratory distress syndrome from Coronavirus Disease 2019. Crit Care Med. 2020;48(8):1129. https://doi.org/10.1097/CCM.0000000000004386.
11. Ball L, Robba C, Herrmann J, Gerard SE, Xin Y, Mandelli M, Battaglini D, Brunetti I, Minetti G, Seitun S, et al. Lung distribution of gas and blood volume in critically ill COVID-19 patients: a quantitative dual-energy computed tomography study. Crit Care. 2021;25:214.
12. Tonelli R, Busani S, Tabbì L, Fantini R, Castaniere I, Biagioni E, Mussini C, Girardis M, Clini E, Marchioni A. Inspiratory effort and lung mechanics in spontaneously breathing patients with acute respiratory failure due to COVID-19: a matched control study. Am J Respir Crit Care Med. 2021;204:725–8.
13. Agarwal A, Basmaji J, Muttalib F, Granton D, Chaudhuri D, Chetan D, Hu M, Fernando SM, Honarmand K, Bakaa L, et al. High-flow nasal cannula for acute hypoxemic respiratory failure in patients with COVID-19: systematic reviews of effectiveness and its risks of aerosolization, dispersion, and infection transmission. Can J Anaesth. 2020;67:1217–48.
14. Tobin MJ, Laghi F, Jubran A. Caution about early intubation and mechanical ventilation in COVID-19. Ann Intensive Care. 2020;10:78.
15. Battaglini D, Robba C, Ball L, Silva PL, Cruz FF, Pelosi P, Rocco PRM. Noninvasive respiratory support and patient self-inflicted lung injury in COVID-19: a narrative review. Br J Anaesth. 2021;127:353–64.
16. Akoumianaki E, Maggiore SM, Valenza F, Bellani G, Jubran A, Loring SH, Pelosi P, Talmor D, Grasso S, Chiumello D, et al. The application of esophageal pressure measurement in patients with respiratory failure. Am J Respir Crit Care Med. 2014;189:520–31.
17. Botta M, Tsonas AM, Pillay J, Boers LS, Algera AG, Bos LDJ, Dongelmans DA, Hollmann MW, Horn J, Vlaar APJ, et al. Ventilation management and clinical outcomes in invasively ventilated patients with COVID-19 (PRoVENT-COVID): a national, multicentre, observational cohort study. Lancet Respir Med. 2021;9:139–48.
18. Grasselli G, Tonetti T, Protti A, Langer T, Girardis M, Bellani G, Laffey J, Carrafiello G, Carsana L, Rizzuto C, et al. Pathophysiology of COVID-19-associated acute respiratory distress syndrome: a multicentre prospective observational study. Lancet Respir Med. 2020;8(12):1201–8. https://doi.org/10.1016/S2213-2600(20)30370-2.
19. Chiumello D, Busana M, Coppola S, Romitti F, Formenti P, Bonifazi M, Pozzi T, Palumbo MM, Cressoni M, Herrmann P, et al. Physiological and quantitative CT-scan characterization of COVID-19 and typical ARDS: a

matched cohort study. Intensive Care Med. 2020;46(12):2187–96. https://doi.org/10.1007/s00134-020-06281-2.

20. Protti A, Santini A, Pennati F, Chiurazzi C, Cressoni M, Ferrari M, Iapichino GE, Carenzo L, Lanza E, Picardo G, et al. Lung response to a higher positive end-expiratory pressure in mechanically ventilated patients with COVID-19. Chest. 2021;161(4):979–88. https://doi.org/10.1016/j.chest.2021.10.012.
21. Lavinio A, Ercole A, Battaglini D, Magnoni S, Badenes R, Taccone FS, Helbok R, Thomas W, Pelosi P, Robba C, et al. Safety profile of enhanced thromboprophylaxis strategies for critically ill COVID-19 patients during the first wave of the pandemic: observational report from 28 European intensive care units. Crit Care. 2021;25:155.
22. Ball L, Barisione E, Mastracci L, Campora M, Costa D, Robba C, Battaglini D, Micali M, Costantino F, Cittadini G, et al. Extension of collagen deposition in COVID-19 post mortem lung samples and computed tomography analysis findings. Int J Mol Sci. 2021;22:7498.

3 Radiological Patterns and Lung Ultrasound

Davide Orlandi, Denise Battaglini,
Ezio Lanza, and Giulio Bergamaschi

3.1 Introduction

The early diagnosis of coronavirus disease 2019 (COVID-19) is one of the crucial points in order to reduce virus spread, also containing morbidity and mortality of the pandemic. Despite the utility of specific molecular tests (such as real time polymerase chain reaction, RT-PCR), imaging is considered one of the key strategies for an early diagnostic typing of the disease, and to individualize patient management [1–3].

D. Orlandi · G. Bergamaschi
Department of Radiology, Ospedale Evangelico Internazionale, Genoa, Italy

D. Battaglini (✉)
Anesthesia and Intensive Care, San Martino Policlinico Hospital, IRCCS for Oncology and Neurosciences, Genoa, Italy

E. Lanza
Department of Radiology, IRCCS Humanitas Research Hospital, Milan, Italy

D. Battaglini, P. Pelosi (eds.), *COVID-19 Critical and Intensive Care Medicine Essentials*, https://doi.org/10.1007/978-3-030-94992-1_3

3.1.1 Imaging Strategy

The presence of respiratory failure, confirmed of coronavirus-2 infection by molecular diagnostic test, and a detrimental blood gas analysis represent the main discriminating parameters to hospitalize a suspected or confirmed COVID-19 patient. Hospitalization should be followed by an early radiographic framework in order to classify the disease progression, and to individualize the patients' care. Besides, the ideal imaging strategy for COVID-19 is still currently debated because it frequently requires the patients' transport to a radiological unit, thus increasing the risk of exposing to the virus the healthcare staff, other patients, and environments [4–6].

3.2 Diagnostic Imaging

3.2.1 Radiological Imaging

Despite of first-line, chest radiographic examination (CXR) is characterized by low sensitivity in the identification of the earliest pulmonary changes of COVID-19, characterized by "ground glass" opacity (GGO). Therefore, CXR is not the most suitable radiological examination, except for excluding alveolar bacterial pneumonia. Additionally, a time interval of at least 12–24 h from the onset of symptoms should be considered before chest X-ray in order to avoid false-negative examinations.

In spite of its limitations, CXR may diagnose various stages of COVID-19 pneumonia. Lung opacities may coalesce creating a diffuse pattern, peaking at 6–12 days from symptom onset (Fig. 3.1a). Reticular opacities may be seen accompanying the GGO, while pleural effusions, cavitation and pneumothorax are considered atypical for COVID-19 pneumonia [7–13].

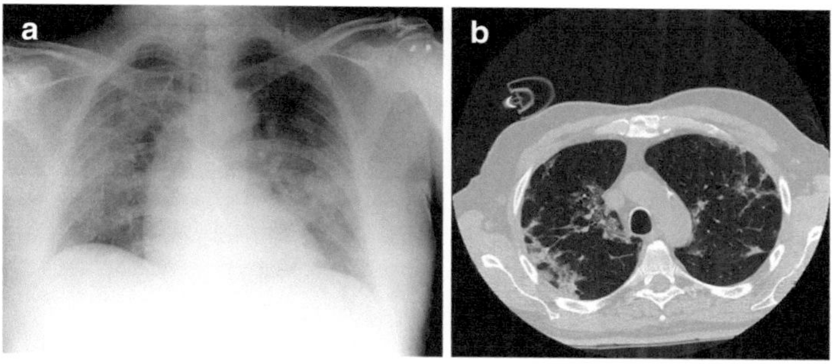

Fig. 3.1 (**a**) Chest X-ray (CXR) and (**b**) high resolution computed tomography (HRCT) of a 67-year-old male patient affected by COVID-19. (**a**) CXR shows low lung volumes with diffuse bilateral alveolar and interstitial opacities. (**b**) HRCT shows bilateral ground-glass opacities, interstitial thickening and consolidations, mainly in the posterior-subpleural lung zones

3.2.2 Chest High Resolution Computed Tomography (HRCT)

High-resolution chest computed tomography (HRCT) has a higher diagnostic sensitivity even in the early stages of the disease process. However, HRCT presents low specificity, especially for patterns which are very similar to other interstitial pneumoniae, such as Influenza A (H1N1), Cytomegalovirus, and other coronaviruses (SARS, MERS). Besides, HRCT is useful for assessing the course and severity of the disease, and therefore in guiding the patient's clinical management, although it is not suitable for a timely dynamic assessment of patients, particularly in critically ill cases.

In the initial stages, there is often evidence at HRCT of bilateral peripheral ground glass opacities, while in a more advanced picture of the disease, the segments involved increase in number, with extension of the ground glass, until involving an ever greater percentage of the parenchyma, switching between only peripheral to more and more centralized lesions, associated with consolidated areas with patchy distribution, mainly peripheral/subpleural, and with greater involvement of the posterior regions and lower lobes (Fig. 3.1b). GGOs may be pure (more commonly) or be accompanied by consolidations (mixed pattern). Intralobular and interlobular septal thickening, likely a combination of interstitial inflammation and fluid, is seen in 27% of cases. Superimposed GGOs giving a crazy-paving pattern is seen in 12% and may be a sign of more severe lung injury and disease progression. Consolidations, seen in up to 32% of cases, have a subpleural or peri-broncho-vascular distribution and may or may not have air-bronchograms. They are associated with more severe disease requiring management in the ICU [14–17].

Subsegmental vascular enlargement (greater than 3 mm) within parenchymal abnormalities has been described in up to 64–89% of patients. Although the exact pathogenesis is uncertain, it is thought to be related to hyperemia or thrombotic microangiopathy [18–22].

3.2.3 COVID-19 Chest CT Phenotypes

COVID-19 chest CT patterns have been classified according to three main phenotypes (1) multiple, focal, possibly overperfused ground-glass opacities with crazy paving appearance; (2) inhomogeneously distributed atelectasis and peribronchial opacities with predominant lung consolidations, and (3) a patchy, ARDS-like pattern". These patterns could be found as isolated or associated, usually following the temporal changes of COVID-19 pneumonia:

- Limited value of chest CT during the first 48 h from symptom onset;
- Early stage within 4 days from symptom onset, with growing GGOs;
- Progressive phase (peak at day 9–13 after symptom onset), with extensive GGOs with multifocal consolidations, septal thickening and crazy-paving
- Late or absorption phase (after 14 days), gradual clearance of GGOs and consolidations. In this phase signs of fibrosis could be observed together with parenchymal bands, subpleural lines, interlobular septal distortion and traction bronchiectasis.

Acute respiratory distress syndrome (ARDS) may occur in one third of hospitalized patients with COVID-19 pneumonia representing one of the more alarming complications of this condition. COVID-related ARDS usually develops slightly later than typical ARDS and could be often related to diffuse alveolar damage and microvascular thrombosis [23–26].

3.2.4 Quantitative Computed Tomography (QCT)

Visual comparison of lung damage on CT scans can be useful to assess the prognostic implications and a timely therapeutic management. Li et al. recently described a visual, quantitative analysis of lung damage, based on a "total severity score" based on the degrees of parenchymal loss, and associated with a score of clinical severity. However, these visual characterizations are mainly subjective, being unsuitable for a systematic disease evaluation.

Computer-aided quantitative analysis of the CT exam (quantitative computed tomography [qCT]) can also be used for this purpose, as already demonstrated by the research on the acute respiratory distress syndrome (ARDS). The areas in which qCT imaging can be potentially involved include the improved accuracy of diagnosis, identification of clinically distinct phenotypes, improvement of disease prognosis, stratification of care, and early objective evaluation of intervention response (Fig. 3.2). There is also a potential role for qCT in evaluating an increasing population of post-COVID-19 lung parenchymal changes such as fibrosis [27–29].

3.2.5 Lung Ultrasound

Lung ultrasound (LUS) is of great value in COVID-19 clinical scenario thanks to its intrinsic features, including high machines and bedside availability and portability, fast and non-invasive examination, readily repeatable, and does not involve ionizing radiation. In this setting, LUS should be considered a valid alternative to other imaging modalities in the follow-up of critically ill patients in intensive care unit (ICU) setting and for long-term

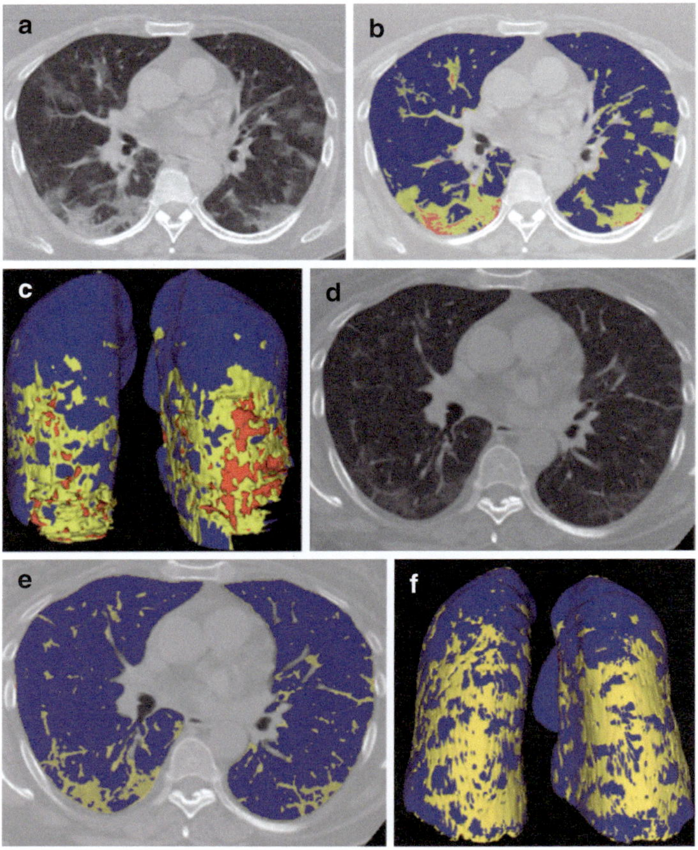

Fig. 3.2 CT scans of a 57 years old lady affected by COVID-19 pneumonia, treated with non-invasive oxygenation during 11 days of hospitalization. (**a**) Non-contrast CT scan ad admission showing typical bilateral ground-glass consolidation (**b**) qCT of the same scan highlighting in yellow the poorly aerated and in red the non-aerated lung volumes (**c**) three-dimensional view of the whole lungs. After 44 days, a CT scan shows significant improvement (**d**) with subtle residual ground-glass opacities and linear scarring, better outlined at qCT (**e**) and using 3D reconstruction (**f**). The patient lamented persisting labored breathing and abrupt intermittent coughing

follow-up of patients discharged from the hospital. The main drawback of LUS is represented by the increased risk of viral exposure for healthcare professionals [30, 31]. Moreover, specificity of lung US is poor due to overlap with other pathologies. The main LUS finding is represented by the B-lines, which are vertical echogenic comet-tail artifacts originating from the pleura and extending to the bottom of the screen. They represent thickened subpleural interlobular septa or fluid-filled alveoli (e.g., cardiogenic or non-cardiogenic pulmonary edema). Another important LUS finding are consolidations, which appear as subpleural hypoechoic areas with an irregular border (shred sign) and a "white lung" pattern posteriorly [32, 33] (Fig. 3.3).

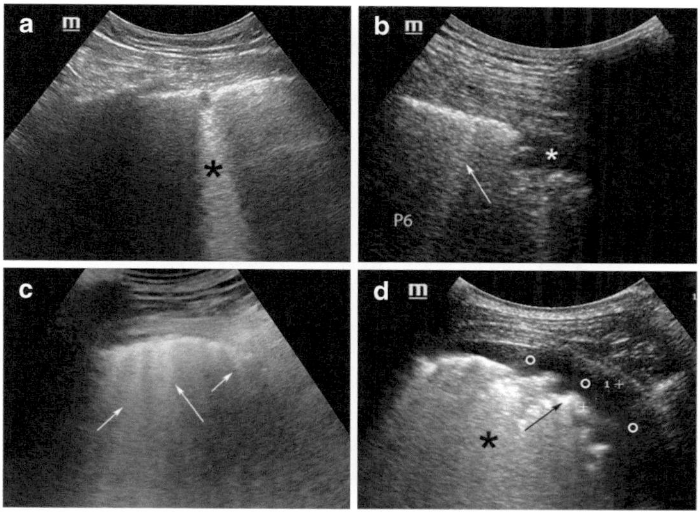

Fig. 3.3 Lung ultrasonography (LUS) images obtained with a convex probe. (**a**) Septal thickening correlating with isolated B-lines (*). (**b**, **c**) Nonconfluent B lines (white arrows) reflecting interstitial involvement of lung parenchyma and spared areas of normal lung parenchyma showing A lines. (*) Parenchymal consolidation area. (**d**) Confluent B lines with "white lung" pattern (*); irregular and thickened pleural line (black arrow) with moderate pleural effusion (circles)

The main LUS patterns in COVID-19 are represented by

- mild disease, with discrete scattered B-lines and small consolidations (<1 cm).
- moderate disease, with confluent and multifocal B-lines, larger consolidations (>1 cm), and irregular and thickened pleural lines.
- critical disease with "white lung" appearance and tissue-like pattern consolidations.
- recovery phase with gradually disappearance of consolidations and B-lines, while normal horizontal reverberation artefacts (A-lines) become prominent.

Various scoring systems have been suggested to quantitate the severity of findings. A good compromise between reproducibility and execution time is represented by a 12-zone protocol where each intercostal space of upper and lower parts of the anterior, lateral, and posterior regions of the left and right chest wall is carefully examined, and findings (pleural effusion, confluent and isolated B-lines, irregular pleural line, consolidations) are recorded on 10-s video clips and then scored accordingly. The total "LUS Score" is calculated by summing the scores of all 12 zones (ranging from 0 to 36, where 0 stands for no lesions, while 36 stands for maximal score). Scores from 1 to 10 were rated as mild, 10–20 as moderate, and more than 20 as severe [34–38].

References

1. World Health Organization. Coronavirus (COVID-19). Updated July 19, 2021. https://covid19.who.int. Accessed 24 Jul 2021.
2. Huang C, Wang Y, Li X, et al. Clinical features of patients infected with 2019 novel coronavirus in Wuhan, China. Lancet. 2020;395(10223):497–506. https://doi.org/10.1016/S0140-6736(20)30183-5.
3. Fang Y, Zhang H, Xie J, et al. Sensitivity of chest CT for COVID-19: comparison to RT-PCR. Radiology. 2020;296(2):E115–7. https://doi.org/10.1148/radiol.2020200432.
4. Sverzellati N, Milone F, Balbi M. How imaging should properly be used in COVID-19 outbreak: an Italian experience. Diagn Interv Radiol. 2020;26(3):204–6. https://doi.org/10.5152/dir.2020.30320.

5. Larici AR, Cicchetti G, Marano R, Merlino B, Elia L, Calandriello L, Del Ciello A, Farchione A, Savino G, Infante A, Larosa L, Colosimo C, Manfredi R, Natale L. Multimodality imaging of COVID-19 pneumonia: from diagnosis to follow-up. A comprehensive review. Eur J Radiol. 2020;131:109217.
6. Sideris GA, Nikolakea M, Karanikola AE, Konstantinopoulou S, Giannis D, Modahl L. Imaging in the COVID-19 era: lessons learned during a pandemic. World J Radiol. 2021;13(6):192–222. https://doi.org/10.4329/wjr.v13.i6.192.
7. Rubin GD, Ryerson CJ, Haramati LB, et al. The role of chest imaging in patient management during the COVID-19 pandemic: a multinational consensus statement from the Fleischner Society. Chest. 2020;158(1):106–16. https://doi.org/10.1016/j.chest.2020.04.003.
8. Schiaffino S, Tritella S, Cozzi A, et al. Diagnostic performance of chest X-ray for COVID-19 pneumonia during the SARS-CoV-2 pandemic in Lombardy, Italy. J Thorac Imaging. 2020;35(4):W105–6. https://doi.org/10.1097/RTI.0000000000000533.
9. Akl EA, Blazic I, Yaacoub S, et al. Use of chest imaging in the diagnosis and management of COVID-19: a WHO rapid advice guide. Radiology. 2020;298(2):E63–9. https://doi.org/10.1148/radiol.2020203173.
10. Wong HYF, Lam HYS, Fong AH, et al. Frequency and distribution of chest radiographic findings in COVID-19 positive patients. Radiology. 2020;296(2):E72–8. https://doi.org/10.1148/radiol.2020201160.
11. Vancheri SG, Savietto G, Ballati F, et al. Radiographic findings in 240 patients with COVID-19 pneumonia: time-dependence after the onset of symptoms. Eur Radiol. 2020;30:1–9. https://doi.org/10.1007/s00330-020-06967-7.
12. Bandirali M, Sconfienza LM, Serra R, et al. Chest X-ray findings in asymptomatic and minimally symptomatic quarantined patients in Codogno, Italy. Radiology. 2020;295(3):E7. https://doi.org/10.1148/radiol.2020201102.
13. Borghesi A, Maroldi R. COVID-19 outbreak in Italy: experimental chest X-ray scoring system for quantifying and monitoring disease progression. Radiol Med. 2020;125(5):509–13. https://doi.org/10.1007/s11547-020-01200-3.
14. Xu B, Xing Y, Peng J, Zheng Z, et al. Chest CT for detecting COVID-19: a systematic review and meta-analysis of diagnostic accuracy. Eur Radiol. 2020;15:1–8. https://doi.org/10.1007/s00330-020-06934-2.
15. Dai W, Zhang H, Yu J, et al. CT imaging and differential diagnosis of COVID-19. Can Assoc Radiol J. 2020;71(2):195–200. https://doi.org/10.1177/0846537120913033.
16. Sverzellati N, Milanese G, Milone F, et al. Integrated radiologic algorithm for COVID-19 pandemic. J Thorac Imaging. 2020;35(4):228–33. https://doi.org/10.1097/RTI.0000000000000516.

17. Prokop M, van Everdingen W, van Rees Vellinga T, et al. CO-RADS—a categorical CT assessment scheme for patients with suspected COVID-19: definition and evaluation. Radiology. 2020;296(2):E97–E104. https://doi.org/10.1148/radiol.2020201473.
18. Borghesi A, Zigliani A, Golemi S, et al. Chest X-ray severity index as a predictor of in-hospital mortality in coronavirus disease 2019: a study of 302 patients from Italy. Int J Infect Dis. 2020;96:291–3. https://doi.org/10.1016/j.ijid.2020.05.021.
19. Liu Z, Jin C, Wu CC, et al. Association between initial chest CT or clinical features and clinical course in patients with coronavirus disease 2019 pneumonia. Korean J Radiol. 2020;21(6):736–45. https://doi.org/10.3348/kjr.2020.0171.
20. Liu F, Zhang Q, Huang C, et al. CT quantification of pneumonia lesions in early days predicts progression to severe illness in a cohort of COVID-19 patients. Theranostics. 2020;10(12):5613–22. https://doi.org/10.7150/thno.45985.
21. Yu Q, Wang Y, Huang S, et al. Multicenter cohort study demonstrates more consolidation in upper lungs on initial CT increases the risk of adverse clinical outcome in COVID-19 patients. Theranostics. 2020;10(12):5641–8. https://doi.org/10.7150/thno.46465.
22. Lanza E, Mancuso ME, Messana G, et al. Compromised lung volume and hemostatic abnormalities in COVID-19 pneumonia: results from an observational study on 510 consecutive patients. J Clin Med. 2021;10(13):2894. https://doi.org/10.3390/jcm10132894.
23. Ojha V, Mani A, Pandey NN, et al. CT in coronavirus disease 2019 (COVID-19): a systematic review of chest CT findings in 4410 adult patients. Eur Radiol. 2020;30:1–10. https://doi.org/10.1007/s00330-020-06975-7.
24. Robba C, Battaglini D, Ball L, Patroniti N, Loconte M, Brunetti I, Vena A, Giacobbe DR, Bassetti M, Rocco PRM, Pelosi P. Distinct phenotypes require distinct respiratory management strategies in severe COVID-19. Respir Physiol Neurobiol. 2020;279:103455.
25. Ball L, Robba C, Maiello L, Herrmann J, Gerard SE, Xin Y, Battaglini D, Brunetti I, Minetti G, Seitun S, Vena A, Giacobbe DR, Bassetti M, Rocco PRM, Cereda M, Castellan L, Patroniti N, Pelosi P, GECOVID (GEnoa COVID-19) Group. Computed tomography assessment of PEEP-induced alveolar recruitment in patients with severe COVID-19 pneumonia. Crit Care. 2021;25:81.
26. Xu Z, Shi L, Wang Y, et al. Pathological findings of COVID-19 associated with acute respiratory distress syndrome. Lancet Respir Med. 2020;8(4):420–2. https://doi.org/10.1016/S2213-2600(20)30076-X.
27. Li K, Fang Y, Li W, et al. CT image visual quantitative evaluation and clinical classification of coronavirus disease (COVID-19). Eur Radiol. 2020;30(8):4407–16. https://doi.org/10.1007/s00330-020-06817-6.

28. Ball L, Robba C, Herrmann J, et al. Lung distribution of gas and blood volume in critically ill COVID-19 patients: a quantitative dual-energy computed tomography study. Crit Care. 2021;25(1):214. https://doi.org/10.1186/s13054-021-03610-9.
29. Lanza E, Muglia R, Bolengo I, et al. Quantitative chest CT analysis in COVID-19 to predict the need for oxygenation support and intubation. Eur Radiol. 2020;30(12):6770–8. https://doi.org/10.1007/s00330-020-07013-2.
30. Colombi D, Petrini M, Maffi G, Villani GD, Bodini FC, Morelli N, Milanese G, Silva M, Sverzellati N, Michieletti E. Comparison of admission chest computed tomography and lung ultrasound performance for diagnosis of COVID-19 pneumonia in populations with different disease prevalence. Eur J Radiol. 2020;133:109344.
31. Orlandi D, Battaglini D, Robba C, et al. COVID-19 phenotypes, lung ultrasound, chest computed tomography, and clinical features in critically ill mechanically ventilated patients. Ultrasound Med Biol. 2021;47(12):3323–32.
32. Volpicelli G, Gargani L. Sonographic signs and patterns of COVID-19 pneumonia. Ultrasound J. 2020;12:22.
33. Bernheim A, Mei X, Huang M, et al. Chest CT findings in coronavirus disease-19 (COVID-19): relationship to duration of infection. Radiology. 2020;295(3):200463. https://doi.org/10.1148/radiol.2020200463.
34. Cantinotti M, Giordano R, Scalese M, Marchese P, Franchi E, Viacava C, Molinaro S, Assanta N, Koestenberger M, Kutty S, Gargani L, Ait-Ali L. Prognostic value of a new lung ultrasound score to predict intensive care unit stay in pediatric cardiac surgery. Ann Thorac Surg. 2020;109(1):178–84.
35. Mento F, Perrone T, Macioce VN, Tursi F, Buonsenso D, Torri E, Smargiassi A, Inchingolo R, Soldati G, Demi L. On the impact of different lung ultrasound imaging protocols in the evaluation of patients affected by coronavirus disease 2019: how many acquisitions are needed? J Ultrasound Med. 2020;40(10):2235–8. https://doi.org/10.1002/jum.15580.
36. Perrone T, Soldati G, Padovini L, Fiengo A, Lettieri G, Sabatini U, Gori G, Lepore F, Garolfi M, Palumbo I, Inchingolo R, Smargiassi A, Demi L, Mossolani EE, Tursi F, Klersy C, Di Sabatino A. A new lung ultrasound protocol able to predict worsening in patients affected by severe acute respiratory syndrome Coronavirus 2 pneumonia. J Ultrasound Med. 2020;40(8):1627–35. https://doi.org/10.1002/jum.15548.
37. Soldati G, Smargiassi A, Inchingolo R, Buonsenso D, Perrone T, Briganti DF, Perlini S, Torri E, Mariani A, Mossolani EE, Tursi F, Mento F, Demi L. Is there a role for lung ultrasound during the COVID-19 pandemic? J Ultrasound Med. 2020;39(7):1459–62.

38. Soldati G, Smargiassi A, Inchingolo R, Buonsenso D, Perrone T, Briganti DF, Perlini S, Torri E, Mariani A, Mossolani EE, Tursi F, Mento F, Demi L. Proposal for international standardization of the use of lung ultrasound for patients with COVID-19: a simple, quantitative. Reprod Method J Ultrasound Med. 2020;39(7):1413–9.

Noninvasive Mechanical Ventilation and Conventional Oxygen Therapy

4

Carla Speziale, Enric Barbeta, and Antoni Torres

4.1 Introduction

COVID-19 pneumonia often presents with severely impaired oxygenation. In patients presenting with hypoxemic acute respiratory failure (ARF), one of the most important goals is to avoid invasive mechanical ventilation. Therefore, in this chapter, we will review the current evidence and rationale for using noninvasive oxygenation and ventilation strategies in patients presenting with COVID-19 and hypoxemic ARF.

4.2 Noninvasive Ventilation in Non-COVID-19 ARF

ARF causes a third of intensive care unit (ICU) admissions and has a high mortality rate [1]. It has been reported that up to 61% of these patients ultimately require endotracheal intubation and

C. Speziale · E. Barbeta · A. Torres (✉)
Servei de Pneumologia Hospital Clinic, University of Barcelona, IDIPAPS, CIBERES, ICREA, Barcelona, Spain
e-mail: ATORRES@clinic.cat

D. Battaglini, P. Pelosi (eds.), *COVID-19 Critical and Intensive Care Medicine Essentials*, https://doi.org/10.1007/978-3-030-94992-1_4

invasive mechanical ventilation [2]. Unfortunately, this invasive respiratory support therapy is associated with several adverse events such as ventilator-associated pneumonia, delirium, ICU-acquired muscle weakness, and venous thromboembolism. Hospital mortality of patients requiring invasive mechanical ventilation due to respiratory failure is 38.6% [3]. As a result of the complications related to invasive mechanical ventilation, noninvasive methods such as noninvasive mechanical ventilation (NIV) have been developed to deliver respiratory support in ARF and to avoid intubation. The rationale for using NIV in hypoxemic ARF is to ameliorate gas exchange and pulmonary mechanics through positive end-expiratory pressure (PEEP) and to decrease inspiratory effort as well as muscle fatigue with adequate pressure support [4]. However, except in patients with acute cardiogenic pulmonary edema, the use of NIV in patients with hypoxemic ARF is controversial. For example, despite initial impressive results in immunocompromised patients [5], enthusiasm for it was reduced after the emergence of negative results from another randomized clinical trial [6]. In nonimmunocompromised patients, several randomized clinical trials demonstrated that NIV was effective in reducing intubation and mortality rates in patients presenting with hypoxemic ARF. However, as all these studies had several limitations, the extrapolation of their results to guide treatment for ARF caused by COVID-19 pneumonia may not be correct. The most important limitation was that the studies included a heterogeneous population [7–9], with the causes of hypoxemic respiratory failure including acute cardiogenic pulmonary edema, community-acquired pneumonia, and acute respiratory distress syndrome (ARDS), among others. This limitation was significant as some of the etiologies of ARF were protective factors, while others were risk factors for intubation in the multivariate analyses. For example, while ARDS was an independent risk factor for intubation, acute cardiogenic pulmonary edema was a protective factor [8]. Chronic respiratory or cardiovascular diseases may benefit from the application of positive pressure, especially in patients with airflow limitation and air trapping, such as those with chronic obstructive pulmonary disease (COPD), or in those with a high left ventricular preload, such as patients with chronic heart failure. In the abovementioned studies, most of the patients had prior cardiovascular and respiratory comorbidities that may have interacted with the final outcome (i.e., intubation). In COVID-19 patients, COPD or asthma is not as common as in patients with other viral infections such as influenza [10, 11]. On the contrary, a significant proportion of critically ill COVID-19 patients present with cardiovascular risk factors such as diabetes mellitus and hypertension [11].

De novo hypoxemic respiratory failure is an interesting concept, as it excludes patients with prior chronic respiratory disorders or heart failure. In this population, NIV has been shown to be hazardous as it may be associated with higher mortality due to ventilator-induced lung injury (VILI) and patient self-inflicted lung injury (P-SILI) [12]. Most patients with hypoxemic ARF undergoing NIV breathe with tidal volumes that are considered nonprotective or iatrogenic [13]. Furthermore, spontaneous ventilation is known to increase lung injury in ARDS as a result of high transpulmonary pressures and the Pendelluft phenomenon alongside high regional strain and stress [14]. Observational studies have also pointed out that NIV might be dangerous in patients with moderate-to-severe ARDS [15]. As most of the patients with COVID-19 pneumonia meet the definition of de novo respiratory failure and ARDS, some studies argue that NIV might delay intubation and prevent the application of protective mechanical ventilation [16]. This has promoted the application of clinical scores such as the HACOR score to identify patients with a high likelihood of requiring intubation during the early course of ARF [17].

High-flow nasal cannulas (HFNC) provide heated and humidified gas (i.e., a mixture of oxygen and air) at a maximal flow reaching up to 60 L/min. This flow, which is higher than that of conventional oxygen therapies, has multiple beneficial effects on respiratory physiology in patients presenting with ARF. It improves oxygenation as the alveolar FiO_2 is similar to the set FiO_2, decreases $PaCO_2$ as a result of the tracheal washout effect, increases the end-expiratory lung volume, and ameliorates lung inhomogeneities. All these factors contribute to the decrease in the work of breathing, prevent respiratory fatigue, and possibly reduce P-SILI [18]. The most important differences with NIV are that the HFNC does not provide pressure support during inspiration and that the level of PEEP probably does not exceed 0–5 cmH_2O at the tracheal level [19].

The FLORALI study [12] demonstrated that HFNC reduced the need for endotracheal intubation and 90-day mortality in patients with moderate-to-severe ARF compared to conventional oxygen therapy and NIV. Interestingly, the population in the FLORALI study showed similarities to patients with COVID-19 pneumonia, presenting de novo respiratory failure, with most of them showing bilateral infiltrates. The effectiveness of HFNC in avoiding intubation has also been challenged by other studies, particularly one that focused on immunocompromised patients [20]. However, a recent meta-analysis analyzing a heterogeneous population with ARF pointed toward its effectiveness [21].

As with NIV, one of the main concerns with HFNC is the delay in intubation and increased mortality [22]. Predictors of HFNC therapy failure that are evaluated early after the beginning of therapy are useful in deciding whether to continue or stop with HFNC treatment. Roca et al. identified the ROX index [23], defined as the ratio of oxygen saturation (as measured by pulse oximetry/FiO_2) to the respiratory rate, as a useful tool to predict failure of HFNC therapy during the first 12 h of its application. In contradistinction to NIV, the evidence suggesting an association between mortality and a delay in intubation as a result of HFNC therapy comes from observational studies assessing a population in whom this noninvasive strategy failed. Although P-SILI is a concept with a strong physiological rationale [14], its precise definition, effectors, monitoring variables, and attributable mortality are not well known [24].

4.3 Noninvasive Ventilation and Oxygenation Strategies in COVID-19 Pneumonia Presenting with Hypoxemic ARF

High-quality evidence supporting the use of HFNC or NIV in COVID-19 pneumonia is limited. Most of the evidence is generated from observational studies [25–34]. After 1 year of the pandemic, only one randomized clinical trial comparing NIV plus HFNC vs. HFNC alone has been published [35].

Landmark epidemiological studies from Asia, Europe, and the USA have revealed scarce use of NIV and HFNC [36–38]. This might have been related to the initial fear and uncertainty regarding the airborne transmission of SARS-CoV-2 promoted by noninvasive respiratory support therapies. Furthermore, as commented above, previous studies on non–COVID-19-related ARF discouraged the use of NIV in patients presenting with de novo respiratory failure with bilateral infiltrates. For that reason, several experts recommended against the use of noninvasive ventilation and oxygenation strategies and advocated early intubation to reduce VILI or P-SILI and delayed intubation [16]. This has attracted a lot of debate and many clinicians, including ourselves, had raised concerns about starting invasive mechanical ventilation guided only by the degree of oxygenation impairment [24]. However, in the first weeks of the pandemic, a lack of ICU beds as well as ventilators prompted the initiation of noninvasive strategies, even outside ICU facilities such as respiratory intermediate care units [34].

Clinicians supporting noninvasive therapies have argued that the intubation rates reported in large series of patients undergoing noninvasive ventilation or oxygenation strategies are lower than in cohorts of patients in whom invasive mechanical ventilation is directly used when the clinical condition has deteriorated. For example, the intubation rate in a cohort of patients in whom NIV or HFNC was seldom used was almost 90% [11]. On the other hand, the intubation rate in a cohort of patients in whom NIV or continuous positive airway pressure (CPAP) was part of the initial respiratory support therapy was significantly lower (i.e., 22–26.6%) [34, 39]. In that study [39], a comparison between the periods in which CPAP or conventional oxygen therapy was used showed that CPAP was associated with lower intubation rates. In another observational study [40], NIV was also found to be associated with a higher probability of survival compared to invasive mechanical ventilation without prior noninvasive support. Furthermore, patients in whom NIV had failed, at a median of 3 days from its start, did not seem to have higher mortality. Another meta-analysis gave similar results and questioned prior beliefs about NIV failure being linked to higher mortality [41]. This must be interpreted with caution as delayed intubation is an arbitrary concept when analyzed as the number of days from ICU admission or as the number of days from the start of noninvasive respiratory support therapy to intubation. In our opinion, a deterioration in clinical status rigorously analyzed on a case-by-case basis should trigger the application of invasive mechanical intubation and determine whether intubation is delayed or not. In most patients with COVID-19 undergoing NIV or CPAP, a high PEEP is set (i.e., >10 cmH_2O). One of the drawbacks of noninvasive respiratory support strategies is that apart from the respiratory rate and gas exchange, it is difficult to monitor the effects of different ventilator settings on lung recruitment, respiratory drive, and pulmonary mechanics.

Other studies have analyzed the use of HFNC in a similar fashion. Compared to an early invasive strategy, the use of HFNC has been reported to be associated with a higher number of ventilation-free days despite the same mortality risk, with the results suggesting that the benefit in this composite outcome (days free from invasive mechanical ventilation and survival at day 28) is mainly driven by a reduction in the need for intubation [42].

With all that said, the evidence supporting NIV, CPAP and HFNC in hypoxemic ARF has gone back and forth and we do not expect this to be any different for COVID-19-induced ARF. Patients with ARF are likely to have heterogeneous conditions and many factors, such as age, impaired respiratory physiology, comorbidities, and ARF etiology, among others, might interact and determine the success or failure of noninvasive therapies. Another critical factor that could predict the success of NIV or HFNC therapy is the response to etiological treatments. Noninvasive respiratory support therapies are used to treat ARF, but not its cause. Therefore, in COVID-19 pneumonia, the main factor for successful treatment is whether immunomodulator and antiviral treatments are effective or not. For example, we do not know whether NIV or HFNC therapy was effective in reducing endotracheal intubation prior to the widespread use of dexamethasone and tocilizumab or if its effectiveness will be enhanced as new treatment options become available.

In light of the results reported for patients with COVID-19-induced hypoxemic ARF, it seems logical to start with a noninvasive oxygenation or ventilation strategy since the risks associated with invasive mechanical ventilation probably outweigh the theoretical lung damage caused by NIV or HFNC. However, if the clinical status of the patient deteriorates despite the best use of such therapies, prompt intubation should be offered. That being said, what are the differences between HFNC and NIV in COVID-19? One observational study found no differences between CPAP, NIV, and HFNC [34]. However, NIV or CPAP is usually started in patients with more severe disease, making it difficult to interpret the results of such studies. Although this might be addressed by adjusting for confounding factors in regression analyses or other statistical models, only a randomized clinical trial can eliminate this bias (i.e., indication bias) as treatment allocation is decided by chance. The abovementioned randomized clinical trial [35] that compared HFNC vs. helmet NIV plus HFNC therapy in COVID-19-induced ARF showed no effect on primary outcome (days free from high-flow nasal oxygen, and noninvasive and invasive ventilation at day 28), but found beneficial effects in several relevant secondary outcomes such as intubation requirement. Any medical act should comprise a multimodal assessment that is performed rigorously and methodologically. The benefits and potential risks of inserting an endotracheal tube or starting noninvasive ventilation or oxygenation strategies should be considered. In our opinion, systematically denying NIV, CPAP, and HFNC in patients with hypoxemic ARF is not advised.

4.4 Safety

Since HFNC and NIV may reduce the need for mechanical ventilation in hypoxemic COVID-19 patients and as these procedures involve the risk of aerosol transmission, recommendations for the safest and most appropriate way of performing them are mandatory.

The Society of Critical Care Medicine (SCCM), the Surviving Sepsis Campaign guidelines and the World Health Organization

(WHO) guidelines for COVID-19 recommend the use of HFNC and/or NIV in acute hypoxemic respiratory failure due to COVID-19. However, the WHO recommends that HFNC and NIV should be used with airborne precautions due to the uncertainty about their potential for being an aerosol-generating medical procedure (AGMP) [43].

We propose the following recommendations based on updated evidence, with airborne precautions to be used to limit the aerosol transmission of the disease both to patients and health-care workers:

- Personal protective equipment, including FFP2 masks or FFP3 masks if available, safety glasses, tied hair or the use of surgical caps, gloves, and antimicrobial surgical gowns, should be worn.
- If available, the patient should be placed in a negative pressure room. When this is not available, an individual room with a private bathroom should be used. In all cases, the doors must remain closed at all times.
- Oxygen should be administered through exhaled air filters. If not available, a surgical mask could be used on the nasal cannula to limit the dispersion of the virus [44, 45].
- A minimum distance of 2 m between the patient and health-care workers is recommended when one is not appropriately protected [46].
- NIV should be used with double-arm configurations when available in order to provide a hermetic circuit and a high-efficacy antimicrobial filter in the expiratory arm. If a double-arm configuration is not available, a high-efficacy low-resistance filter must be used to minimize the dispersion of the exhaled gases. An alternative is the use of a one-arm configuration involving an active valve with a filter at the exit of the valve. Nonvented interfaces with an antibacterial or antiviral filter between the patient and the expiratory port may reduce environmental contamination [44].
- A helmet interface should be the first option if possible [44, 45, 47]. It is mandatory to pay special attention to and watch for

leak points, avoid skin lesions and keep the system hermetic. Skin protection patches, which increase leaks, should be avoided.

– Nebulizers generate aerosol particles that can carry the virus to the lungs. Thus, nebulizer therapies should only be used if they are deemed extremely necessary and jet systems should be avoided.
– It is known that the risk of generating and dispersing bioaerosols is similar for HFNC and standard oxygen masks. Therefore, the use of an HFNC with a surgical mask on the patient's face is reasonable [48].

References

1. Vincent J-L, Akça S, De Mendonça A, Haji-Michael P, Sprung C, Moreno R, Antonelli M, Suter PM, SOFA Working Group. The epidemiology of acute respiratory failure in critically ill patients. Chest. 2002;121(5):1602–9.
2. Thille AW, Contou D, Fragnoli C, Córdoba-Izquierdo A, Boissier F, Brun-Buisson C. Non-invasive ventilation for acute hypoxemic respiratory failure: intubation rate and risk factors. Crit Care. 2013;17(6):R269.
3. Pham T, Pesenti A, Bellani G, Rubenfeld G, Fan E, Bugedo G, Lorente JA, do Vale Fernandes A, Van Haren F, Bruhn A, Rios F, Esteban A, Gattinoni L, Larsson A, McAuley DF, Ranieri M, Thompson BT, Wrigge H, Brochard LJ, Laffey JG, LUNG SAFE Investigators and the European Society of Intensive Care Medicine Trials Group. Outcome of acute hypoxaemic respiratory failure. Insights from the lung safe study. Eur Respir J. 2020;57(6):2003317.
4. Kallet RH, Diaz JV. The physiologic effects of noninvasive ventilation. Respir Care. 2009;54(1):102–15.
5. Antonelli M, Conti G, Bufi M, Costa MG, Lappa A, Rocco M, Gasparetto A, Meduri GU. Noninvasive ventilation for treatment of acute respiratory failure in patients undergoing solid organ transplantation: a randomized trial. JAMA. 2000;283(2):235–41.
6. Lemiale V, Mokart D, Resche-Rigon M, Pène F, Mayaux J, Faucher E, Nyunga M, Girault C, Perez P, Guitton C, Ekpe K, Kouatchet A, Théodose I, Benoit D, Canet E, Barbier F, Rabbat A, Bruneel F, Vincent F, Klouche K, Loay K, Mariotte E, Bouadma L, Moreau A-S, Seguin A, Meert A-P, Reignier J, Papazian L, Mehzari I, Cohen Y, Schenck M, Hamidfar R,

Darmon M, Demoule A, Chevret S, Azoulay E, Groupe de Recherche en Réanimation Respiratoire du patient d'Onco-Hématologie (GRRR-OH). Effect of noninvasive ventilation vs oxygen therapy on mortality among immunocompromised patients with acute respiratory failure: a randomized clinical trial. JAMA. 2015;314(16):1711–9.

7. Wysocki M, Tric L, Wolff MA, Millet H, Herman B. Noninvasive pressure support ventilation in patients with acute respiratory failure. A randomized comparison with conventional therapy. Chest. 1995;107(3):761–8.
8. Ferrer M, Esquinas A, Leon M, Gonzalez G, Alarcon A, Torres A. Noninvasive ventilation in severe hypoxemic respiratory failure: a randomized clinical trial. Am J Respir Crit Care Med. 2003;168(12):1438–44.
9. Brambilla AM, Aliberti S, Prina E, Nicoli F, Forno MD, Nava S, Ferrari G, Corradi F, Pelosi P, Bignamini A, Tarsia P, Cosentini R. Helmet CPAP vs. oxygen therapy in severe hypoxemic respiratory failure due to pneumonia. Intensive Care Med. 2014;40(7):942–9.
10. Nguyen-Van-Tam JS, Openshaw PJM, Hashim A, Gadd EM, Lim WS, Semple MG, Read RC, Taylor BL, Brett SJ, McMenamin J, Enstone JE, Armstrong C, Nicholson KG, Influenza Clinical Information Network (FLU-CIN). Risk factors for hospitalisation and poor outcome with pandemic A/H1N1 influenza: United Kingdom first wave (May–September 2009). Thorax. 2010;65(7):645–51.
11. Grasselli G, Zangrillo A, Zanella A, Antonelli M, Cabrini L, Castelli A, Cereda D, Coluccello A, Foti G, Fumagalli R, Iotti G, Latronico N, Lorini L, Merler S, Natalini G, Piatti A, Ranieri MV, Scandroglio AM, Storti E, Cecconi M, Pesenti A, COVID-19 Lombardy ICU Network, et al. Baseline characteristics and outcomes of 1591 patients infected with SARS-CoV-2 admitted to ICUs of the Lombardy Region, Italy. JAMA. 2020;323(16):1574–81.
12. Frat JP, Thille AW, Mercat A, Girault C, Ragot S, Perbet S, Prat G, Boulain T, Morawiec E, Cottereau A, Devaquet J, Nseir S, Razazi K, Mira J-P, Argaud L, Chakarian J-C, Ricard J-D, Wittebole X, Chevalier S, Herbland A, Fartoukh M, Constantin J-M, Tonnelier J-M, Pierrot M, Mathonnet A, Béduneau G, Delétage-Métreau C, Jean-Christophe MR, Brochard L, Robert R, FLORALI Study Group; REVA Network. High-flow oxygen through nasal cannula in acute hypoxemic respiratory failure. N Engl J Med. 2015;372(23):2185–96.
13. Carteaux G, Millán-Guilarte T, De Prost N, Razazi K, Abid S, Thille AW, Schortgen F, Brochard L, Brun-Buisson C, Dessap AM. Failure of noninvasive ventilation for de novo acute hypoxemic respiratory failure: role of tidal volume. Crit Care Med. 2016;44(2):282–90.
14. Yoshida T, Torsani V, Gomes S, De Santis RR, Beraldo MA, Costa ELV, Tucci MR, Zin WA, Kavanagh BP, Amato MBP. Spontaneous effort

causes occult pendelluft during mechanical ventilation. Am J Respir Crit Care Med. 2013;188(12):1420–7.
15. Bellani G, Laffey JG, Pham T, Madotto F, Fan E, Brochard L, Esteban A, Gattinoni L, Bumbasirevic V, Piquilloud L, Van Haren F, Larsson A, McAuley DF, Bauer PR, Arabi YM, Ranieri M, Antonelli M, Rubenfeld GD, Thompson BT, Wrigge H, Slutsky AS, Pesenti A, LUNG SAFE Investigators; ESICM Trials Group. Noninvasive ventilation of patients with acute respiratory distress syndrome. Insights from the LUNG SAFE Study. Am J Respir Crit Care Med. 2017;195(1):67–77.
16. Marini JJ, Gattinoni L. Management of COVID-19 respiratory distress. JAMA. 2020;323(22):2329–30.
17. Duan J, Han X, Bai L, Zhou L, Huang S. Assessment of heart rate, acidosis, consciousness, oxygenation, and respiratory rate to predict noninvasive ventilation failure in hypoxemic patients. Intensive Care Med. 2017;43(2):192–9.
18. Mauri T, Turrini C, Eronia N, Grasselli G, Volta CA, Bellani G, Pesenti A. Physiologic effects of high-flow nasal cannula in acute hypoxemic respiratory failure. Am J Respir Crit Care Med. 2017;195(9):1207–15.
19. Groves N, Tobin A. High flow nasal oxygen generates positive airway pressure in adult volunteers. Aust Crit Care. 2007;20(4):126–31.
20. Azoulay E, Lemiale V, Mokart D, Nseir S, Argaud L, Pène F, Kontar L, Bruneel F, Klouche K, Barbier F, Reignier J, Berrahil-Meksen L, Louis G, Constantin J-M, Mayaux J, Wallet F, Kouatchet A, Peigne V, Théodose I, Perez P, Girault C, Jaber S, Oziel J, Nyunga M, Terzi N, Bouadma L, Lebert C, Lautrette A, Bigé N, Raphalen J-H, Papazian L, Darmon M, Chevret S, Demoule A. Effect of high-flow nasal oxygen vs standard oxygen on 28-day mortality in immunocompromised patients with acute respiratory failure: the HIGH randomized clinical trial. JAMA. 2018;320(20):2099–107.
21. Ferreyro BL, Angriman F, Munshi L, Del Sorbo L, Ferguson ND, Rochwerg B, Ryu MJ, Saskin R, Wunsch H, da Costa BR, Scales DC. Association of noninvasive oxygenation strategies with all-cause mortality in adults with acute hypoxemic respiratory failure: a systematic review and meta-analysis. JAMA. 2020;324(1):57–67.
22. Kang BJ, Koh Y, Lim CM, Huh JW, Baek S, Han M, et al. Failure of high-flow nasal cannula therapy may delay intubation and increase mortality. Intensive Care Med. 2015;41(4):623–32.
23. Roca O, Caralt B, Messika J, Samper M, Sztrymf B, Hernández G, García-de-Acilu M, Frat J-P, Masclans JR, Ricard J-D. An index combining respiratory rate and oxygenation to predict outcome of nasal high-flow therapy. Am J Respir Crit Care Med. 2019;199(11):1368–76.
24. Tobin MJ, Jubran A, Laghi F. Noninvasive strategies in COVID-19: epistemology, randomised trials, guidelines, physiology. Eur Respir J. 2021;57(2):2004247.

25. Ferrando C, Mellado-Artigas R, Gea A, COVID-19 Spanish ICU Network, et al. Awake prone positioning does not reduce the risk of intubation in COVID-19 treated with high-flow nasal oxygen therapy: a multicenter, adjusted cohort study. Crit Care. 2020;24:597.
26. Zucman N, Mullaert J, Roux D, Roca O, Ricard J-D, Contributors. Prediction of outcome of nasal high flow use during COVID-19-related acute hypoxemic respiratory failure. Intensive Care Med. 2020;46:1924–6.
27. Xia J, Zhang Y, Ni L, et al. High-flow nasal oxygen in coronavirus disease 2019 patients with acute hypoxemic respiratory failure: a multicenter, retrospective cohort study. Crit Care Med. 2020;48:e1079–86.
28. Panadero C, Abad-Fernández A, Rio-Ramirez MT, et al. High-flow nasal cannula for acute respiratory distress syndrome (ARDS) due to COVID-19. Multidiscip Respir Med. 2020;15:693.
29. Vianello A, Arcaro G, Molena B, et al. High-flow nasal cannula oxygen therapy to treat patients with hypoxemic acute respiratory failure consequent to SARS-CoV-2 infection. Thorax. 2020;75:998–1000.
30. Guy T, Créac'hcadec A, Ricordel C, et al. High-flow nasal oxygen: a safe, efficient treatment for COVID-19 patients not in an ICU. Eur Respir J. 2020;56:2001154.
31. Duan J, Chen B, Liu X, et al. Use of high-flow nasal cannula and noninvasive ventilation in patients with COVID-19: a multicenter observational study. Am J Emerg Med. 2020;46:276–81.
32. Wang K, Zhao W, Li J, Shu W, Duan J. The experience of high-flow nasal cannula in hospitalized patients with 2019 novel coronavirus-infected pneumonia in two hospitals of Chongqing, China. Ann Intensive Care. 2020;10:37.
33. Demoule A, Vieillard Baron A, Darmon M, et al. High-flow nasal cannula in critically ill patients with severe COVID-19. Am J Respir Crit Care Med. 2020;202:1039–42.
34. Franco C, Facciolongo N, Tonelli R, Dongilli R, Vianello A, Pisani L, Scala R, Malerba M, Carlucci A, Negri EA, Spoladore G, Arcaro G, Tillio PA, Lastoria C, Schifino G, Tabbì L, Guidelli L, Guaraldi G, Ranieri VM, Clini E, Nava S. Feasibility and clinical impact of out-of-ICU noninvasive respiratory support in patients with COVID-19-related pneumonia. Eur Respir J. 2020;56(5):2002130.
35. Grieco DL, Menga LS, Cesarano M, Rosà T, Spadaro S, Bitondo MM, Montomoli J, Falò G, Tonetti T, Cutuli SL, Pintaudi G, Tanzarella ES, Piervincenzi E, Bongiovanni F, Dell'Anna AM, Cese LD, Berardi C, Carelli S, Bocci MG, Montini L, Bello G, Natalini D, De Pascale G, Velardo M, Volta CA, Ranieri VM, Conti G, Maggiore SM, Antonelli M, COVID-ICU Gemelli Study Group. Effect of helmet noninvasive ventilation vs. high-flow nasal oxygen on days free of respiratory sup-

port in patients with COVID-19 and moderate to severe hypoxemic respiratory failure: the HENIVOT randomized clinical trial. JAMA. 2021;325(17):1731–43.
36. Grasselli G, Zangrillo A, Zanella A, Antonelli M, Cabrini L, Castelli A, COVID-19 Lombardy ICU Network, et al. Baseline characteristics and outcomes of 1591 patients infected with SARS-CoV-2 admitted to ICUs of the Lombardy region, Italy. JAMA. 2020;323(16):1574–81.
37. Cummings MJ, Baldwin MR, Abrams D, Jacobson SD, Meyer BJ, Balough EM, et al. Epidemiology, clinical course, and outcomes of critically ill adults with COVID-19 in New York City: a prospective cohort study. Lancet. 2020;395:1763–70.
38. Zhou F, Yu T, Du R, Fan G, Liu Y, Liu Z, et al. Clinical course and risk factors for mortality of adult inpatients with COVID-19 in Wuhan, China: a retrospective cohort study. Lancet. 2020;395:1054–62.
39. Oranger M, Gonzalez-Bermejo J, Dacosta-Noble P, Llontop C, Guerder A, Trosini-Desert V, Faure M, Raux M, Decavele M, Demoule A, Morélot-Panzini C, Similowski T. Continuous positive airway pressure to avoid intubation in SARS-CoV-2 pneumonia: a two-period retrospective case-control study. Eur Respir J. 2020;56(2):2001692.
40. Grasselli G. Risk factors associated with mortality among patients with COVID-19 in intensive care units in Lombardy, Italy. JAMA Intern Med. 2020;180(10):1345–55.
41. Papoutsi E, Giannakoulis VG, Xourgia E, Routsi C, Kotanidou A, Siempos II. Effect of timing of intubation on clinical outcomes of critically ill patients with COVID-19: a systematic review and meta-analysis of non-randomized cohort studies. Crit Care. 2021;25:121.
42. Mellado-Artigas R, Ferreyro BL, Angriman F, Hernández-Sanz M, Arruti E, Torres A, Villar J, Brochard L, Ferrando C, for the COVID-19 Spanish ICU Network. High-flow nasal oxygen in patients with COVID-19-associated acute respiratory failure. Crit Care. 2021;25:58.
43. Mitra AR, Ronco JJ, Ayas NT. High-flow nasal cannula and infection control precautions in COVID-19. Can J Respir Crit Care Sleep Med. 2020;4(4):279–80.
44. Gómez CC, Rodríguez ÓP, Torné ML, et al. Clinical consensus recommendations regarding non-invasive respiratory support in the adult patient with acute respiratory failure secondary to SARS-CoV-2 infection. Rev Esp Anestesiol Reanim. 2020;67(5):261–70.
45. World Health Organization. Rational use of personal protective equipment for coronavirus disease 2019 (COVID-19): interim guidance, vol. 23. Geneva: World Health Organization; 2020.
46. Leung CCH, Joynt GM, Gomersall CD, Wong WT, Lee A, Ling L, et al. Comparison of high-flow nasal cannula versus oxygen face mask for environmental bacterial contamination in critically ill pneumonia

patients: a randomized controlled crossover trial. J Hosp Infect. 2019;101:84–7.
47. CDC. Coronavirus Disease 2019 (COVID-19). Atlanta: Centers for Disease Control and Prevention; 2020.
48. Li J, Fink JB, Ehrmann S. High-flow nasal cannula for COVID-19 patients: low risk of bio-aerosol dispersion. Eur Respir J. 2020;55(5):2000892.

Indications for Intubation in COVID-19

5

Lorenzo Ball, Elena Ciaravolo, and Chiara Robba

5.1 Introduction

Intubation and invasive mechanical ventilation are often unavoidable in most severe cases of COVID-19 pneumonia; however, deciding the optimum timing and best practices of intubation is challenging [1, 2]. While most hospitalized patients with COVID-19 can be managed with conventional oxygen therapy [3], a certain percentage will require escalation to high-flow nasal cannulas (HFNC), continuous positive airway pressure (CPAP) or bilevel noninvasive positive pressure ventilation (NIV) [4]. These measures can avoid intubation in selected patients. Nonetheless, the proportion of hospitalized COVID-19 patients requiring invasive mechanical ventilation varies across studies, ranging from 5

L. Ball (✉) · C. Robba
Department of Surgical Sciences and Integrated Diagnostics (DISC), University of Genoa, Genoa, Italy

Anesthesia and Intensive Care, Ospedale Policlinico San Martino, IRCCS per l'Oncologia e le Neuroscienze, Genoa, Italy
e-mail: lorenzo.ball@unige.it

E. Ciaravolo
Department of Surgical Sciences and Integrated Diagnostics (DISC), University of Genoa, Genoa, Italy

D. Battaglini, P. Pelosi (eds.), *COVID-19 Critical and Intensive Care Medicine Essentials*, https://doi.org/10.1007/978-3-030-94992-1_5

to 30% [3, 5, 6]. This chapter discusses the clinical, technical, and safety aspects that deserve to be considered when considering intubation in patients with severe COVID-19 related acute respiratory failure.

5.2 Technical Aspects and Operator Safety Concerns

Aerosolized particles exhaled by COVID-19 patients in the acute viral phase are highly infectious [7]. Factors influencing contagiousness include patient's viral load, use of personal protection equipment (PPE) and distance between the patient and the operator [8, 9]. For these reasons, intubation in COVID-19 patients is in intrinsically a risky procedure for the operator [10]. Adequate PPE during intubation include appropriate gown, eye protection, full face shields, and N95, N99, FFP2, FFP3 respirators or powered air-purifying respirators (PAPR). Bag-valve mask ventilation is a highly aerosol-generating procedure; therefore, it should be avoided whenever feasible or its duration should be limited as much as possible using rapid sequence intubation protocols. The possibility of using video laryngoscopes instead of direct laryngoscopy to allow increased distance from the operator to the patient's mouth has been widely discussed, but definitive data on safety and success rate when used in conjunction with COVID-19 grade PPE is lacking [11]. Pilot randomized studies conducted in simulation context before the COVID-19 pandemic highlighted that the use of high-grade PPE could increase the intubation procedure duration [12, 13] and possibly reduce the success rate [13].

5.3 Clinical Context and Rationale for Intubation

The possibility to manage mild–moderate cases of acute hypoxemic respiratory failure (AHRF) refractory to conventional oxygen therapy was introduced in relatively recent times [14]. The most recent definition of acute respiratory distress syndrome

(ARDS) recognizes the possibility of classifying spontaneously breathing patients as having ARDS, provided that they receive at least 5 cmH_2O of CPAP or positive end-expiratory pressure (PEEP) [15]. Both AHRF and ARDS definitions include a broad spectrum of disease, with different prognosis and possibly different responses to noninvasive respiratory support. Regardless of the underlying cause, these patients have severe acute hypoxemia, as reflected by a PaO_2/FiO_2 ratio below 300 mmHg, and signs of respiratory distress and elevated respiratory drive. The $PaCO_2$ will be normal in an initial phase, may be decreased in an intermediate phase in which patients react to hypoxemia increasing minute ventilation, and finally increased in advanced stages when compensation mechanisms fail to maintain the clearance of carbon dioxide. In a large observational study in 2016, noninvasive respiratory support was reported in 14.4% of patients meeting the criteria for ARDS [16]. Regardless of the type of noninvasive respiratory support, prepandemic recommendations suggested the use of noninvasive support in a narrow window of severity of AHRF/ARDS: while it can support efficiently the respiratory function in a patient with moderate and possibly resolving disease, noninvasive assistance could delay an unavoidable intubation and expose patients to an increased risk of death [14].

An approach to intubation limited to the evaluation of hypoxemia is simplistic and possibly results in unnecessary intubations, due to the dissociation between severity of hypoxia and respiratory system compliance in COVID-19 [17]. While in the early phases of COVID-19 patients may present with hypoxemia in absence of dyspnea, advanced severe COVID-19 invariably presents with increased respiratory drive, thus exposing the patients to risk of worsening of the respiratory function due to patient self-inflicted lung injury [18]. Early stages could benefit from noninvasive respiratory support with high FiO_2, as gas exchange impairment is heavily influenced by the extension of regions of low ventilation to perfusion ratio, corresponding to radiological ground glass lesions [19]. However, in advanced stages consolidation and shunt overlap to ground glass, resulting in a pattern similar to conventional ARDS [1, 19]. Benefits of intubation over noninvasive respiratory support include reduction or suppression of the respiratory drive, reduction of the basal metabolism, and allowance of maintaining protective mechanical ventilation. On the other hand, risks are related to the need for sedation, the presence of an artificial airway and exposure to mechanical ventilation, which may result in overlapping ventilator-associated bacterial pneumonia, which often complicates the course of critically ill COVID-19 patients [20] and eventually ventilator-induced lung injury. While in the early phases of the pandemic early intubation was often advocated [21], questions have been raised toward the risks of liberal early intubation based on physiological arguments [22] but also facing the burden of ICU workload characterizing the surges of the pandemic, which is associated with increased mortality [23]. Balancing between risks and benefits of intubation in this context is challenging, and the optimum timing of intubation remains largely an open question.

5.4 Criteria for Intubation in COVID-19

Most patients requiring intubation are receiving, at the time of the procedure, noninvasive respiratory support. Common criteria considered for intubation are the severity of hypoxemia evaluated with the PaO_2/FiO_2 ratio, the respiratory rate, the presence of dyspnea with signs of increased inspiratory effort, including low $PaCO_2$. However, different types of noninvasive respiratory support affect differently these physiologic parameters; therefore, it is difficult to define absolute cutoff values that fit for all patients. The decision to intubate should be individualized taking into account patient history, severity of hypoxemia and dyspnea, and logistic aspects specific to the hospital setting and the degree of concurrent overload of health-care resources. In fact, in the context of pandemic surges, the availability of ICU beds and ventilators has been often a factor contributing to delayed intubation which is associated with increased mortality [24]. In a multicenter study focusing on COVID-19 patients treated with CPAP outside of the ICU, risk factors associated with CPAP failure and intubation were age, lactate dehydrogenase levels and the trajectory of PaO_2/FiO_2 during CPAP treatment [25]. While the PaO_2/FiO_2 ratio alone is often included in algorithms for intubation in patients with ARDS from causes other than COVID-19, the body of evidence accumulated during the pandemic demonstrates that conservative intubation strategies are feasible, since many patients with severe hypoxia can be managed noninvasively especially if no signs of increased respiratory drive are detected [26]. However, this should not be interpreted as a call to avoid intubation at any cost, which is a lifesaving and unavoidable maneuver in most severe cases.

While protocols and indications varied across guidelines and recommendations, respiratory rate above 28–30 breaths per minute, peripheral saturation below 92–95% despite CPAP with at least a FiO_2 of 0.6 are commonly accepted thresholds to consider intubation [1, 25]. In addition to hypoxemia and respiratory rate, several other parameters and condition should be considered as indications to intubation: respiratory acidosis, inability to maintain airway protection reflexes, altered consciousness or psychomotor agitation during noninvasive support, respiratory arrest, uncontrolled vomiting, and hemodynamic instability, in particular when systolic pressure is below 90 mmHg despite adequate volemic status. In addition to purely respiratory acidosis, the presence of elevated lactate levels is a sign of peripheral hypoxia that should be considered. Figure 5.1 resumes a proposed algorithm

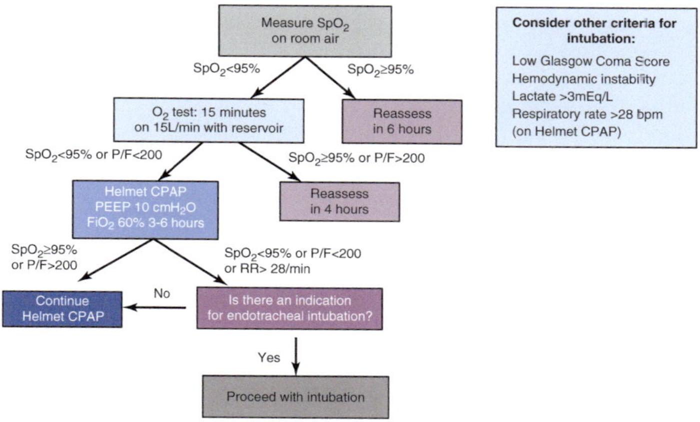

Fig. 5.1 Proposed algorithm for intubation in COVID-19 patients. (Reproduced with permission from [1])

for stepwise management of worsening respiratory failure and possible intubation in COVID-19.

5.5 Conclusions

The decision of intubating a COVID-19 patient is complex and should be based on the integrated evaluation of several clinical parameters, not limited to oxygenation alone. While universal criteria for intubation are difficult to define, several algorithms have been proposed to support the clinician in this challenging decision.

Financial Support and Sponsorship None.

References

1. Robba C, Battaglini D, Ball L, Patroniti N, Loconte M, Brunetti I, Vena A, Giacobbe DR, Bassetti M, Rocco PRM, et al. Distinct phenotypes require distinct respiratory management strategies in severe COVID-19. Respir Physiol Neurobiol. 2020;279:103455.
2. Pisano A, Yavorovskiy A, Verniero L, Landoni G. Indications for tracheal intubation in patients with coronavirus disease 2019 (COVID-19). J Cardiothorac Vasc Anesth. 2021;35:1276–80.
3. Huang C, Wang Y, Li X, Ren L, Zhao J, Hu Y, Zhang L, Fan G, Xu J, Gu X, et al. Clinical features of patients infected with 2019 novel coronavirus in Wuhan, China. Lancet. 2020;395:497–506.
4. Vena A, Giacobbe DR, Di Biagio A, Mikulska M, Taramasso L, De Maria A, Ball L, Brunetti I, Loconte M, Patroniti NA, et al. Clinical characteristics, management and in-hospital mortality of patients with coronavirus disease 2019 in Genoa, Italy. Clin Microbiol Infect. 2020;26:1537–44.
5. Grasselli G, Tonetti T, Protti A, Langer T, Girardis M, Bellani G, Laffey J, Carrafiello G, Carsana L, Rizzuto C, et al. Pathophysiology of COVID-19-associated acute respiratory distress syndrome: a multicentre prospective observational study. Lancet Respir Med. 2020;8(12):1201–8. https://doi.org/10.1016/S2213-2600(20)30370-2.
6. Guan W, Ni Z, Hu Y, Liang W, Ou C, He J, Liu L, Shan H, Lei C, Hui DSC, et al. Clinical characteristics of coronavirus disease 2019 in China. N Engl J Med. 2020;382:1708–20.
7. Li Q, Guan X, Wu P, Wang X, Zhou L, Tong Y, Ren R, Leung KSM, Lau EHY, Wong JY, et al. Early transmission dynamics in Wuhan, China, of novel Coronavirus–infected pneumonia. N Engl J Med. 2020;382:1199–207.

8. Luo M, Cao S, Wei L, Tang R, Hong S, Liu R, Wang Y. Precautions for intubating patients with COVID-19. Anesthesiology. 2020;132:1616–8.
9. Ball L, Alberti S, Belfortini C, Almondo C, Robba C, Battaglini D, Cravero C, Pelosi P, Caratto V, Ferretti M. Effects of distancing and pattern of breathing on the filtering capability of commercial and custom-made facial masks: an in-vitro study. PLoS One. 2021;16:e0250432.
10. Wax RS, Christian MD. Practical recommendations for critical care and anesthesiology teams caring for novel coronavirus (2019-nCoV) patients. Can J Anesth. 2020;67:568–76.
11. Saito T, Taguchi A, Asai T. Videolaryngoscopy for tracheal intubation in patients with COVID-19. Br J Anaesth. 2020;125:e284–6.
12. Shin DH, Choi PC, Na JU, Cho JH, Han SK. Utility of the Pentax-AWS in performing tracheal intubation while wearing chemical, biological, radiation and nuclear personal protective equipment: a randomised crossover trial using a manikin. Emerg Med J. 2013;30:527–31.
13. Castle N, Owen R, Hann M, Clark S, Reeves D, Gurney I. Impact of chemical, biological, radiation, and nuclear personal protective equipment on the performance of low- and high-dexterity airway and vascular access skills. Resuscitation. 2009;80:1290–5.
14. Brochard L, Lefebvre J-C, Cordioli R, Akoumianaki E, Richard J-C. Noninvasive ventilation for patients with hypoxemic acute respiratory failure. Semin Respir Crit Care Med. 2014;35:492–500.
15. ARDS Definition Task Force, Ranieri VM, Rubenfeld GD, Thompson BT, Ferguson ND, Caldwell E, Fan E, Camporota L, Slutsky AS. Acute respiratory distress syndrome: the Berlin definition. JAMA. 2012;307:2526–33.
16. Bellani G, Laffey JG, Pham T, Fan E, Brochard L, Esteban A, Gattinoni L, van Haren F, Larsson A, McAuley DF, et al. Epidemiology, patterns of care, and mortality for patients with acute respiratory distress syndrome in intensive care units in 50 countries. JAMA. 2016;315:788–800.
17. Chiumello D, Busana M, Coppola S, Romitti F, Formenti P, Bonifazi M, Pozzi T, Palumbo MM, Cressoni M, Herrmann P, et al. Physiological and quantitative CT-scan characterization of COVID-19 and typical ARDS: a matched cohort study. Intensive Care Med. 2020;46(12):2187–96. https://doi.org/10.1007/s00134-020-06281-2.
18. Battaglini D, Robba C, Ball L, Silva PL, Cruz FF, Pelosi P, Rocco PRM. Noninvasive respiratory support and patient self-inflicted lung injury in COVID-19: a narrative review. Br J Anaesth. 2021;127:353–64.
19. Ball L, Robba C, Herrmann J, Gerard SE, Xin Y, Mandelli M, Battaglini D, Brunetti I, Minetti G, Seitun S, et al. Lung distribution of gas and blood volume in critically ill COVID-19 patients: a quantitative dual-energy computed tomography study. Crit Care. 2021;25:214.
20. Giacobbe DR, Battaglini D, Enrile EM, Dentone C, Vena A, Robba C, Ball L, Bartoletti M, Coloretti I, Di Bella S, et al. Incidence and prognosis

of ventilator-associated pneumonia in critically ill patients with COVID-19: a multicenter study. J Clin Med. 2021;10:555.
21. Gattinoni L, Marini JJ, Chiumello D, Busana M, Camporota L. COVID-19: scientific reasoning, pragmatism and emotional bias. Ann Intensive Care. 2020;10:134.
22. Tobin MJ, Jubran A, Laghi F. P-SILI as justification for intubation in COVID-19: readers as arbiters. Ann Intensive Care. 2020;10:156.
23. Bravata DM, Perkins AJ, Myers LJ, Arling G, Zhang Y, Zillich AJ, Reese L, Dysangco A, Agarwal R, Myers J, et al. Association of intensive care unit patient load and demand with mortality rates in US Department of Veterans Affairs hospitals during the COVID-19 pandemic. JAMA Netw Open. 2021;4:e2034266.
24. Vaschetto R, Barone-Adesi F, Racca F, Pissaia C, Maestrone C, Colombo D, Olivieri C, De Vita N, Santangelo E, Scotti L, et al. Outcomes of COVID-19 patients treated with continuous positive airway pressure outside the intensive care unit. ERJ Open Res. 2021;7:00541–2020.
25. De Vita N, Scotti L, Cammarota G, Racca F, Pissaia C, Maestrone C, Colombo D, Olivieri C, Della Corte F, Barone-Adesi F, et al. Predictors of intubation in COVID-19 patients treated with out-of-ICU continuous positive airway pressure. Pulmonology. 2021. https://doi.org/10.1016/j.pulmoe.2020.12.010.
26. Voshaar T, Stais P, Köhler D, Dellweg D. Conservative management of COVID-19 associated hypoxaemia. ERJ Open Res. 2021;7:00026–2021.

6 Invasive Mechanical Ventilation in COVID-19

Andrea Berardino and Lorenzo Ball

6.1 Introduction

Since the beginning of the COVID-19 pandemic, peculiar pathophysiological mechanisms have been identified as discussed in the previous chapters [1]. However, while these important aspects improved our understanding of the disease, severe COVID-19 patients often require invasive mechanical ventilation [2]. These patients typically show bilateral lung infiltrates, low arterial oxygen partial pressure to fractional inspired oxygen ratio (PaO_2/FiO_2 < 300 mmHg) and require ventilation with positive end-expiratory pressure (PEEP) above 5 cmH_2O. Therefore, nearly all intubated COVID-19 patients meet the Berlin criteria for ARDS [3]. While in the early phases of the disease a high respiratory

A. Berardino
Department of Surgical Sciences and Integrated Diagnostics (DISC), University of Genoa, Genoa, Italy

L. Ball (✉)
Department of Surgical Sciences and Integrated Diagnostics (DISC), University of Genoa, Genoa, Italy

Anesthesia and Intensive Care, Ospedale Policlinico San Martino, IRCCS per l'Oncologia e le Neuroscienze, Genoa, Italy
e-mail: lorenzo.ball@unige.it

D. Battaglini, P. Pelosi (eds.), *COVID-19 Critical and Intensive Care Medicine Essentials*, https://doi.org/10.1007/978-3-030-94992-1_6

system compliance can be observed [1], most intubated patients present with reduced compliance similarly to conventional ARDS patients [4, 5]. For these reasons, most of the recommendations for titration of mechanical ventilation in these patients are derived from the current knowledge in ARDS [6]. The aims of titrating ventilation settings is to maintain adequate oxygenation, ensure carbon dioxide removal while limiting the risk for ventilator-induced lung injury (VILI) [6]. Commonly recommended gas exchange targets include arterial oxyhemoglobin saturation of 88–95% or a PaO_2 of 55–80 mmHg, tolerating mild hypercapnia provided that the arterial pH remains above 7.25–7.30 [7]. This chapter will discuss the role of different mechanical ventilation settings and rescue strategies in patients invasively ventilated for COVID-19 pneumonia.

6.2 Tidal Volume

The median respiratory system compliance of COVID-19 patients once intubated and admitted to the intensive care unit (ICU) is around 40 mL/cmH_2O, while the total lung weight is increased by 60% compared to a healthy individual [4, 5, 8]. These parameters reflect a reduced size of the "baby lung," namely, the amount of lung tissue available for ventilation, similarly to what occurs in conventional ARDS. This constitutes the pathophysiological rationale for the use of low tidal volume in these patients, which should be kept around 6 mL per kg of predicted body weight (PBW) [9], with an acceptable range between 4 and 8 mL/kg PBW. Higher lung compliance has been reported in a subgroup of intubated COVID-19: in these patients, slightly higher tidal volumes could be tolerated. In fact, when compared to patients with conventional ARDS, COVID-19 have a higher compliance when matched for oxygenation impairment [10]. However, since these patients are at risk of deteriorating respiratory function and worsening of lung elastance and since low tidal volume ventilation is feasible and tolerated in most patients, the general recommendation remains keeping the tidal volume within protective range (6–8 mL/kg of PBW) in all patients receiving invasive mechanical ventilation for COVID-19 pneumonia (Table 6.1).

Table 6.1 Summary of recommendations concerning invasive ventilation settings in COVID-19

Parameter	Target values or ranges	Comments
PaO_2	55–80 mmHg or SpO_2 88–95%	Lower oxygenation targets allow using lower PEEP and/or FiO_2
$PaCO_2$	Tolerate moderate hypercapnia if pH > 7.25	Increase the respiratory rate as first measure to lower $PaCO_2$, values up to 30–35 min^{-1} can be used Attention to intrinsic PEEP
Tidal volume	6–8 mL per kg of predicted body weight	Do not titrate on actual body weight
P_{plat}	Keep below 27–30 cmH_2O	Higher values could be acceptable if chest wall elastance is high
P_{driv}	Keep below 13–15 cmH_2O	Consider further reduction of tidal volume if increased
PEEP	Set individually	Pay attention to deterioration of compliance with high PEEP levels Consider negative hemodynamic Effects of PEEP: monitor central venous oxygenation, arterial–venous gradient of CO_2 and lactates
Recruitment maneuvers	Not as part of routine care	Consider as rescue therapy
Inhaled nitric oxide	Rescue therapy, could improve oxygenation	Unclear effects on mortality
Prone positioning	Improves oxygenation, could reduce mortality	In ARDS better results if applied early in severe cases Potential role of prolonged prone positioning in severe cases
Extracorporeal support	Improve oxygenation and carbon dioxide removal	Patients must be carefully selected

PEEP positive end-expiratory pressure, *FiO_2* fraction of inspired oxygen, P_{plat} plateau pressure, P_{driv} driving pressure (P_{plat} − PEEP)

6.3 Plateau and Driving Pressure

Once a given tidal volume is delivered to the respiratory system of a patient with a certain compliance at a given PEEP level, this results in a specific plateau pressure (P_{plat}). P_{plat} is considered a simple surrogate of stress, namely, the maximum distending force applied to the lungs. This assumption has known limitations, related to the heterogeneous partitioning of respiratory system elastance into its components (lungs and chest wall) in ARDS patients [11], however, since esophageal pressure monitoring is not routinely used in most centers [12] especially in the pandemic context, most guidelines recommend limiting plateau pressure below 28–30 cmH_2O [13]. Lower values might be preferable, while higher values might be tolerated in presence of increased chest wall elastance, as occurs in obese patients and in those with increased intra-abdominal pressure. However, when high plateau pressures are observed, measurement of chest wall elastance with esophageal manometry might be necessary and rescue therapies could be considered.

The difference between P_{plat} and PEEP is referred to as driving pressure (P_{driv}) and defined as:

$$P_{driv} = P_{plat} - \text{PEEP} = \frac{V_T}{C_{rs}},$$

where C_{rs} is the compliance of the respiratory system and V_T the tidal volume. This parameter has been proposed as a surrogate of dynamic strain, being C_{rs} roughly correlated with the end-expiratory lung volume. Values of P_{driv} above 15 cmH_2O have been associated with increased mortality in patients with ARDS [14]. However, a trial in which P_{driv} was lowered through the use of higher PEEP levels plus recruitment maneuvers observed higher mortality in the intervention group [15]. If gas exchange parameters allow, patients with elevated P_{plat} or P_{driv} might benefit from further reduction of tidal volume, as this will lower both pressures at the price of reducing minute ventilation, which might be compensated for increasing the respiratory rate [16].

6.4 Peep and Recruitment Maneuvers

Setting the optimum PEEP level in patients with COVID-19-related ARDS remains one of the most controversial aspects. Observational studies reported that the applied levels of PEEP in COVID-19 were similar to previous reports in ARDS from other causes [4, 17]. However, studies based on lung imaging reported a high variability in response to PEEP [18], with most patients showing limited potential for lung recruitment [8], which might be increased with the concomitant use of recruitment maneuvers [19]. Nonetheless, all studies reported worsening of respiratory system compliance at higher PEEP levels, despite an improvement of lung aeration and oxygenation [8, 18, 19]. This decoupling between oxygenation response and compliance response in COVID-19 poses specific challenges when setting PEEP: patients improving oxygenation at higher PEEP might worsen their respiratory system's elastic properties, therefore increasing P_{driv}, P_{plat} and consequently the risk of VILI. In the absence of new evidence from randomized trials, PEEP settings should be based on current recommendations for ARDS: the use of higher PEEP in most severe patients is commonly advocated [13], but recent meta-analyses failed to show mortality benefits of higher PEEP strategies when compared to strategies aimed at maintaining oxygenation targets with the use of the lowest possible PEEP level [20]. Titration of PEEP should be tailored on an individual basis, considering its effects on oxygenation, respiratory mechanics, and hemodynamics. The use of recruitment maneuvers should be considered as a rescue measure, to overcome an acute impairment of oxygenation unresponsive to increased PEEP and/or fraction of inspired oxygen.

6.5 Fraction of Inspired Oxygen

The fraction of inspired oxygen (FiO_2) is an often-neglected aspect of mechanical ventilation. Experimental studies suggest a potential toxicity of exposure to high FiO_2, especially when translating into high PaO_2 levels. Despite recommendations toward the attainment of moderate–low oxygenation targets, patients with ARDS often show PaO_2 levels higher than those advocated by guidelines and protocols. This also applies to COVID-19 patients [17]. However, recent randomized trials in critically ill patients requiring mechanical ventilation did not observe differences in mortality when comparing restrictive versus conventional oxygen administration strategies [21]. Settings of FiO_2 an PEEP are interconnected, as both could increase oxygenation. However, these act differently, the former increasing alveolar oxygen concentration and the latter recruiting alveoli. Given the relevant role played by areas with low ventilation-perfusion ratio in COVID-19 strategies prioritizing FiO_2 increase over PEEP increase might be acceptable.

6.6 Rescue Strategies

Rescue strategies in severe patients include prone positioning, inhaled nitric oxide, extracorporeal CO_2 removal ($ECCO_2R$) and extracorporeal membrane oxygenation (ECMO). Prone positioning can be helpful in severe COVID-19 to reduce atelectasis, redistribute pulmonary blood flow and ventilation. This improves oxygenation, with a potential beneficial effect on mortality: prone positioning might lead to more homogeneous distribution of regional pleural pressure, possibly reducing VILI. However, in conventional ARDS its benefit on mortality was only shown in a trial applying this measure early and in case of moderate–severe ARDS [22]. In COVID-19, prone positioning was extensively used also for prolonged cycles; most patients respond to pronation improving oxygenation, but the impact on mortality has to be elucidated [23]. Inhaled nitric oxide has been proposed to improve ventilation–perfusion mismatch and oxygenation in ARDS. While most COVID-19 patients improve oxygenation with the administration of inhaled nitric oxide, it is unclear whether mortality is affected [24]. As in any form of respiratory failure, advanced stages might be refractory to conventional therapeutic strategies. In these patients, $ECCO_2R$ or ECMO might be considered.

$ECCO_2R$ does not improve oxygenation, but removing CO_2 could allow reaching protective ventilation parameters, that is, low tidal volume, P_{plat} and P_{driv} in COVID-19 patients with extremely low compliance and refractory hypercapnia [25]. ECMO also improves oxygenation and, when patients are selected appropriately, has outcomes similar to those in ARDS [26]. However, both ECMO and $ECCO_2R$ are expensive and resource-consuming, therefore their use should be limited to selected cases. Objective criteria for ECMO are difficult to ascertain in the context of a pandemic.

6.7 Clinical Message and Conclusions

Despite specific aspects of COVID-19, most ventilation strategies were derived from knowledge in ARDS from other causes. PEEP titration deserves careful consideration, as higher PEEP levels were associated with worse respiratory system compliance in physiological studies in COVID-19. However, randomized trials should clarify the optimal ventilatory strategies in COVID-19 patients.

Financial Support and Sponsorship None.

References

1. Gattinoni L, Chiumello D, Caironi P, Busana M, Romitti F, Brazzi L, Camporota L. COVID-19 pneumonia: different respiratory treatments for different phenotypes? Intensive Care Med. 2020;46(6):1099–102. https://doi.org/10.1007/s00134-020-06033-2.
2. Berlin DA, Gulick RM, Martinez FJ. Severe Covid-19. N Engl J Med. 2020;383:2451–60.
3. ARDS Definition Task Force, Ranieri VM, Rubenfeld GD, Thompson BT, Ferguson ND, Caldwell E, Fan E, Camporota L, Slutsky AS. Acute respiratory distress syndrome: the Berlin definition. JAMA. 2012;307:2526–33.
4. Botta M, Tsonas AM, Pillay J, Boers LS, Algera AG, Bos LDJ, Dongelmans DA, Hollmann MW, Horn J, Vlaar APJ, et al. Ventilation management and clinical outcomes in invasively ventilated patients with

COVID-19 (PRoVENT-COVID): a national, multicentre, observational cohort study. Lancet Respir Med. 2021;9:139–48.

5. Grasselli G, Tonetti T, Protti A, Langer T, Girardis M, Bellani G, Laffey J, Carrafiello G, Carsana L, Rizzuto C, et al. Pathophysiology of COVID-19-associated acute respiratory distress syndrome: a multicentre prospective observational study. Lancet Respir Med. 2020;8(12):1201–8. https://doi.org/10.1016/S2213-2600(20)30370-2.
6. Robba C, Battaglini D, Ball L, Pelosi P, Rocco PRM. Ten things you need to know about intensive care unit management of mechanically ventilated patients with COVID-19. Expert Rev Respir Med. 2021;15:1293–302.
7. Brower RG, Lanken PN, MacIntyre N, Matthay MA, Morris A, Ancukiewicz M, Schoenfeld D, Thompson BT, National Heart, Lung, and Blood Institute ARDS Clinical Trials Network. Higher versus lower positive end-expiratory pressures in patients with the acute respiratory distress syndrome. N Engl J Med. 2004;351:327–36.
8. Ball L, Robba C, Maiello L, Herrmann J, Gerard SE, Xin Y, Battaglini D, Brunetti I, Minetti G, Seitun S, et al. Computed tomography assessment of PEEP-induced alveolar recruitment in patients with severe COVID-19 pneumonia. Crit Care. 2021;25:81.
9. Alhazzani W, Møller MH, Arabi YM, Loeb M, Gong MN, Fan E, Oczkowski S, Levy MM, Derde L, Dzierba A, et al. Surviving sepsis campaign: guidelines on the management of critically ill adults with Coronavirus Disease 2019 (COVID-19). Intensive Care Med. 2020;46:854–87.
10. Chiumello D, Busana M, Coppola S, Romitti F, Formenti P, Bonifazi M, Pozzi T, Palumbo MM, Cressoni M, Herrmann P, et al. Physiological and quantitative CT-scan characterization of COVID-19 and typical ARDS: a matched cohort study. Intensive Care Med. 2020;46(12):2187–96. https://doi.org/10.1007/s00134-020-06281-2.
11. Chiumello D, Carlesso E, Cadringher P, Caironi P, Valenza F, Polli F, Tallarini F, Cozzi P, Cressoni M, Colombo A, et al. Lung stress and strain during mechanical ventilation for acute respiratory distress syndrome. Am J Respir Crit Care Med. 2008;178:346–55.
12. Akoumianaki E, Maggiore SM, Valenza F, Bellani G, Jubran A, Loring SH, Pelosi P, Talmor D, Grasso S, Chiumello D, et al. The application of esophageal pressure measurement in patients with respiratory failure. Am J Respir Crit Care Med. 2014;189:520–31.
13. Fan E, Del Sorbo L, Goligher EC, Hodgson CL, Munshi L, Walkey AJ, Adhikari NKJ, Amato MBP, Branson R, Brower RG, et al. An Official American Thoracic Society/European Society of Intensive Care Medicine/Society of Critical Care Medicine clinical practice guideline: mechanical ventilation in adult patients with acute respiratory distress syndrome. Am J Respir Crit Care Med. 2017;195:1253–63.
14. Amato MBP, Meade MO, Slutsky AS, Brochard L, Costa ELV, Schoenfeld DA, Stewart TE, Briel M, Talmor D, Mercat A, et al. Driving pressure and

survival in the acute respiratory distress syndrome. N Engl J Med. 2015;372:747–55.
15. Writing Group for the Alveolar Recruitment for Acute Respiratory Distress Syndrome Trial (ART) Investigators, Cavalcanti AB, Suzumura ÉA, Laranjeira LN, de Paisani DM, Damiani LP, Guimarães HP, Romano ER, de Regenga MM, LNT T, et al. Effect of lung recruitment and titrated positive end-expiratory pressure (PEEP) vs low PEEP on mortality in patients with acute respiratory distress syndrome: a randomized clinical trial. JAMA. 2017;318:1335–45.
16. Pelosi P, Ball L. Should we titrate ventilation based on driving pressure? Maybe not in the way we would expect. Ann Transl Med. 2018;6:389.
17. Grasselli G, Zangrillo A, Zanella A, Antonelli M, Cabrini L, Castelli A, Cereda D, Coluccello A, Foti G, Fumagalli R, et al. Baseline characteristics and outcomes of 1591 patients infected with SARS-CoV-2 admitted to ICUs of the Lombardy region, Italy. JAMA. 2020;323:1574.
18. Mauri T, Spinelli E, Scotti E, Colussi G, Basile MC, Crotti S, Tubiolo D, Tagliabue P, Zanella A, Grasselli G, et al. Potential for lung recruitment and ventilation–perfusion mismatch in patients with the acute respiratory distress syndrome from Coronavirus Disease 2019. Crit Care Med. 2020;48(8):1129. https://doi.org/10.1097/CCM.0000000000004386.
19. Protti A, Santini A, Pennati F, Chiurazzi C, Cressoni M, Ferrari M, Iapichino GE, Carenzo L, Lanza E, Picardo G, et al. Lung response to a higher positive end-expiratory pressure in mechanically ventilated patients with COVID-19. Chest. 2021;161(4):979–88. https://doi.org/10.1016/j.chest.2021.10.012.
20. Ball L, Serpa Neto A, Trifiletti V, Mandelli M, Firpo I, Robba C, Gama de Abreu M, Schultz MJ, Patroniti N, Rocco PRM, et al. Effects of higher PEEP and recruitment manoeuvres on mortality in patients with ARDS: a systematic review, meta-analysis, meta-regression and trial sequential analysis of randomized controlled trials. Intensive Care Med Exp. 2020;8:39.
21. Mackle D, Bellomo R, Bailey M, et al. The ICU-ROX investigators and the Australian and new Zealand Intensive Care Society clinical trials group: conservative oxygen therapy during mechanical ventilation in the ICU. N Engl J Med. 2020;382:989–98.
22. Guérin C, Reignier J, Richard J-C, Beuret P, Gacouin A, Boulain T, Mercier E, Badet M, Mercat A, Baudin O, et al. Prone positioning in severe acute respiratory distress syndrome. N Engl J Med. 2013;368:2159–68.
23. PRONA-COVID Group, Langer T, Brioni M, Guzzardella A, Carlesso E, Cabrini L, Castelli G, Dalla Corte F, De Robertis E, Favarato M, et al. Prone position in intubated, mechanically ventilated patients with COVID-19: a multi-centric study of more than 1000 patients. Crit Care. 2021;25:128.

24. Abou-Arab O, Huette P, Debouvries F, Dupont H, Jounieaux V, Mahjoub Y. Inhaled nitric oxide for critically ill Covid-19 patients: a prospective study. Crit Care. 2020;24:645.
25. Ding X, Chen H, Zhao H, Zhang H, He H, Cheng W, Wang C, Jiang W, Ma J, Qin Y, et al. $ECCO_2R$ in 12 COVID-19 ARDS patients with extremely low compliance and refractory hypercapnia. Front Med. 2021;8:654658.
26. Diaz RA, Graf J, Zambrano JM, Ruiz C, Espinoza JA, Bravo SI, Salazar PA, Bahamondes JC, Castillo LB, Gajardo AI, et al. ECMO for COVID-19-associated severe ARDS in Chile: a nationwide incidence and cohort study. Am J Respir Crit Care Med. 2021;204(1):34–43. https://doi.org/10.1164/rccm.202011-4166OC.

7 Weaning, Tracheostomy, and Chest Physiotherapy

Carmen Pascale, Giuseppe Servillo, Gennaro Russo, and Maria Vargas

7.1 Weaning from Mechanical Ventilation in COVID-19 Patients

Weaning is gradual reduction of ventilation. A new systematic review suggests that noninvasive ventilation after early extubation helps in reducing the total days spent on invasive mechanical ventilation; also the patients spending less time on invasive ventilation had lower rates of ventilator-associated pneumonia [1, 2]. In some cases this process is rapid and uneventful; however, for some patients the process may be prolonged for days or weeks. Weaning is a term that is used in two separate ways. Firstly, it implies the termination of mechanical ventilation and secondly the removal of any artificial airway [1, 2].

Weaning, the progressive decline in the amount of ventilation support that a patient receives from a ventilator, accounts for approximately 40% of the total time spent on mechanical

C. Pascale · G. Servillo · M. Vargas (✉)
Department of Neurosciences, Reproductive and Odontostomatological Sciences, University of Naples "Federico II", Naples, Italy

G. Russo
Otolaryngology Head and Neck Surgery Unit of "Azienda Ospedaliera di Rilievo Nazionale dei Colli, Ospedale Monaldi", Naples, Italy

D. Battaglini, P. Pelosi (eds.), *COVID-19 Critical and Intensive Care Medicine Essentials*, https://doi.org/10.1007/978-3-030-94992-1_7

ventilation. Patients who wean successfully at the earliest opportunity have less morbidity and mortality and use fewer resources than patients who require mechanical ventilation [1, 2]. The practice of daily sedation interruption (DSI), a method to reduce the complications of prolonged sedation, has been reported to be a safe and beneficial approach to facilitating weaning. However, the best practices in the ICU setting are the daily assessment of a patient's readiness to wean and the gradual decrease in ventilation parameters according to clinical recommendations. Some mechanical ventilation parameters, such as the fraction of inspired oxygen (FiO_2) and the positive end-respiratory pressure (PEEP), are associated with lung injury if higher-than-needed values are used. This means that as long as a patient is ventilated, it is essential to use the lowest values that allow for adequate oxygenation and ventilation [3, 4]. Most patients receiving invasive ventilatory support for acute respiratory failure are readily liberated from the ventilator upon recovery from their acute illness. For a significant minority of patients, however, the transition from mechanical ventilatory support to unassisted breathing proves challenging. Once ventilated patients demonstrate evidence of initial recovery from the cause of acute respiratory failure, they are subjected to a daily trial of spontaneous breathing [1–3]. Difficult weaning is diagnosed by failure of a trial of spontaneous breathing. A consensus panel of experts defined difficult weaning as failure of up to 2 trials of spontaneous breathing, and prolonged weaning as failure of 3 or more trials (114). Using these definitions, estimates of the prevalence of difficult weaning range between 25–40% and 6–20% of patients meet criteria for prolonged weaning [4, 5].

The COVID-19 pandemic has resulted in the implementation of rapidly changing protocols and guidelines related to the indications and protocols for extubation. Both are aerosol-generating procedures, commonly associated with coughing, which necessitates proximity of the physician to the patient.

A meta-analysis of 10 randomized control trials including 3165 patients showed no significant difference in the successful extubation, reintubation rate, ICU mortality, and ICU length of stay between spontaneous breathing trials (SBTs) using low levels of pressure support and a T-piece [6]. Three well-performed trials in resource-rich ICUs clearly showed benefit from early SBTs [7–9]. However, because of much aerosol generating from a T-piece trial, a low-level pressure support is the preferred method for SBTs in COVID-19 patients. Anecdotal evidence demonstrated longer intubation periods, higher volume of secretions, and airway edema in mechanical ventilated COVID-19 patients; all of these factors increase the risk of postextubation respiratory failure. Therefore, we suggest a higher degree of readiness for weaning and direct supplementation of low-flow oxygen after extubation in COVID-19 patients.

To reduce the risk of reintubation, it is preferable a higher degree of extubation readiness in COVID-19 patients. This practice should include higher criteria for passing SBTs, or promote SBTs to last longer, or repeated for confirmation. Nurses and physicians should develop local SBT protocols, and oversedation should be recognized and avoided at the moment the decision is taken to proceed without invasive ventilation. At every extubation, one of the main aims should be the best possible protection of the health-care workers. Personal protective equipment should be used and changed every time, and the extubating sequences should be safe, simple, familiar, and reliable according to available resources. A Canadian group restricted the aerosolization and droplet spraying during extubation with plastic drapes applied over the head and the endotracheal tube [10]. Finally, whenever available, the physiotherapist should be involved in the weaning and extubation process.

In COVID-19 patients as general rules we suggest the following

1. Daily assessments for readiness for weaning by a low-level pressure support (strong recommendation, low quality of evidence).
2. *Against* using a T-piece trial because of contamination risk (weak recommendation, low quality of evidence).
3. Familiar, local extubation protocols to minimize infection risk among health-care workers (weak recommendation, low quality of evidence).

7.2 Tracheostomy in COVID-19 Patients

Tracheostomy is a common procedure for patients admitted to ICUs with acute respiratory distress and with difficult weaning. During the pandemic, many countries published their own guidelines. Nonetheless, guidelines about timing and technical procedures for tracheostomy are still lacking. Current studies suggest that 10–15% of patients hospitalized with COVID-19 require invasive mechanical ventilation [11–13], frequently for prolonged periods. In fact, a recent report from New York City noted that a significant proportion of patients required mechanical ventilation for more than 21 days [14]. Many institutions have recommended a conservative extubation strategy due to a high rate of reintubation and the associated risk of viral spread. This may further stress a limited pool of intensive care resources, including mechanical ventilators and sedative drugs. In this setting, performance of tracheostomy in appropriate candidates has the potential to free up resources across a health system. This may or may not play a role in the decision based on local factors. Tracheostomy is a high-risk procedure for patients with COVID-19 and is considered an aerosol-generating procedure (AGP). Aerosol-generating procedures are associated with high droplet and particle generation, placing health-care providers at increased risk for transmission of respiratory viral infections. Aerosol-generating procedures should be minimized as much as possible to prevent the spread of infection. Some modifications to the well-known percutaneous techniques have been proposed to minimize the risk related to COVID-19 infection [15, 16]. As follows, we suggest a modified technique to improve staff and patient safety during this pandemic.

- The tracheostomy team should be made by two expert ICU physician in airway procedures and one nurse.
- All personnel should be equipped with the proper personnel protective equipment (PPE), including an N99 mask, eye goggles, transparent full-face shield, gown, and double gloves.
- Before the procedure, patients were anesthetized and paralyzed.

- Before the beginning of the procedures, volume control ventilation should be set.
- Five minutes of preoxygenation is needed before the procedure.
- The ICU physician should replace the endotracheal tube (ETT) in place with a smaller ETT, with an internal diameter of 6 mm or less, by using a videolaryngoscope.
- The endotracheal tube should be cuffed at the level of the carina. Then the ventilator will be connected and switched on.
- By using the videolaryngoscope to visualize the glottis, the fiberoptic bronchoscope with an external diameter of 5 mm should be passed through the vocal cords.
- The fiberoptic bronchoscope should be kept just under the level of vocal cords outside the ETT to control the different tracheostomy steps.
- Perform the percutaneous tracheostomy with the technique you know best.
- The puncture of the anterior tracheal wall, Seldinger insertion, dilatation, and cannula positioning will be all performed with the smaller endotracheal tube cuffed and positioned at the carina
- When the cannula will be positioned, the ventilator will be switched off and the smaller ETT may be removed.
- The fiberoptic bronchoscope will be removed after the removal of the ETT.

The decision to perform tracheostomy should include potential risks and benefits for the patient, risks of infection spread to health-care workers, other patients and family and available health-care resources. Criteria has included failed extubation, a failed sedation hold, and anticipated prolonged respiratory wean [17]. A multidisciplinary expert opinion recommended that tracheostomy be delayed until at least day 10 of mechanical ventilation and considered only when patients are showing signs of clinical improvement to tolerate the procedure [18]. Tracheostomy is not recommended in patients who still need high fractions of inspired oxygen, have high ventilator requirements, and might require prone positioning as part of their ventilatory strategy. Prone positioning is more difficult to achieve for patients with tracheostomy due to a higher risk of dislodgement, displacement or occlusion [18]. There is still controversy around the timing of viral load reduction; testing for SARS-CoV-2 using PCR or NAAT does not distinguish between viable and nonviable virus, and virus can be detected using these methods for weeks to months after clinical illness [19]. The timing of the tracheostomy should be based on the clinical indication, and should not be deferred on the basis of PCR test positivity [19]. There is no consistent guidance to help clinical staff plan the most appropriate time to perform a tracheostomy in the critically ill. Outside of the COVID pandemic, there are some groups who would clearly benefit from an early tracheostomy. There is evidence that some neurosurgical patients or some with short/medium-term neurological conditions can reduce ICU and hospital length of stay with an early tracheostomy. Patients who need medium-term respiratory support also benefit, but this group is difficult to characterize early in their ICU stay. The data available from international colleagues and from the literature available suggests that the acute lung injury phase of those patients with COVID-19 pneumonitis lasts around 10–14 days [20]. For those patients who are invasively ventilated, those who tolerate critical illness and the necessary support, can anticipate an ICU stay of at least 10–14 days, probably longer in many. These estimates may change as the pandemic unfolds, but the clinical experience in Europe supports these observations from other countries.

7.3 Chest Physiotherapy in COVID-19

Physiotherapists in an ICU setting have focused to treat functional impairment especially in the patient on mechanical ventilation support. The physiotherapeutic care begins with a detailed assessment and scheduling goals of treatment. This care involves the use of techniques such as endotracheal suction of bronchial secretions, mobilization, and positioning of the patient. The physiotherapy treatment is addressed to prevent and reduce potential pulmonary complications such as hypoventilation, hypoxemia and infection in order to restore muscular and pulmonary function as fast as possible [21, 22]. Physical therapy consists of services provided by physical therapists to individuals and populations to develop, maintain and restore maximum movement and functional ability throughout the lifespan [23]. In the ICU physical therapy aims to prevent physical impairments and to promote physical functioning. In the ICU, the physical therapist is an indispensable member of the multidisciplinary team, who aims to preserve or improve physical function with respect to among other, muscle strength, exercise tolerance, and the performance of physical activities. With physical impairments being predominantly contributing to post–intensive care syndrome (PICS), it has been proposed to start as early as possible with physical therapy in the ICU [24, 25]. Several studies showed the positive effects of physical therapy interventions (such as cycling, physical exercises, mobilization in and out of the bed, and ambulation) on muscle strength, physical functioning, and quality of life, as well as delirium, the duration of mechanical ventilation, and length of ICU and hospital stay [22, 26–28]. The effects of physical therapy treatment strategies on different aspects of functioning and disabilities can be measured and classified according to the domains of the International Classification of Functioning, Disability and Health (ICF). To implement physical therapy in an ICU setting, safe treatment strategies and accurate assessment of physical functioning based on the ICF framework are required. Because physical therapy goals differ between the different phases of recovery aiming at different domains of body functions and structures (muscle atrophy, strength, and exercise capacity) and activities (transfers and walking capacity). Although the different physical therapy interventions are applied in daily clinical practice in the ICU, questions remain regarding the optimum dosage and intensity [24, 25]. Physiotherapists in the ICU interact closely with medical, nursing and other allied health professionals regarding the patient's condition, progression and treatment plans, as well as aid in service integration through collaboration with multiple providers, playing an essential role in the continuum of care when transitioning patients from the ICU [23]. Furthermore, the collaboration between team members promotes and optimizes the active participation of all health care professionals in clinical decision making, focusing on patient needs while ensuring respect for each team members contributions [25]. The optimal management of patients in the ICU is achieved through a multidisciplinary approach, which requires teamwork with clear individual roles, sharing of knowledge, skills, and best practices. The effectiveness of teamwork is considered to be a significant factor that influences the quality of care provided in the ICU.

Physiotherapy plays an integral part in critical care and rehabilitation of the COVID-19 patient. The success of rehabilitation depends upon acute care physiotherapy received by the patient in the ICU. As an essential member of the critical care team, planning and executing an individually tailored rehabilitation program, comes under the purview of a physiotherapist. In addition to providing airway clearance in ventilated patients, physiotherapy provides strategies to optimize oxygenation. COVID-19 patients are at high risk of developing ICU acquired weakness (ICU-AW) [29], thus high morbidity and mortality. It is hence essential to initiate early rehabilitation in order to limit the severity of ICU AW and promote rapid functional recovery [29].

The methods of rehabilitating COVID-19 patients who stayed in the ICU differ only slightly from the techniques of daily rehabilitation implemented in other wards. Every patient should be approached individually and therapy plans should be dynamically adjusted to a patient's changing condition. Frequently applied technique for physiotherapy in COVID-19 patients may include the following:

1. Exercises for thromboprophylaxis—SARS-CoV-2 increases the risk of thromboembolic complications and patients in the ICU are mostly lying in beds.
2. Vibrating chest massage—a device inducing vibrations of the chest facilitates detachment of airway secretions in the lungs and stimulates its relocation to the upper respiratory tract, where it can be evacuated.
3. Chest tapping—facilitates evacuation of airway secretions.

4. Positioning patients on their stomach—very important, according to some research this position promotes regeneration of lungs both in patients who are mechanically ventilated and those who breathe spontaneously. A physiotherapist's role involves placing the patient in the right position and correcting his/her posture while he or she lies on the stomach, in order to prevent complications.
5. Passive exercises—maintenance of mobility in joints—from the very beginning of a patient's stay in the ICU.
6. Passive–active exercises for patients in analgosedation or conscious.
7. Active exercises—for conscious patients.
8. Education on using the TriFlow device—practicing breathing with resistance on inhalation and exhalation.
9. Verticalization.
10. Mobilization.

References

1. Ely EW, Baker AM, Dunagan DP, Burke HL, Smith AC, Kelly PT, Johnson MM, Browder RW, Bowton DL, Haponik EF. Effect on the duration of mechanical ventilation 165 of identifying patients capable of breathing spontaneously. N Engl J Med. 1996;335:1864–9.
2. Esteban A, Ferguson ND, Meade MO, Frutos-Vivar F, Apezteguia C, Brochard L, Raymondos K, Nin N, Hurtado J, Tomicic V, González M, Elizalde J, Nightingale P, Abroug F, Pelosi P, Arabi Y, Moreno R, Jibaja M, D'Empaire G, Sandi F, Matamis D, Montañez AM, Anzueto A. Evolution of mechanical ventilation in response to clinical research. Am J Respir Crit Care Med. 2008;177:170–7.
3. Boles J-M, Bion J, Connors A, Herridge M, Marsh B, Melot C, Pearl R, Silverman H, Stanchina M, Vieillard-Baron A, Welte T. Weaning from mechanical ventilation. Eur Respir J. 2007;29:1033–56.
4. Peñuelas O, Frutos-Vivar F, Fernández C, Anzueto A, Epstein SK, Apezteguia C, González M, Nin N, Raymondos K, Tomicic V, Desmery P, Arabi Y, Pelosi P, Kuiper M, Jibaja M, Matamis D, Ferguson ND, Esteban A, For the Ventila Group. Characteristics and outcomes of ventilated patients according to time to liberation from mechanical ventilation. Am J Respir Crit Care Med. 2011;184:430–7.
5. Funk G-C, Anders S, Breyer M-K, Burghuber OC, Edelmann G, Heindl W, Hinterholz G, Kohansal R, Schuster R, Schwarzmaier-D'Assie A,

Valentin A, Hartl S. Incidence and outcome of weaning from mechanical ventilation according to new categories. Eur Respir J. 2010;35:88–94.
6. Li Y, Li H, Zhang D. Comparison of T-piece and pressure support ventilation as spontaneous breathing trials in critically ill patients: a systematic review and meta-analysis. Crit Care. 2020;24:67.
7. Ely EW, Baker AM, Dunagan DP, Burke HL, Smith AC, Kelly PT, Johnson MM, Browder RW, Bowton DL, Haponik EF. Effect on the duration of mechanical ventilation of identifying patients capable of breathing spontaneously. N Engl J Med. 1996;335:1864–9.
8. Girard TD. Efficacy and safety of a paired sedation and ventilator weaning protocol for mechanically ventilated patients in intensive care (awakening and breathing controlled trial): a randomised controlled trial. Lancet. 2008;371:126–34.
9. Kress JP, Pohlman AS, O'Connor MF, Hall JB. Daily interruption of sedative infusions in critically ill patients undergoing mechanical ventilation. N Engl J Med. 2000;342:1471–7.
10. Matava CT, Yu J, Denning S. Clear plastic drapes may be effective at limiting aerosolization and droplet spray during extubation: implications for COVID-19. Can J Anaesth. 2020;67:902–4.
11. Wang D, Hu B, Hu C, Zhu F, Liu X, Zhang J, et al. Clinical characteristics of 138 hospitalized patients with 2019 novel Coronavirus-infected pneumonia in Wuhan, China. JAMA. 2020;323(11):1061–9.
12. Richardson S, Hirsch JS, Narasimhan M, Crawford JM, McGinn T, Davidson KW, et al. Presenting characteristics, comorbidities, and outcomes among 5700 patients hospitalized with COVID-19 in the New York City area. JAMA. 2020;323(20):2052–9.
13. Docherty AB, Harrison EM, Green CA, Hardwick HE, Pius R, Norman L, et al. Features of 20 133 UK patients in hospital with Covid-19 using the ISARIC WHO clinical characterisation protocol: prospective observational cohort study. BMJ. 2020;369:m1985.
14. Argenziano MG, Bruce SL, Slater CL, Tiao JR, Baldwin MR, Barr RG, et al. Characterization and clinical course of 1000 patients with Coronavirus disease 2019 in New York: retrospective case series. BMJ. 2020;369:m1996.
15. Vargas M, Servillo G. Improving staff safety during tracheostomy in COVID-19 patients. Head Neck. 2020;42(6):1278–9.
16. Vargas M, Russo G, Iacovazzo C, Servillo G. Modified percutaneous tracheostomy in COVID-19 critically ill patients. Head Neck. 2020;42(7):1363–6.
17. McGrath B, Brenner M, Warrillow S, et al. Tracheostomy in the COVID-19 era: global and multidisciplinary guidance. Lancet. 2020;8:717–25.
18. David A, Russel M, El-Sayed I, et al. Tracheostomy guidelines developed at a large academic medical center during the COVID-19 pandemic. Head Neck. 2020;42:1291–6.

19. The RECOVERY Collaborative Group. Dexamethasone in hospitalized patients with Covid-19 preliminary report. N Engl Med. 2020;384:693–704. https://doi.org/10.1056/NEJMoa2021436.
20. Vargas M, Sutherasan Y, Antonelli M, et al. Tracheostomy procedures in the intensive care unit: an international survey. Crit Care. 2015;19(1):291.
21. Bailey P, George T, Vick S, et al. Early activity is feasible and safe in respiratory failure patients. Crit Care Med. 2007;35:139–45.
22. Burtin C, Clerckx B, Robbeets C, et al. Early exercise in critically ill patients enhances short-term functional recovery. Crit Care Med. 2009;37(9):2499–505.
23. World Confederation for Physical Therapy. Policy statement: description of physical therapy. http://www.wcpt.org/policy/ps-descriptionPT.
24. Kayambu G, Boots R, Paratz J. Physical therapy for the critically ill in the ICU: a systematic review and meta-analysis. Crit Care Med. 2013;41:1543–54.
25. Sommers J, Engelbert RH, Dettling-Ihnenfeldt D, et al. Physiotherapy in the intensive care unit: an evidence-based, expert driven, practical statement and rehabilitation recommendations. Clin Rehabil. 2015;29:1051–63.
26. Bourdin G, Barbier J, Burle JF, et al. The feasibility of early physical activity in intensive care unit patients: a prospective observational one-center study. Respir Care. 2010;55:400–7.
27. Calvo-Ayala E, Khan BA, Farber MO, et al. Interventions to improve the physical function of ICU survivors: a systematic review. Chest. 2013;144:1469–80.
28. Gerovasili V, Stefanidis K, Vitzilaios K, et al. Electrical muscle stimulation preserves the muscle mass of critically ill patients: a randomized study. Crit Care. 2009;13:R161.
29. Hodgson CL, Tipping CJ. Physiotherapy management of intensive care unit-acquired weakness. J Physiother. 2017;63(1):4–10.

Part III

Neurological Manifestations of COVID-19

8 Neuropathogenesis and Neurological Manifestations of SARS-CoV-2

Lavienraj Premraj, Rakesh C. Arora, and Sung-Min Cho

Abbreviations

ACE-2	Angiotensin converting enzyme-2 cellular receptor
BBB	Blood–brain-barrier
B-CSF-B	Blood–cerebrospinal fluid-barrier
COVID-19	Coronavirus Disease 2019

L. Premraj
Griffith University School of Medicine, Gold Coast, QLD, Australia

R. C. Arora
Cardiac Science Program, St Boniface General Hospital Research Centre, Winnipeg, MB, Canada

University of Manitoba, Winnipeg, MB, Canada

University of Toronto, Toronto, ON, Canada

S.-M. Cho (✉)
Neuroscience Critical Care and Cardiac Surgery Division, Departments of Neurology, Neurosurgery, Surgery, and Anaesthesiology and Critical Care Medicine, Johns Hopkins University School of Medicine, Baltimore, MD, USA
e-mail: csungmi1@jhmi.edu

D. Battaglini, P. Pelosi (eds.), *COVID-19 Critical and Intensive Care Medicine Essentials*, https://doi.org/10.1007/978-3-030-94992-1_8

CSF	Cerebrospinal fluid
CNS	Central nervous system
ICH	Intracranial hemorrhage
MRI	Magnetic resonance imaging
OSNs	Olfactory sense neurons
OE	Olfactory epithelium
SARS-CoV-2	Severe acute respiratory syndrome Coronavirus 2
TMPRSS-2	Transmembrane protease, serine 2

8.1 Current Neuropathogenic Hypotheses

8.1.1 Transcribial Spread

The spread of the SARS-CoV-2 (COVID-19) virus to the brain via the nose (i.e., transcribial spread) remains a commonly discussed theory of neuroinvasion. Neuronal entry of SARS-CoV-2 relies upon spike (S) protein binding to angiotensin converting enzyme 2 (ACE-2). The cleavage of viral spike protein by transmembrane serine protease 2 (TMPRSS2) activates the virus [1]. It is argued that SARS-CoV-2 may infect the central nervous system (CNS) by ACE-2–mediated entry into olfactory sense neurons (OSNs) of the olfactory epithelium. From here, it may enter second-order neurons along the olfactory nerve and then brain tissue [2, 3]. Anosmia, which is highly associated with COVID-19, is commonly attributed to this mechanism. However, recent in vitro animal and autopsy studies challenged the transcribial spread mechanism by showing OSNs may not express ACE-2 or TMPRSS [1, 3–6]. Therefore, infection of susceptible cells in the olfactory epithelium (OE) alone may better reflect symptoms in COVID-19.

Interestingly, single cell RNA sequencing finds high level ACE-2 expression in sustentacular cells, Bowman's gland cells and olfactory bulb (olfactory bulb) pericytes of mouse and human neuroepithelium [5, 7, 8]. Infection of these cell types may be a nonneuronal mechanism for anosmia in COVID-19. Furthermore, interferon, usually released by cells to heighten viral defenses, upregulates ACE-2 expression in vitro, potentially increasing susceptibility of ACE-2 expressing olfactory epithelial cell types [9]. As in vitro data argues against infection of OSNs, the prevalence of anosmia (85%) requires mechanistic explanation unreliant upon viral entry into OSNs [10–12].

Anosmia can be caused by viral entry and dysfunction of other neuroepithelial cell types. Specifically, SARS-CoV-2 entry into sustentacular cells (ACE-2 expressing support cells that enwrap the mature OSN dendrites, Fig. 8.1) can produce anosmia [13]. In human-ACE-2 expressing mice, SARS-CoV-2 infection produced transient anosmia marked by cytotoxic T cell infiltration and decreased OE uniformity. Here, sustentacular cells and Bowman's gland cells in OE were major targets of SARS-CoV-2 [14]. As in human-COVID-19, anosmia in animal models resolved within weeks [14, 15].

Occasionally, anosmia in COVID-19 patients persists up to 3–6 months post infection [11]. In these patients, stems cells located at the base of the olfactory epithelium (Fig. 8.1) must repopulate extensively damaged neuroepithelium. Unlike traditional viral anosmia, incomplete recovery of olfactory function is not uncommon in COVID-19, which may be due to infection of the stem cells themselves that express ACE-2 at low levels [7, 16].

Findings of histopathological studies that detect viral RNA in the olfactory bulb must be reconciled with the aforementioned inflammatory etiology of anosmia. As a number of studies verified the absence of ACE-2 in the olfactory bulb [17–19], it is more likely that olfactory bulb pericytes (ACE-2 expressing) are infected by SARS-CoV-2 virions within the CSF of the subperineural and arachnoid spaces (Fig. 8.1). This is consistent with reduced olfactory bulb volume observed in COVID-19 patients [20, 21].

While previously, SARS-CoV-1 may have invaded the brain by the transcribial route [2], recent evidence, though inconclusive, fails to verify this mechanism in COVID-19. Therefore, anosmia is likely due to inflammatory damage of neuroepithelium rather than direct neuronal infection. The possibility of viral entry via alternative receptors expressed on neuronal membranes should be further studied.

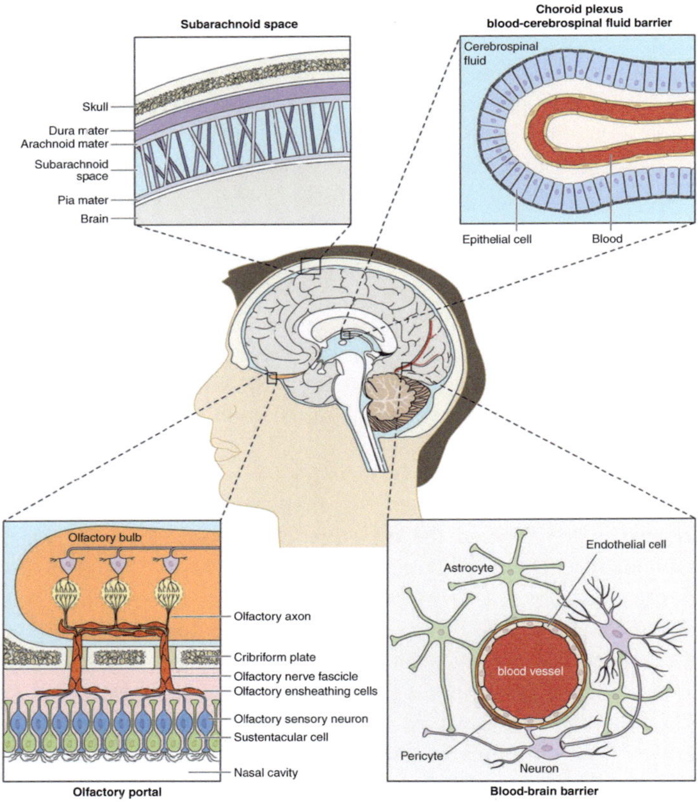

Fig. 8.1 Anatomical description of potential sites of SARS-CoV-2 entry (reproduced from Dando et al.)

8.1.2 Hematogenous Pathway

The hematogenous pathway allows for viral invasion through the blood–brain barrier (B–BB) and or blood–CSF barrier (B–CSF-B) endothelial cells (Fig. 8.1). The frequency of viremia in COVID-19 patients varies widely (1–41%) [22–25]. Circulating SARS-CoV-2 can bind to B–BB/B–CSF-B endothelial cells where host proteases cleave SARS-CoV-2 spike protein into S1 and S2 fragments [26, 27].

Mechanistic studies indicate that the spike protein S1 fragment crosses the B–BB by ACE-2–mediated transcytosis [28]. Specifically, studies using human brain endothelial cells to model the B–BB find that SARS-CoV-2 spike protein triggers immune activation and increases B–BB permeability [29]. The subsequent inflammatory response is specific for matrix metalloproteinases, causing B–BB membrane degeneration and elevation of cytokines IL-6, IL-1β, and CXCL10 in the brain (Fig. 8.2b) [29]. SARS-CoV-2 also can infect mature ACE-2 expressed in human choroid plexus cells in vitro but it is important to recognize that this model failed to demonstrate tropism for neurons or glia [30]. However, when infection of the choroid plexus epithelium and leakage of the B–CSF-B was observed, there was no viral spread to proximal cortical regions despite a 44% reduction in B–CSF-B integrity [30, 31]. In vitro, neuroinflammation was a key feature of COVID-19 pathogenesis in the brain, despite the absence of direct SARS-CoV-2 neuronal entry.

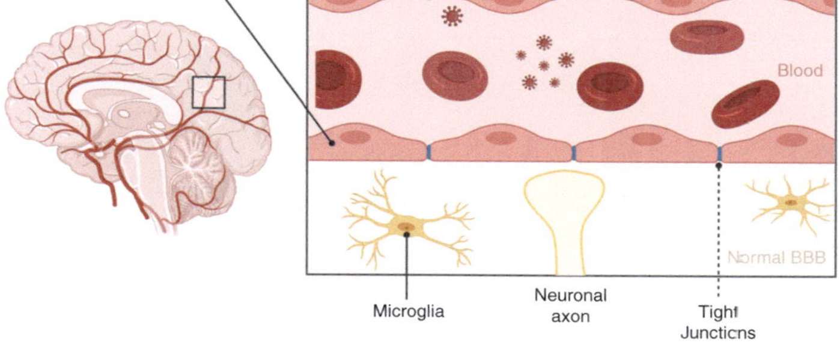

Fig. 8.2 Blood–brain barrier disruption at the cellular level

To date, the presence of SARS-CoV-2 in CSF was rare in the literature; one study found in those with neurological symptoms, only 6% had SARS-CoV-2 PCR positive CSF [32]. Instead, elevated inflammatory markers without viral particles or viral RNA in CSF was commonly observed [33–37]. Therefore, neurological complications of COVID-19 appear to be precipitated by the host immune response, rather than direct viral replication in the brain based on current available literature. Furthermore, comorbidities associated with COVID-19 severity (hypertension, previous neurological injury, and infection) may exacerbate B–BB, B–CSF-B degeneration and inflammation [38]. Cytokine storm from inflammatory response can also significantly decrease B–BB integrity.

In summary, it is mechanistically possible for SARS-CoV-2 to enter through endothelial/choroid plexus cells, crossing a severely leaky and inflamed B–BB/B–CSF-B, which then, circulates within the CSF and localizes in brain regions of ACE-2 (and TMPRSS) expression (Fig. 8.2). Thus, midline structures (e.g., circumventricular organs and the median eminence) may be more likely to be affected as they are relatively unprotected by the B–B-B [21]. Viral spread within the brain parenchyma is limited by the absence ACE-2 expression in adjacent regions [30]. Therefore, it is not surprising that clinical studies attempting to quantify SARS-CoV-2 presence on autopsy have showed either low-level or absent viral RNA in brain tissue as prior studies have focused on cortex and brainstem. Figure 8.3 illustrates the correlation between ACE-2 expressing brain regions and neuropathological findings. Additionally, the neurodegenerative sequalae of inflammation and glial activation may explain links between COVID-19 and cognitive impairment [39]. Ultimately, autopsy and in vitro studies appear to be more consistent with the hematogenous hypothesis.

8.2 Mechanisms of Neurological Complications

Generally, neurological complications likely result from the systemic response to infection or COVID-19 hospitalization rather than SARS-CoV-2 presence in the CNS. Common neurological

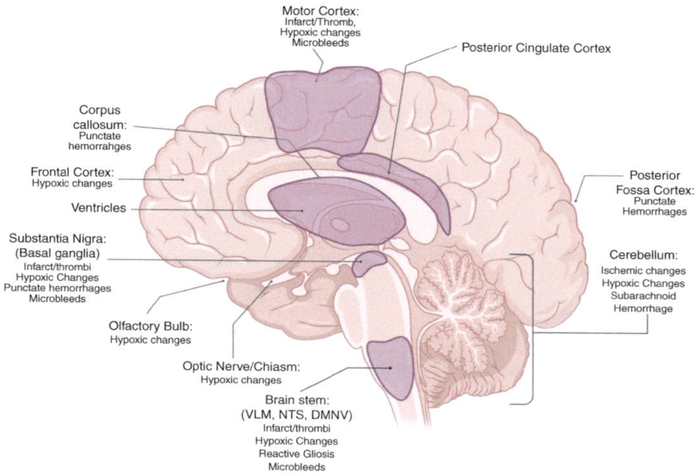

Fig. 8.3 Location of histopathological findings (arrowed) and ACE-2 expressing brain regions (purple)

complications include ischemic stroke, intracranial hemorrhage (ICH), encephalopathy, delirium, and peripheral nerve injury [40, 41] (Table 8.1). Herein, we provide a concise summary of potential mechanisms of common neurological complications in COVID-19.

8.2.1 Ischemic Stroke

Ischemic stroke is a rare but serious complication of COVID-19 occurring in in 1–3% in hospitalized patients and 0.7% of critically ill patients [42, 43]. Understanding incidence of stroke as a complication of COVID-19 proves troublesome. Given the high prevalence of COVID-19 disease, patients who present with ischemic stroke clinically may be incidentally SARS-CoV-2 positive. Further, hospitalization and systemic response to infection result in hypercoagulability and increased risk of arrhythmia. These factors predispose ischemic stroke that is not directly SARS-CoV-2 mediated. CSF pro-inflammatory cytokines (IL-6, TNFα, IL-

Table 8.1 Neurological disease associated with COVID-19

Central nervous system
Encephalitis
– Infectious
– Autoimmune
Transverse myelitis
Acute disseminated encephalomyelitis
Cerebrovascular disease
Ischemic stroke
Intracranial hemorrhage
– Intracerebral hemorrhage
– Subarachnoid hemorrhage
– Subdural hematoma
Peripheral nervous system
GBS
– GBS variants
Peripheral neuropathy
– Sensory
– Autonomic
Anosmia
Ageusia
Other
Seizure
Delirium
Encephalopathy

12p70, IL-10) were not significantly elevated in stroke patients with concurrent COVID-19 compared to nonstroke patients, suggesting stroke may not be from neuroinvasion and rather, a complication of COVID-19 hospitalization [44]. SARS-CoV-2 induced hypercoagulable state is marked by increased D-Dimer, prothrombin time, disseminated intravascular coagulation via common inflammatory pathways (kinin, complement, and intrinsic coagulation pathways) [45]. Specifically, the downregulation of endothelial nitric oxide synthase pathways and impairment of heparan sulfate expression on vascular endothelium [46, 47] creates a prothrombotic state. SARS-CoV-2 over activates the sympathetic nervous system (due to renin–angiotensin–aldosterone system (RAAS) dysregulation), exacerbating traditional stroke risk factors. Microthrombi and hypoxic changes detected upon autopsy corroborate the aforementioned etiology of ischemic stroke.

8.2.2 Intracranial Hemorrhage

Although mechanisms underlying ICH with COVID-19 infection are not well discussed, it is postulated that viral entry into the sub-intimal ACE-2 expressing smooth muscle weakens arterial walls [48]. Additionally, RAAS dysfunction, cytokine storm, SARS-CoV-2–mediated endothelialitis, vasculitis, and B–BB/B–SCF-B degeneration are all plausible inflammatory etiologies of ICH in COVID-19 [49, 50]. COVID-19 associated ICH is usually linked to at least one known ICH risk factor as well as severe pneumonia [51]. Broadly, ICH frequently involves deep parenchymal areas (e.g., basal ganglia) or the ventricles, while olfactory gyrus hemorrhage is only reported once [51, 52]. Such findings are consistent with the understanding that midline brain structures may be more prone to damage in COVID-19. The prevalence of COVID-19 associated ICH is estimated to be 0.7% but is difficult to verify given the prolonged hospitalization of patients with severe COVID-19 [53]. Administration of high-intensity prophylactic or full-dose anticoagulation therapy elevates bleeding risk [54]. Similar to ischemic stroke, patients presenting with ICH, who are incidentally SARS-CoV-2 positive, may lead to an over-estimation of ICH prevalence.

8.2.3 Delirium

The pathophysiology of delirium in patients with COVID-19 has not well defined but remains highly prevalent, in particular in those patients require admission to the ICU. Inflammatory damage may result in neuronal dysfunction of cholinergic circuits while cardiovascular and respiratory insufficiency increases brain dopamine and decrease acetylcholine synthesis [55]. Metabolic abnormalities (e.g., uremic or hepatic encephalopathy) and regional energy deprivation are suggested pathways for delirium [56]. In addition, acute hospitalization with COVID-19 can cause metabolic encephalopathy, most often due to hypoxemia, sepsis, and uremia, which was independently associated with a 24% increased risk of in-hospital mortality [57]. Also, SARS-CoV-2 genomic scripts hijack the mitochondrial genome impairing cerebral oxygen availability and utilization [58, 59]. Clinically, use of mechanical ventilation, benzodiazepines, opioids, vasopressor infusions, steroids and antipsychotics increased risk of delirium the day after administration [60, 61]. Not surprisingly, Kennedy et al. demonstrated that delirium can present in older adults as the primary symptom of COVID-19 [62]. Given its prevalence and multifactorial etiology, appropriate precautions should be taken to minimize risk of delirium in COVID-19 patients.

8.2.4 Immune-Mediated Diseases: Autoimmune Encephalitis, Guillain–Barré Syndrome, Transverse Myelitis, and Neuropathy

Reports of Guillain–Barré syndrome (GBS) and Miller–Fisher variant appear to confirm that immune-mediated polyneuropathy is a complication of COVID-19 infection, with disease pattern and treatment typical of post-infectious GBS. GBS is traditionally preceded by a nonspecific upper respiratory infection up to 4 weeks prior to the onset of weakness. In acute COVID-19 illness associated GBS, CSF showed classic albuminocytologic dissociation in the absence of SARS-CoV-2 and detection of serum antiganglioside antibodies (Anti-Gs) was uncommon [63]. Given the typical clinical presentation and classical demyelinating electrodiagnostic pattern, it is unlikely COVID-19-GBS is from direct viral invasion of peripheral nerves. In molecular simulations, SARS-CoV-2 binds to sialic acid residues on monosialotetrahexosylganglioside (GM-1) [64]. Therefore, similarities between viral protein–associated gangliosides and peripheral nerve gangliosides may allow autoantibody-mediated peripheral nerve damage.

As not all patients demonstrate Anti-Gs [63], GBS may be mediated by novel autoantibodies yet to be characterized in COVID-19.

8.2.5 Direct Infection—Encephalitis

Only few case reports of COVID-19 associated encephalitis have emerged; in a large observational study of 841 hospitalized COVID-19 patients, one developed encephalitis (0.1%) [65]. Immunotherapy (as well as corticosteroids and plasmapheresis) in these patients may reduce length of hospital stay significantly [66]. Although these small reports suggest inflammatory etiology, further CSF studies are required to confirm.

8.3 Conclusions and Clinical Considerations

Evidence regarding the neuropathogenesis of COVID-19 infection largely appears to refute the theory of transcribial spread. Conversely, increased B–BB/B–CSF-B permeability after endothelial cell infection/inflammation may allow SARS-CoV-2 to enter the CNS. A lack of consensus among CSF and autopsy studies, however, limits conclusions about pathogenesis despite relative consensus in vitro studies. Even without clear viral CNS presence, the effect of neuroinflammation due to systemic illness should not be underestimated. As neurological complications are attributed to severe disease, prophylaxis ought to minimize the brain's exposure to pathogen-associated molecular patterns, cytokine storm, and hypoxia. To this end, steroid immunosuppression reduces mortality in severe COVID-19 and may protect against acute inflammatory CNS damage [67]. Though long-term and delayed neurological complications are of concern, especially in the ICU, few studies establish exact causes or empirical treatments. Statistically robust CSF and MRI studies, especially those that apply stratification to neurological outcome and ICU admission, would allow for a more clinically relevant understanding of COVID-19 neuropathogenesis.

Source of Funding None.

Conflicts of Interest/Disclosures Sung-Min Cho has nothing to disclose. Rakesh C. Arora has received an unrestricted educational grant from Pfizer Canada Inc. and honoraria from Abbott Nutrition, Edwards Lifesciences, and Mallinckrodt Pharmaceuticals for work unrelated to this chapter. Lavien Premraj has nothing to disclose.

References

1. Hoffmann M, et al. SARS-CoV-2 cell entry depends on ACE2 and TMPRSS2 and is blocked by a clinically proven protease inhibitor. Cell. 2020;181(2):271–80.
2. Netland J, et al. Severe acute respiratory syndrome coronavirus infection causes neuronal death in the absence of encephalitis in mice transgenic for human ACE2. J Virol. 2008;82(15):7264–75.
3. Zubair AS, et al. Neuropathogenesis and neurologic manifestations of the coronaviruses in the age of coronavirus disease 2019. JAMA Neurol. 2020;77(8):1018.
4. Bilinska K, et al. Expression of the SARS-CoV-2 entry proteins, ACE2 and TMPRSS2, in cells of the olfactory epithelium: identification of cell types and trends with age. ACS Chem Nerosci. 2020;11(11):1555–62.
5. Brann DH, et al. Non-neuronal expression of SARS-CoV-2 entry genes in the olfactory system suggests mechanisms underlying COVID-19-associated anosmia. Sci Adv. 2020;6(31):eabc5801.
6. Qiu C, et al. Olfactory and gustatory dysfunction as an early identifier of COVID-19 in adults and children: an international multicenter study. Otolaryngol Head Neck Surg. 2020;163(4):714–21.
7. Chen M, et al. Elevated ACE-2 expression in the olfactory neuroepithelium: implications for anosmia and upper respiratory SARS-CoV-2 entry and replication. Eur Respir J. 2020;56(3):2001948.
8. Klingenstein M, et al. Evidence of SARS-CoV2 entry protein ACE2 in the human nose and olfactory bulb. Cells Tissues Organs. 2021;209(4–6):155–64.
9. Ziegler CGK, et al. SARS-CoV-2 receptor ACE2 is an interferon-stimulated gene in human airway epithelial cells and is detected in specific cell subsets across tissues. Cell. 2020;181(5):1016–35.
10. Lechien JR, et al. Olfactory and gustatory dysfunctions as a clinical presentation of mild-to-moderate forms of the coronavirus disease (COVID-19): a multicenter European study. Eur Arch Otorhinolaryngol. 2020;277(8):2251–61.
11. Touisserkani SK, Ayatollahi A. Oral corticosteroid relieves post-COVID-19 anosmia in a 35-year-old patient. Case Rep Otolaryngol. 2020;2020:5892047.

12. Vaira LA, et al. Anosmia and Ageusia: common findings in COVID-19 patients. Laryngoscope. 2020;130(7):1787.
13. Heydel J-M, et al. Odorant-binding proteins and xenobiotic metabolizing enzymes: implications in olfactory perireceptor events. Anat Rec. 2013;296(9):1333–45.
14. Ye Q, et al. SARS-CoV-2 infection causes transient olfactory dysfunction in mice. Cold Spring Harbor: Cold Spring Harbor Laboratory; 2020.
15. Abdelalim AA, et al. Corticosteroid nasal spray for recovery of smell sensation in COVID-19 patients: a randomized controlled trial. Am J Otolaryngol. 2021;42(2):102884.
16. Schwob JE. Neural regeneration and the peripheral olfactory system. Anat Rec. 2002;269(1):33–49.
17. Meinhardt J, et al. Olfactory transmucosal SARS-CoV-2 invasion as a port of central nervous system entry in individuals with COVID-19. Nat Neurosci. 2021;24(2):168–75.
18. Tsivgoulis G, et al. Olfactory bulb and mucosa abnormalities in persistent COVID-19-induced anosmia: a magnetic resonance imaging study. Eur J Neurol. 2021;28(1):e6.
19. Yao L, et al. Olfactory cortex and olfactory bulb volume alterations in patients with post-infectious olfactory loss. Brain Imaging Behav. 2018;12(5):1355–62.
20. da Silva Júnior PR, et al. Anosmia and COVID-19: perspectives on its association and the pathophysiological mechanisms involved. Egypt J Neurol Psychiatry Neurosurg. 2021;57(1):8.
21. Pajo AT, et al. Neuropathologic findings of patients with COVID-19: a systematic review. Neurol Sci. 2021;42(4):1255–66.
22. Chen W, et al. Detectable 2019-nCoV viral RNA in blood is a strong indicator for the further clinical severity. Emerg Microbes Infect. 2020;9(1):469–73.
23. Huang C, et al. Clinical features of patients infected with 2019 novel coronavirus in Wuhan, China. Lancet (London, England). 2020;395(10223):497–506.
24. Wang W, et al. Detection of SARS-CoV-2 in different types of clinical specimens. JAMA. 2020;323(18):1843–4.
25. Zhang W, et al. Molecular and serological investigation of 2019-nCoV infected patients: implication of multiple shedding routes. Emerg Microbes Infect. 2020;9(1):386–9.
26. Berger I, Schaffitzel C. The SARS-CoV-2 spike protein: balancing stability and infectivity. Cell Res. 2020;30(12):1059–60.
27. Cai Y, et al. Distinct conformational states of SARS-CoV-2 spike protein. Science. 2020;369(6511):1586–92.
28. Rhea EM, et al. The S1 protein of SARS-CoV-2 crosses the blood–brain barrier in mice. Nat Neurosci. 2021;24(3):368–78.
29. Buzhdygan TP, et al. The SARS-CoV-2 spike protein alters barrier function in 2D static and 3D microfluidic in-vitro models of the human blood–brain barrier. Neurobiol Dis. 2020;146:105131.

30. Pellegrini L, et al. SARS-CoV-2 infects the brain choroid plexus and disrupts the blood–CSF barrier in human brain organoids. Cell Stem Cell. 2020;27(6):951–61.
31. Jacob F, et al. Human pluripotent stem cell-derived neural cells and brain organoids reveal SARS-CoV-2 neurotropism predominates in choroid plexus epithelium. Cell Stem Cell. 2020;27(6):937–50.
32. Lewis A, et al. Cerebrospinal fluid in COVID-19: a systematic review of the literature. J Neurol Sci. 2021;421:117316.
33. Bellon M, et al. Cerebrospinal fluid features in SARS-CoV-2 RT-PCR positive patients. Clin Infect Dis. 2020;73(9):e3102–5.
34. Destras G, et al. Systematic SARS-CoV-2 screening in cerebrospinal fluid during the COVID-19 pandemic. Lancet Microbe. 2020;1(4):e149.
35. de Espíndola OM, et al. Patients with COVID-19 and neurological manifestations show undetectable SARS-CoV-2 RNA levels in the cerebrospinal fluid. Int J Infect Dis. 2020;96:567–9.
36. Franke C, et al. High frequency of cerebrospinal fluid autoantibodies in COVID-19 patients with neurological symptoms. Brain Behav Immun. 2020;93:415–9.
37. Neumann B, et al. Cerebrospinal fluid findings in COVID-19 patients with neurological symptoms. J Neurol Sci. 2020;418:117090.
38. Ellul MA, et al. Neurological associations of COVID-19. Lancet Neurol. 2020;19(9):767–83.
39. Meier IB, et al. Neurological and mental health consequences of COVID-19: potential implications for well-being and labour force. Brain Commun. 2021;3(1):fcab012.
40. Helms J, et al. Delirium and encephalopathy in severe COVID-19: a cohort analysis of ICU patients. Crit Care. 2020;24(1):1.
41. Mao L, et al. Neurologic manifestations of hospitalized patients with coronavirus disease 2019 in Wuhan, China. JAMA Neurol. 2020;77(6):683.
42. Merkler AE, et al. Risk of ischemic stroke in patients with coronavirus disease 2019 (COVID-19) vs patients with influenza. JAMA Neurol. 2020;77(11):1366–72.
43. Fanning JP, Barnett A, Premraj L, Whitman G, Arora R, Battaglini D, Huth S, Porto DB, Choi H, Suen J, Bassi GL, Fraser MG. Stroke complicating critically-ill patients with SARS-CoV-2: analysis of the COVID-19 Critical Care Consortium (CCCC) International, Multicentre Observational Study. Minneapolis, MN: American Academy of Neurology; 2021.
44. Garcia MA, et al. Cerebrospinal fluid in COVID-19 neurological complications: no cytokine storm or neuroinflammation. Cold Spring Harbor: Cold Spring Harbor Laboratory; 2021.
45. Iadecola C, Anrather J, Kamel H. Effects of COVID-19 on the nervous system. Cell. 2020;183(1):16–27.
46. Kumar A, et al. SARS-CoV-2 cell entry receptor ACE2 mediated endothelial dysfunction leads to vascular thrombosis in COVID-19 patients. Med Hypotheses. 2020;145:110320.

47. Nugent MA, et al. Perlecan is required to inhibit thrombosis after deep vascular injury and contributes to endothelial cell-mediated inhibition of intimal hyperplasia. Proc Natl Acad Sci U S A. 2000;97(12):6722–7.
48. Gupta A, et al. Extrapulmonary manifestations of COVID-19. Nat Med. 2020;26(7):1017–32.
49. Lawton MT, et al. Coronavirus disease 2019 (COVID-19) can predispose young to intracerebral hemorrhage: a retrospective observational study. BMC Neurol. 2021;21(1):83.
50. Muhammad S, et al. Letter to editor: severe brain haemorrhage and concomitant COVID-19 infection: a neurovascular complication of COVID-19. Brain Behav Immun. 2020;87:150–1.
51. Mishra S, et al. Intracranial hemorrhage in COVID-19 patients. J Stroke Cerebrovasc Dis. 2021;30(4):105603.
52. Thu SS, Matin N, Levine SR. Olfactory gyrus intracerebral hemorrhage in a patient with COVID-19 infection. J Clin Neurosci. 2020;79:275–6.
53. Cheruiyot I, et al. Intracranial hemorrhage in coronavirus disease 2019 (COVID-19) patients. Neurol Sci. 2021;42(1):25–33.
54. Zahid MJ, et al. Hemorrhagic stroke in setting of severe COVID-19 infection requiring extracorporeal membrane oxygenation (ECMO). J Stroke Cerebrovasc Dis. 2020;29(9):105016.
55. Trzepacz PT. Is there a final common neural pathway in delirium? Focus on acetylcholine and dopamine. Semin Clin Neuropsychiatry. 2000;5(2):132–48.
56. Maclullich AMJ, et al. Unravelling the pathophysiology of delirium: a focus on the role of aberrant stress responses. J Psychosom Res. 2008;65(3):229–38.
57. Frontera JA, et al. Toxic metabolic encephalopathy in hospitalized patients with COVID-19. Neurocrit Care. 2021;35:1–14.
58. Singh KK, et al. Decoding SARS-CoV-2 hijacking of host mitochondria in COVID-19 pathogenesis. Am J Physiol Cell Physiol. 2020;319(2):C258–67.
59. Wu K, Zou J, Chang HY. RNA-GPS predicts SARS-CoV-2 RNA localization to host mitochondria and nucleolus. bioRxiv. 2020;2020:065201. https://doi.org/10.1101/2020.04.28.065201.
60. Kotfis K, et al. COVID-19: ICU delirium management during SARS-CoV-2 pandemic. Crit Care. 2020;24(1):176.
61. Pun BT, et al. Prevalence and risk factors for delirium in critically ill patients with COVID-19 (COVID-D): a multicentre cohort study. Lancet Respir Med. 2021;9(3):239–50.
62. Kennedy M, et al. Delirium in older patients with COVID-19 presenting to the emergency department. JAMA Netw Open. 2020;3(11):e2029540.
63. Caress JB, et al. COVID-19—associated Guillain–Barré syndrome: the early pandemic experience. Muscle Nerve. 2020;62(4):485–91.
64. Garg RK, Paliwal VK, Gupta A. Encephalopathy in patients with COVID-19: a review. J Med Virol. 2021;93(1):206–22.

65. Romero-Sánchez CM, et al. Neurologic manifestations in hospitalized patients with COVID-19: the ALBACOVID registry. Neurology. 2020;95(8):e1060–70.
66. Cao A, et al. Severe COVID-19-related encephalitis can respond to immunotherapy. Brain. 2020;143(12):e102.
67. RECOVERY Collaborative Group. Dexamethasone in hospitalized patients with Covid-19. N Engl J Med. 2021;384(8):693–704.

9 Clinical Characteristics

Jonathon P. Fanning

9.1 Clinical Characteristics of COVID-19

Neurological symptoms are reported by more than 80% of hospitalised COVID-19 patients at some point during their disease [1]. These neurological manifestations range from transient, non–life-threatening symptoms to severe and potentially fatal disease states (Table 9.1). Despite being the most commonly reported neurological symptoms, the often subjective, non-specific, and transient neurological symptoms will not be discussed further in this chapter. Instead, we will focus on severe acute infectious/para-infectious central and peripheral nervous system manifestations that have frequently been reported in hospitalized patients with active SARS-CoV-2 infection and may either be the primary reason for, or a complicating factor contributing to intensive care unit (ICU) admission [2]. While the same neurological manifestations have been identified worldwide, their frequency has varied both

J. P. Fanning (✉)
Faculty of Medicine, University of Queensland,
Brisbane, QLD, Australia

Nuffield Department of Population Health, University of Oxford,
Oxford, UK
e-mail: j.fanning@uq.edu.au

D. Battaglini, P. Pelosi (eds.), *COVID-19 Critical and Intensive Care Medicine Essentials*, https://doi.org/10.1007/978-3-030-94992-1_9

Table 9.1 Neurological sequelae of COVID-19

Transient neurological symptoms
Fatigue
Myalgia/asthenia
Headache
Altered smell (anosmia) and/or taste (dysgeusia)
Nausea
Central nervous system disorders
Ischaemic stroke
Intracranial haemorrhage
Various encephalopathies
Encephalitis and meningoencephalitis
Myelitis
Seizures
Peripheral nervous system disorders
Guillain–Barré syndrome and variants (e.g. Miller Fisher syndrome)
Nerve palsies (e.g. facial nerve, brachial nerve)
Peripheral neuropathies
Myasthenia gravis Myopathy

within and between populations. Additionally, most reported studies failed to control for confounding factors or differentiate between levels of care or the severity of infection. These differences are not further explored in the summary below; however, they are an important factor to keep in mind.

9.2 Central Nervous System Manifestations of COVID-19

9.2.1 Ischaemic Stroke

Stroke is relatively infrequent in COVID-19, with incidence rates ranging between 1.3% among all hospitalised COVID-19 patients and 2.8% in those admitted to ICUs [3–7]. Cerebral venous thrombosis has also been reported with an estimated frequency of

0.08% [8]. Overall, patients who are older, more severely ill, and/or have comorbid illness or some other risk factor predisposing them to stroke appear to be at increased risk of ischaemic stroke [9–11]. Reports of acute ischaemic stroke also exist in a second population consisting of younger COVID-19 patients without pre-existing cardiovascular risk factors [3]. These patients also are more likely to suffer strokes of indeterminate aetiology (so-called cryptogenic stroke) and have higher risks of severe disability and death [3–6], though these risks are often not evident in those patients who develop ischaemic stroke following admission to an ICU for COVID-19 [7].

Among hospitalized patients, the average time to ischaemic stroke detection following admission is approximately 10 days [4]. Among patients being treated in an ICU for other COVID-related complications, like severe acute respiratory distress, the diagnosis and treatment of a stroke may be delayed, especially when patients are sedated and/or paralysed, and because of the commonplace stretching of resources required during pandemic surges.

9.2.2 Intracranial Haemorrhage (ICH)

The prevalence of ICH in COVID-19 patients has been estimated at 0.2–0.9%, though rates up to 2.6% have been documented [2, 12]. Most patients are in their 50s, but ages range from young adulthood to the very old. As with ischaemic strokes, the interval between the onset of COVID-19 symptoms and appearance of neurological signs and/or symptoms from an ICH varies considerably. Rarely, an ICH occurs very early in the course of COVID-19, documented as early as 3 days following the onset of coryzal symptoms, and to be the reason for hospital admission in some patients [13]. However, an ICH is most often diagnosed 2 weeks after COVID-19 symptom onset, following a patient's admission to an ICU and the initiation of mechanical ventilation [7]. In this setting, ICH triples the cumulative hazard of death [7].

The ICHs themselves range greatly in appearance, on either computed tomography (CT) or magnetic resonance imaging

(MRI), from large focal haemorrhages causing a mass effect to multiple microhemorrhages associated with vasogenic oedema. Their clinical presentation also may vary considerably, depending on their size, nature, and location. Atypical presentations like haemorrhagic posterior reversible encephalopathy syndrome (PRES) and bilateral thalamic microhaemorrhages have been reported [14–16]. As with ischaemic strokes, diagnosis and, therefore, treatment in ICU settings can be appreciably delayed.

9.2.3 Encephalopathy

In critically ill COVID-19 patients, encephalopathy is the most common neurological manifestation, reported in up to 80% of ICU and 32% of hospitalised patients [11, 17]. Symptoms typically develop over hours to days; though, in exceptional circumstances, they have been the presenting feature. Clinically, encephalopathy can manifest as changes in personality or behaviour, a dysexecutive syndrome, and/or altered level of consciousness, including frank delirium and coma. Over one-third of patients present with encephalopathy in the absence of typical COVID symptoms [18]. In critically ill COVID patients with such neurological changes, the breadth of causes to consider is extensive, including encephalitis (either infectious or immune-mediated), hypoxia, drugs, toxins, and metabolic derangements. Patients with encephalopathy tend to be older and male, to have had a more rapid course from symptom onset to hospitalization, to smoke cigarettes, and to have a range of comorbid illnesses, including prior neurological disorders, cancer, cardiovascular disease, diabetes, and renal failure [11].

Investigations typically reveal the following

- Normal CSF: no pleocytosis; RT-PCR negative for SARS-CoV-2.
- MRI: non-specific leukoencephalopathy (T2 symmetric and confluent hyperintensity of bilateral deep and subcortical white

matter with mild restricted diffusion) and scattered micro-haemorrhages [19].
- EEG abnormalities are frequent but variably described and confounded by sedation. Most EEGs reveal unspecified abnormalities or diffuse, especially bifrontal, slowed activity [17].

9.2.4 Encephalitis and Meningitis

Encephalitis is diagnosed whenever encephalopathic clinical symptoms occur in association with evidence of brain inflammation. As such, CSF is a key differentiator, and relative to encephalopathic patients, those with encephalitis show evidence of at least one of the following: CSF pleocytosis, protein elevation, or viral detection. Prevalence estimates for COVID-19-related encephalitis are limited and varied, spanning from 0.1–4.5% [20, 21]. Relative to most COVID-19 patients with encephalopathy, encephalitis patients often are younger [20, 21]. Nuchal rigidity indicating meningeal inflammation, Kernig's sign, and Brudzinski's sign are all consistent with encephalomyelitis. The diagnosis of SARS-COV-2 encephalitis is principally made after other conditions are excluded and based on the patient's response to antiviral therapy. Numerous forms of atypical encephalitis are documented in patients with COVID-19 (Table 9.2).

Acute demyelinating encephalomyelitis (ADEM)—which classically follows a viral or bacterial infection or, less frequently, certain vaccinations—consists of rapidly evolving, diffuse inflammation in the brain and spinal cord causing myelin injury. It has been described in several COVID-19 patients, most commonly among patients in their 50s [22]. Symptoms evolve rapidly, sometimes progressing quickly to seizures and/or coma. Given widespread myelin damage, patients may develop weakness to the point of paralysis, difficulty coordinating voluntary muscle movements, and unilateral or bilateral blindness, such that multiple sclerosis (MS) must be considered. The white matter injury detected in brain images may also appear similar to MS, which would be the favoured diagnosis in the presence of older brain

Table 9.2 Forms of encephalopathy/encephalitis diagnosed in COVID-19 patients

Non-specific COVID-19 related encephalopathy
Acute demyelinating encephalomyelitis (ADEM)
Acute necrotizing encephalopathy (ANE)
Limbic encephalitis
Bickerstaff's brainstem encephalitis
Encephalopathy with focal or diffuse leptomeningeal abnormalities
Miscellaneous encephalopathies with other imaging findings
Encephalitis with akathisia and chorea
Cytotoxic lesion of the corpus callosum
Focal or multifocal FLAIR hyperintensities
White matter and/or basal ganglia lesions without ADEM or ANE
Generalized myoclonus and hypersomnia
Acute Parkinsonian syndrome
Ophthalmoparesis with hypothalamic and pituitary stalk involvement

lesions on MRI, though there is no established association with SARS-CoV-2.

9.2.5 Transverse Myelitis

Most notable among the spinal cord complications of COVID-19 are single case reports of transverse myelitis, with patients ranging from 3 to 69 years old [23]. Manifestations range from patchy paraesthesia or progressive headaches (the latter with spinal involvement only diagnosed on MRI) to complete quadriplegia and coma. Weakness (67%), bladder and/or bowel dysfunction (50%), and sensory deficits and/or autonomic dysfunction (38%) are common, with ataxia comparatively rare. Though fever is reported in most, the upper and lower respiratory characteristics that are so predominant in hospitalized COVID-19 patients are either uncommon or mild. CSF abnormalities are common (especially elevated protein), though identification of SARS-CoV-2 in CSF is infrequent. While the majority (>80%) of cases involve isolated myelitis, concomitant brain and/or brainstem involvement, especially ADEM, must be considered.

9.2.6 Seizures

Seizures have only rarely (<1%) been reported as a neurological symptom of COVID-19 [1, 3, 24]. However, these reports represent only incidentally observed seizures with explicit screening for seizures sparse. Limited data suggest that the incidence of de novo seizures increases to near 10% with rigorous continuous electroencephalography [25]. Hence, it might be that seizures are more common in COVID-19 patients than currently recognized, though more robust screening methods are necessary to detect them.

9.3 Peripheral Nervous System Manifestations of COVID-19

9.3.1 Guillain–Barré Syndrome and Miller Fisher Syndrome

Guillain–Barré syndrome (GBS) is an acute polyradiculopathy characterized by rapidly progressive, symmetrical limb weakness, areflexia, and sensory symptoms with variants (most notably the Miller Fisher variant) characterized by facial weakness. The incidence of GBS in patients with COVID-19 is estimated at 0.4–0.5%, though the degree to which GBS is associated with COVID-19 remains unclear. In fact, the overall incidence of GBS cases has declined during the pandemic, presumably due to the reduced transmission of other more strongly associated viruses [26, 27]. Patient ages range from 23 to 77 (median age 55) and males predominate (70%). The initial clinical presentation is highly variable, ranging from development during inpatient treatment for severe infection through isolated neurological symptoms numerous weeks post infection. Typically, neurological symptoms start 2–3 weeks after respiratory symptoms. Some reports suggest that symptoms may appear more rapidly and be more severe than typical for GBS, though a causative association is not excessively apparent [26].

9.3.2 Other Peripheral Neuropathies

A small number of case reports have been published describing nonspecific peripheral neuropathies developing over the course of COVID-19. These have varied in timing, including onsets days prior to the onset of respiratory symptoms, occasionally as the only symptom. In such cases, it is unclear if this represents a clinically isolated neurological presentation of COVID-19 or if its appearance is coincident.

9.3.3 Myasthenia Gravis

New-onset myasthenia gravis (MG)—an autoimmune disease in which largely IgG-1 and IgG-3 antibodies attack nicotinic acetylcholine receptors at neuromuscular junctions, resulting in progressive weakness—has been described in a small number of COVID-19 patients [28], but its relationship to COVID-19 remains uncertain, given the sparsity of reports. What has been reported more extensively is sudden, progressive worsening of already-diagnosed MG after patients contract COVID-19.

9.4 Conclusions

While early reports indicated exceedingly high rates of neurological complications in critically ill COVID-19 patients, the true rates of stroke, haemorrhage, and delirium are likely comparable to those of other critical illnesses and previous coronavirus pandemics. Currently published data are inadequate to either accurately estimate the prevalence of many central and peripheral nervous system manifestations observed in COVID-19 patients or establish any firm causative link between SARS-CoV-2 and neurological disease. Nonetheless, it is imperative that clinicians remain hypervigilant to detect neurological complications in COVID-19 patients, given both their frequency and the difficulties inherent detecting impaired neurological function in critically ill patients who are often mechanically ventilated and sedated.

References

1. Huth S, Cho SM, Robba C, Highton D, Battaglini D, Bellapart J, Suen JY, Li Bassi G, Taccone FS, Arora R, Whitman G, Fraser JF, Fanning JP. Neurological manifestations of coronavirus disease 2019: a comprehensive review and meta-analysis. Front Neruol. 2021;12:664599.
2. Mao L, Jin H, Wang M, Hu Y, Chen S, He Q, Chang J, Hong C, Zhou Y, Wang D, et al. Neurologic manifestations of hospitalized patients with coronavirus disease 2019 in Wuhan, China. JAMA Neurol. 2020;77(6):683–90.
3. Oxley TJ, Mocco J, Majid S, Kellner CP, Shoirah H, Singh IP, De Leacy RA, Shigematsu T, Ladner TR, Yaeger KA, Skliut M, Weinberger J, Danagayach NS, Bederson JB, Tuhrim S, Fifi JT. Large-vessel stroke as a presenting feature of COVID-19 in the young. N Engl J Med. 2020;382(20):e60.
4. Beyrouti R, Adams ME, Benjamin L, Cohen H, Farmer SF, Goh YY, Humphries F, Jager HR, Losseff NA, Perry RJ, Shah S, Simister RJ, Turner D, Chandratheva A, Werring DJ. Characteristics of ischemic stroke associated with COVID-19. J Neurol Neurosurg Psychiatry. 2020;91(8):889.
5. Bekelis K, Missios S, Ahmad J, Labropoulos N, Schimer CM, Calnan DR, Skinner J, MacKenzie TA. Ischemic stroke occurs less frequently in patients with COVID-19: a multicentre cross-sectional study. Stroke. 2020;51:3570–6.
6. Qureshi AI, Baskett WI, Huang W, Shyu D, Myers D, Raju M, Lobanova I, Suri MFK, Naqvi SH, French BR, Siddiq F, Gomez CR, Shyu CR. Acute ischemic stroke and Covid 19: an analysis of 27,676 patients. Stroke. 2021;52(3):905–12.
7. Cho SM, Premraj L, Fanning J, Huth S, Barnett A, Whitman G, Arora R, Battaglini D, Bastos Porto D, Choi HM, Suen J, Li Bassi G, Fraser J, Robba C, Griffee M. Ischemic and hemorrhagic stroke among critically ill patients with COVID-19: an international multicenter COVID-19 Critical Care Consortium Study. Crit Care Med. 2021;49(12):e1223–33.
8. Baldini T, Asioli GM, Romoli M, Carvalho DM, Schulte EC, Hauer L, Aguiar De Sousa D, Seliner J, Zini A. Cerebral venous thrombosis and severe acute respiratory syndrome coronavirus-2 infection: a systematic review and meta-analysis. Eur J Neurol. 2021;28:1–13.
9. Helms J, Tacquard C, Severac F, Leonard-Lorant I, Ohana M, Delabranche X, Merdji H, Clere-Jehl R, Schenck M, Fagot Gandet F, et al. High risk of thrombosis in patients with severe SARS-CoV-2 infection: a multicenter prospective cohort study. Intensive Care Med. 2020;46(6):1089–98.
10. Li Y, Li M, Wang M, Zhou Y, Chang J, Xian Y, Wang D, Mao L, Jin H, Hu B. Acute cerebrovascular disease following COVID-19: a single center,

retrospective, observational study. Stroke Vasc Neurol. 2020;5(3):279–84.

11. Helms J, Kremer S, Merdji H, Clere-Jehl R, Schenck M, Kummerlen C, Collange O, Boulay C, Fafi-Kremer S, Ohana M, et al. Neurologic features in severe SARS-CoV-2 infection. N Engl J Med. 2020;382(23):2268–70.
12. Klok FA, Kruip M, van der Meer N, Arbous M, Gommers D, Kant K, Kaptein F, Paassen J, Stals M, Huisman M, Endeman H. Incidence of thrombotic complications in critically ill ICU patients with COVID-19. Thromb Res. 2020;191:145–7.
13. Avula A, Nalleballe K, Narula N, Sapozhnikov S, Dandu V, Toom S, Glaser A, Elsayegh D. COVID-19 presenting as stroke. Brain Behav Immun. 2020;87:115–9.
14. Dixon L, Varley J, Gontsarova A, Mallon D, Tona F, Muir D, Luqmani A, Jenkins IH, Nicholas R, Jones B, et al. COVID-19-related acute necrotizing encephalopathy with brain stem involvement in a patient with aplastic anemia. Neurol Neuroimmunol Neuroinflamm. 2020;7(5):e789.
15. Franceschi AM, Ahmed O, Giliberto L, Castillo M. Hemorrhagic posterior reversible encephalopathy syndrome as a manifestation of COVID-19 infection. AJNR Am J Neuroradiol. 2020;41(7):1173–6. https://doi.org/10.3174/ajnr.A6595.
16. Kaya Y, Kara S, Akinci C, Kocaman AS. Transient cortical blindness in COVID-19 pneumonia; a PRES-like syndrome: case report. J Neurol Sci. 2020;413:116858.
17. Helms J, Kremer S, Merdji H, Schenck M, Severac F, Clere-Jehl R, et al. Delirium and encephalopathy in severe COVID-19: a cohort analysis of ICU patients. Crit Care. 2020;24:491.
18. Kennedy M, Helfand BK, Gou RY, Gartaganis SL, Webb M, Moccia JM, et al. Delirium in older patients with COVID-19 presenting to the emergency department. JAMA Netw Open. 2020;3(11):e2029540.
19. Radmanesh A, Derman A, Lui Y, Raz E, Loh J, Hagiwara M, Borja M, Zan E, Fatterpekar G. COVID-19-associated diffuse leukoencephalopathy and microhemorrhages. Radiology. 2020;297(1):E223–7.
20. Romero-Sánchez CM, Díaz-Maroto I, Fernández-Díaz E, Sánchez-Larsen Á, Layos-Romero A, García-García J, González E, Redondo-Peñas I, Perona-Moratalla AB, Del Valle-Pérez JA, et al. Neurologic manifestations in hospitalized patients with COVID-19: the ALBACOVID registry. Neurology. 2020;95(8):e1060–70.
21. Varatharaj A, Thomas N, Ellul MA, Davies NWS, Pollak TA, Tenorio EL, Sultan M, Easton A, Breen G, Zandi M, et al. Neurological and neuropsychiatric complications of COVID-19 in 153 patients: a UK-wide surveillance study. Lancet Psychiatry. 2020;7(10):875–82.
22. Paterson RW, Brown RL, Benjamin L, Nortley R, Wiethoff S, Bharucha T, Jayaseelan DL, Kumar G, Raftopoulos RE, Zambreanu L, et al. The

emerging spectrum of COVID-19 neurology: clinical, radiological and laboratory findings. Brain J Neurol. 2020;143(10):3104–20.
23. Mondal R, Deb S, Shome G, Ganguly U, Lahiri D, Benito-León J. COVID-19 and emerging spinal cord complications: a systematic review. Mult Scler Relat Disord. 2021;51:102917.
24. Lu L, Xiong W, Liu D, Liu J, Yang D, Li N, Mu J, Guo J, Li W, Wang G, et al. New onset acute symptomatic seizure and risk factors in coronavirus disease 2019: a retrospective multicenter study. Epilepsia. 2020;61(6):e49–53.
25. Louis S, Dhawan A, Newey C, Nair D, Jehi L, Hantus S, Punia V. Continuous electroencephalography characteristics and acute symptomatic seizures in COVID-19 patients. Clin Neurophysiol. 2020;131(11):2651–6.
26. Toscano G, Palmerini F, Ravaglia S, Ruiz L, Invernizzi P, Cuzzoni MG, Franciotta D, Baldanti F, Daturi R, Postorino P, et al. Guillain–Barré syndrome associated with SARS-CoV-2. N Engl J Med. 2020;382(26):2574–7.
27. Keddie S, Pakpoor J, Mousele C, Pipis M, Machado P, Foster M, et al. Epidemiology and cohort study finds no association between COVID-19 and Guillain–Barré syndrome. Brain. 2021;144(2):682–93.
28. Restivo DA, Centonze D, Alesina A, Marchese-Ragona R. Myasthenia gravis associated with SARS-CoV-2 infection. Ann Intern Med. 2020;173(12):1027–8.

10 The Role of Noninvasive Multimodal Neuromonitoring

Marco Micali, Judith Bellapart, and Denise Battaglini

10.1 Background

The pathophysiology of neurological injury related to Coronavirus disease-2019 (COVID-19) is multifactorial. Several pathophysiological pathways have been described in patients with COVID-19 infection presenting neurological complications. Microangiopathy has been shown to be an important underlying process causing small vessel cerebral infarct [1] or hemorrhagic transformations;

M. Micali
Anesthesia and Intensive Care, San Martino Policlinico Hospital, IRCCS for Oncology and Neuroscience, Genoa, Italy

Department of Surgical Science and Integrated Diagnostics, University of Genoa, Genoa, Italy

J. Bellapart
Critical Care Research Group (CCRG), Brisbane, QLD, Australia

Royal Brisbane and Women's Hospital, Brisbane, QLD, Australia

D. Battaglini (✉)
Anesthesia and Intensive Care, San Martino Policlinico Hospital, IRCCS for Oncology and Neuroscience, Genoa, Italy

Department of Medicine, University of Barcelona, Barcelona, Spain

D. Battaglini, P. Pelosi (eds.), *COVID-19 Critical and Intensive Care Medicine Essentials*, https://doi.org/10.1007/978-3-030-94992-1_10

endotheliitis, has been reported in the context of systemic inflammatory response (SIRS) which is shared among other COVID-19 related clinical presentations [2]. Direct viral cytopathic injury has been described in anatomopathological samples in patients with encephalitis. Autoimmune processes leading to peripheral or central neuritis have also been described with COVID infection [3]. Therefore, neurological injury related to COVID-19 may present with a variety of overlapping syndromes. This pathological myriad impacts in the monitoring of these patients as there is no specific surveillance that can be used for the screening of evolving neurological complications. Early detection of new neurological involvement is warranted to prevent and manage complications. Being not available a concrete monitoring to apply to each of these scenarios, physicians need to be guided by high level clinical suspicion and an approach of diagnostic exclusion in the daily management of these patients. In this context, the role of noninvasive multimodal neuromonitoring acquires a new perspective in COVID-19. This chapter overviews the possible ways to detect patients at risk of neurological complications, highlighting the possible role of multimodal neuromonitoring systems.

10.2 Clinical Features

Several studies have shown that the most frequent neurological presentations of COVID-19 are headache, anosmia, ageusia, myalgia, myositis, encephalopathy, ischemic stroke, and intracerebral hemorrhage [4]. The most commonly affected anatomical regions by ischemia are the cerebrum and cerebellum, with MRI studies highlighting the possible development of posterior reversible encephalopathy syndrome (PRES), hypoxic encephalopathy and exacerbation of preexisting demyelinating disease [4].

In addition, studies have found that infection with COVID-19 can accelerate the progression of acute stroke and that elderly patients with COVID-19 may be more likely to develop cerebrovascular disease, while those with a previous cerebrovascular history are 2.5 times more likely to develop severe COVID-19 [5]. SARS-CoV-2 has also been reported to trigger autoimmune diseases such as multiple sclerosis, acute disseminated encephalomyelitis, acute encephalitis, acute autoimmune polyneuropathy, and critical illness polyneuropathy as well as cerebrovascular events [4].

Another important manifestation in COVID-19 patient is delirium. According to literature, delirium prevalence ranges from 27 to 74% among hospitalized patients with COVID-19 [4, 6]. Therefore, the prompt recognition of patients at risk of neurological manifestation become essential for patients' management.

10.3 Noninvasive Multimodal Neuromonitoring in COVID-19

As above mentioned, SARS-CoV-2 may damage important brain structures essential for brain homeostasis. At this point, diagnostic methods play a crucial role to early identify those patients who may suffer of brain damage. The role of noninvasive neuromonitoring in non-primarily brain damaged patients can be pivotal since invasive neuromonitoring may not be indicated. This offers the advantage to facilitate the screening of silent neurological complications. Moreover, critical COVID-19 patients require of mechanical ventilation and are sedated and paralyzed to optimize ventilation; this situation limits the possibility of wake-up tests for neurological examination. Therefore, noninvasive neuromonitoring can be considered attractive diagnostic and prognostic tools for patients with high clinical suspicious of neurological involvement and limited diagnostic options. Well known diagnostic and screening interventions adjusted to the monitoring of COVID-19 patients include:

10.3.1 Brain Ultrasonography

Brain ultrasonography is a bedside, noninvasive and safe tool to assess brain anatomic dysfunction, pathophysiology, and cerebral blood flow [7]. Transcranial doppler (TCD) and, in particular transcranial color-coded duplex ultrasonography, is a powerful tool for the assessment of brain anatomical features, cerebral blood flow (CBF), cerebral flow autoregulation, and intracranial pressure (ICP). It can also allow the detection of new onset hemorrhages that may lead to mass effect, by the identification of midline shift or ventriculomegaly [7]. Brain ultrasonography is usually performed with a 2–2.5 MHz ultrasound probe through four main acoustic windows (transtemporal, transorbital, occipital, and submandibular) [7]. According to the Poiseuille theorem, CBF can be estimated from the cerebral blood flow centerline velocity, and the angle of insonation of the ultrasound beam. According to the principle of conservation of energy, the velocity will remain constant if the area of the insonated vessel is unchanged. Based on these two classical principles, TCD allows the quantification of CBF through the entire circle of Willis. The impairment of cerebrovascular hemodynamic (CVH) and intracranial compliance (ICC), due to the elevation of ICP is frequent in COVID-19 admitted to ICU and could predict poor outcome [8]. Several factors can potentially increase ICP and impair CVH in COVID-19 patients with respiratory distress, including increased partial pressure of carbon dioxide causing cerebral vasodilatation, or the use of higher ventilatory pressures consequently increasing intrathoracic pressure [4]. ICP value >20–22 mmHg is considered indicative of intracranial hypertension [9]. ICP can be noninvasively calculated as follows:

$$\mathrm{CPPe}_{\mathrm{TCD}} = \mathrm{MAP}\left(\text{mean arterial pressure}\right) * d\mathrm{FV} / \mathrm{mFV} + 14$$

$$\mathrm{nICP}_{\mathrm{TCD}} = \mathrm{MAP} - \mathrm{CPPe}$$

This method can accurately exclude intracranial hypertension with a sensitivity of 100% and a specificity of 91.2% in critically ill patients [10]. The association between eCPP abnormalities and delirium in sepsis is well known, with a decrease in flow velocity at TCD probably due to increased resistances and impaired autoregulation [11]. This can also be considered for COVID-19, who showed a great prevalence of delirium and cerebral dysfunction very similar to those associated with sepsis during ICU stay [4, 6]. Indeed, altered eCPP was found in several COVID-19 patients:

low cerebral perfusion pressure (eCPP) was defined as eCPP ≤ 45 mmHg, while high eCPP was defined as eCPP ≥ 75 mmHg [8].Another useful tool for estimating ICP is the technique of pulsatility index (PI). PI is an index of variation of the eCPP, which is strictly correlated, positively, with the increase of the nICP. PI was defined as altered in COVID-19 as any value ≥1.2 [8]:

$$\mathrm{PI} = \left(\mathrm{sFV} - d\mathrm{FV}\right) / \mathrm{mFV}$$

$$\mathrm{mFV} = \left(\mathrm{sFV} + 2 * d\mathrm{FV}\right) / 3$$

[mFV, mean flow velocity; sFV, systolic flow velocity; *d*FV, diastolic flow velocity].

$$\mathrm{nICP\,calculated\,from\,PI: nICPPI} = \left(10.93^{*}\,\mathrm{PI}\right) - 1.28$$

Based on this formula, a PI of > 2.13 would correlate to an ICP > 22 mmHg as for the most recent guidelines, whereas a PI of <1.2 corresponds to <12 mmHg of ICP [12] (Fig. 10.1).The waveform analysis allows the identification of pathological processes through pattern recognition. ICP waveform analysis can provide information on the state of cerebrovascular reactivity, compensatory reserve, can be used to estimate individualized optimal CPP levels [13], and to predict and identify cerebral circulatory arrest [12]. Alterations in intracranial compliance were found with the B4C tool in several COVID-19 patients with a $P2/P1$ ratio > 1 (i.e., $P2 > P1$) [14], where $P1$ is the percussion wave that represents arterial pulsation and $P2$ is the tidal wave that represents intracranial compliance [14, 15]. However, this monitoring system is highly specific of neurointensive care units and might be difficult to perform for a daily bedside examination in a pandemic setting.

Other peculiar TCD findings among COVID-19 patients have been found: the presence of microemboli at the level of the cerebral circulation was investigated by some authors. Microemboli are commonly monitored in patients with patent foramen ovale or conditions that increase the patency of intrapulmonary shunts. Indeed, the presence of underlying microangiopathy in COVID-19

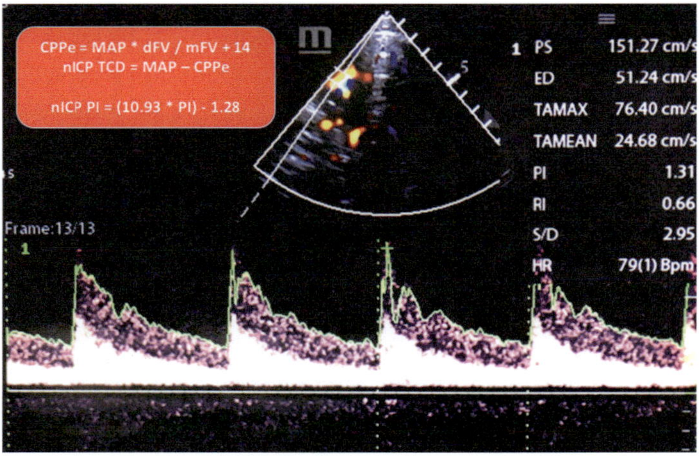

Fig. 10.1 TCD waveforms in the middle cerebral artery and ICP calculation. Non-invasive ICP calculation by using two different formulas: (1) CPPe = MAP * *d*FV/mFV + 14; nICP TCD = MAP − CPPe; (2) nICP PI = (10.93 * PI) − 1.28. Calculated values in this patient: (1) CPPe = 84 * 5 1.24/76.40 + 14 = 70.33 mmHg; nICP TCD = 84–70.33 = 13.66 mmHg; (2) nICP PI = (10.93 * 1.31) − 1.28 = 13.04 mmHg

may lead to an increase in microembolic signal [16]. Salazar et al. detected high intensity signals by TCD in 26% and pulmonary shunt in 23% of COVID-19 patients [17], while Ziai et al. did not detect any microembolism with TCD in patients with severe COVID-19 [18]. Reynolds et al. found microbubbles in the 83% of examined patients, whose presence was inversely correlated with the partial pressure of oxygen (PaO_2)/fraction of inspired oxygen (FiO_2) fraction and lung compliance [19].

Cerebral midline shift (MLS) is a life-threatening condition associated with poor neurological outcome, that is commonly diagnosed via computed tomography (CT). A recent meta-analysis, although with huge methodological limitations, concluded that brain ultrasonography may be a reliable alternative to brain CT-scan for the rapid evaluation of MLS [20]. The detection of MLS has been described in stroke and intracranial hemorrhage among non-COVID-19 patients [21], and being COVID-19 at higher risk of stroke [22] this tool could be helpful in selected cases of high suspicious of cerebral derangement. This methodic at bedside is really simple to perform with an ultrasound probe: after identifying the MCA in the circle of Willis, the insonation window should be adjusted with the midbrain in the center of the screen and contralateral skull visible. From this position, the transducer should be tilted upward by 10° to identify the third ventricle that presents with hyperechoic margins, the pineal gland, and the surrounding hypoechogenic thalamus. The distances ($d1$ and $d2$) between the center of the third ventricle and the bone at both sides of the head are used for calculating the MLS, according to the formula [12]: $\text{MLS} = (d1 - d2)/2$ or from the ipsilateral side of the probe to the third ventricle (distance $d3$), and the full distance from the ipsilateral temporal bone to the contralateral temporal bone ($d4$), according to the formula [12]: $\text{MLS} = d3 - (d4/2)$. Of note, no correlation between high ICP and MLS has been found, suggesting that MLS might be nonuniform across the subfalcine space [21].

The optic nerve sheath diameter (ONSD) is one of the most valid methods to noninvasively calculate the ICP. A cutoff of >5 mm correlates well with an ICP of >20 mmHg [23]. The optic nerve is surrounded by the subarachnoid space. If the pressure of the cerebrospinal fluid increases, the retrobulbar part of the optic nerve expands. The increases in ICP, in the perioptic cerebrospinal fluid causes a greater enlargement of the retrobulbar segment of the optic nerve sheath, 3 mm behind the globe, compared to the posterior segment. Czosnyka et al. demonstrated that nICP derived from ONSD measurements is the strongest parameter correlated with invasive ICP. Furthermore, the latter is correlated with mortality at discharge [24]. The study of ICP in COVID-19 patients is becoming increasingly popular. From the first studies it emerges that in several of these patients there is an increase of the $\text{nICP}_{\text{ONSD}}$ of about 5–6 mm; this suggests that an increased nICP is a common finding in COVID-19. The increase of nICP [$\text{nICP ONSD} = 5 \times \text{ONSD} - 14$] [24] was also associated with increased ICU length of stay. This type of neuromonitoring might be therefore important to detect patients who may have an increased risk of longer ICU-stay, with subsequent complications and difficult recovery [4] (Fig. 10.2).

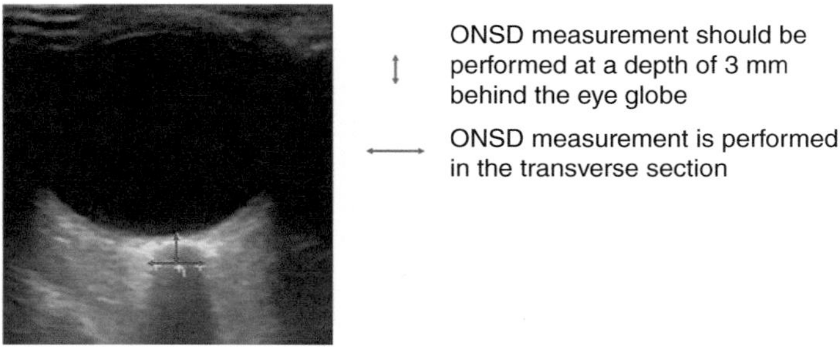

Fig. 10.2 Optic nerve sheath diameter. How to calculate the diameter of optic nerve sheath

10.3.2 Near Infrared Spectroscopy

The use of near-infrared spectroscopy (NIRS), to provide continuous monitoring of the percentage of oxygenated hemoglobin and tissue saturation, allows the detection of changes in regional brain oxygenation over time. This could be particularly relevant for COVID-19 who showed marked hypoxemia and ventilation/perfusion mismatch. NIRS uses sensors placed on the patient's forehead, emitting optical radiation (infrared waves). Thanks to the different absorption of oxygenated and deoxygenated hemoglobin, NIRS allows information on regional cortical tissue perfusion (rSO_2) and cerebral flow. Furthermore, since tissue hypoperfusion is associated with an increase in oxygen extraction and a reduction in hemoglobin saturation, the saturation provided by NIRS can be considered an indicator of regional tissue perfusion. Tissue hypoxia was defined as a regional cerebral saturation of oxygen (rSO_2), measured by NIRS <60% in COVID-19 [25].

Some studies have shown that rSO_2, measured by NIRS, is reduced in patients with delirium compared to healthy patients [11]. NIRS might be adopted in COVID-19 for assessing the effects on cerebral oxygenation of ventilator rescue therapies and hemodynamic assessments. After recruitment maneuvers (RMs), cerebral oxygenation decreased significantly; while after prone position, PaO_2 and rSO_2 significantly increased. The use of inhaled nitric oxide (iNO) increased PaO_2 and rSO_2 significantly, while they were significantly reduced using extracorporeal-CO_2 removal ($ECCO_2R$). A significant relationship was found between peripheral saturation of oxygen and rSO_2 and between PaO_2 and rSO_2 [26]. Again, Robba et al. [25] investigated rSO_2 at baseline and after a passive leg raising test, fluid challenge, and/or norepinephrine bolus. All tests resulted in increased MAP and rSO_2 at NIRS with different responses, suggesting that passive leg raising acts increasing intrathoracic pressure and help detecting between fluid challenge and norepinephrine needs, while norepinephrine shows more autoregulatory and oxygenator effects than fluid challenge in COVID-19 because of its intrinsic properties on cerebral vessels and brain barrier. Hence, NIRS should be applied in mechanically ventilated patients with COVID-19 as an early-warning indicator of inadequate brain oxygen delivery, to increase the systemic delivery of oxygen and to prevent hypoxic complications. Within this context an adequate oxygen delivery could be obtained by modulating either the cardiac output, hemoglobin concentration, or, if possible, pulmonary gas exchange [3].

10.3.3 Automated Pupillometer

Automated infrared pupillometry may be a valid noninvasive tool to investigate nervous system dysfunction, in particular brain stem reflexes [7]. Pupillary light reactivity is measured by using an infrared camera to record a video footage of the changes in the pupillary surface in both eyes. Pupillary light reactivity is assessed by a calibrated light stimulation. Quantitative reactivity is express as the percentage of pupillary light response, and baseline pupil size is express in millimeters. The pupillary constriction velocity is express in mm/s. Abnormal pupillary reactivity is defined as an abnormal pupillary light reflex as reported by the pupillometer defined as a pupillary constriction rate $< 13\%$ [4, 27–29]. The pupillary light reflex, and the sizes and differences between pupils may provide information regarding the functional status of oculomotor and optic nerves. The changes in pupillary reactivity showed a good accuracy to predict delirium in ventilated critically ill patients [30]. Of note, many drugs (such as opioids and sedatives), alcohol and hypothermic condition can alter pupillary activity, but despite adjusting the doses, the association between delirium and impaired pupillary activity remains high. The abnormally low quantitative pupillary constriction variables may trigger interventions targeted at limiting delirium risk or complement available composite scores for predicting delirium [30]. In a series of COVID-19 patients, approximately 40% of all patients exhibited altered pupillary reactivity and a higher proportion of them manifest with delirium [4]; although the underlying pathophysiological mechanisms in COVID-19 are still unclear. Despite the confirmed utility of automated pupillometry for detecting patients at higher risk of delirium, its value has been corroborated also for prognostication after cardiac arrest, outcome after traumatic brain injury, and pain assessment of unconscious patients [7].

10.3.4 Electroencephalogram

Electroencephalogram (EEG) can provide diagnostic and prognostic information in critically ill patients. Variable patterns of EEG activity can be associated to encephalopathy, seizures, hypoxic brain injury, cerebral structural abnormalities and coma. EEG can be also used for determining the depth of anesthesia and the achievement of burst-suppression for the treatment of status epilepticus [31]. During the COVID-19 pandemic EEG has been a useful monitoring tool in patients with prolonged periods of ventilation [32]. Among COVID-19 patients with neurological involvement, commonly reported EEG patterns have been slow wave activity, delta activity, triphasic waves, periodic discharges, and burst suppressions. In this scenario, EEG has contributed to neurological prognostication by the exclusion of reversible causes [31]. In a recent meta-analysis in COVID-19, typical EEG patterns include abnormal background activity (96%) and generalized slowing. Around 20% have an epileptiform discharge (60% of them with known epileptiform activity), although the proportion of seizures and status epilepticus on EEG is relatively low in COVID-19 (2% and <1%) [32].

10.4 Conclusions

The pathogenicity of COVID-19 has shown a specific neurotropism. Neurological manifestations such as delirium, increased ICP, and stroke have been reported among COVID-19 patients. Noninvasive neuromonitoring strategies might be helpful for the detection of new brain derangements in COVID-19 critically ill patients. However, the role of neuromonitoring in COVID-19 remains not clear and should be further investigated.

References

1. Qureshi AI, Baskett WI, Huang W, et al. Acute ischemic stroke and COVID-19. Stroke. 2021;52(3):905–12. https://doi.org/10.1161/STROKEAHA.120.031786.
2. Azizi SA, Azizi S-A. Neurological injuries in COVID-19 patients: direct viral invasion or a bystander injury after infection of epithelial/endothelial cells. J Neurovirol. 2020;26(5):631–41. https://doi.org/10.1007/s13365-020-00903-7.
3. Battaglini D, Brunetti I, Anania P, et al. Neurological manifestations of severe SARS-CoV-2 infection: potential mechanisms and implications of individualized mechanical ventilation settings. Front Neurol. 2020;11:845. https://doi.org/10.3389/fneur.2020.00845.
4. Battaglini D, Santori G, Chandraptham K, et al. Neurological complications and noninvasive multimodal neuromonitoring in critically ill mechanically ventilated COVID-19 patients. Front Neurol. 2020;11:602114. https://doi.org/10.3389/fneur.2020.602114.
5. Li Y, Li M, Wang M, et al. Acute cerebrovascular disease following COVID-19: a single center, retrospective, observational study. Stroke Vasc Neurol. 2020;5(3):279–84. https://doi.org/10.1136/svn-2020-000431.
6. Pun BT, Badenes R, Heras La Calle G, et al. Prevalence and risk factors for delirium in critically ill patients with COVID-19 (COVID-D): a multicentre cohort study. Lancet Respir Med. 2021;9(3):239–50. https://doi.org/10.1016/S2213-2600(20)30552-X.
7. Rasulo FA, Togni T, Romagnoli S. Essential noninvasive multimodality neuromonitoring for the critically ill patient. Crit Care. 2020;24(1):100. https://doi.org/10.1186/s13054-020-2781-2.
8. Brasil S, Taccone FS, Wahys SY, et al. Cerebral hemodynamics and intracranial compliance impairment in critically ill COVID-19 patients: a pilot study. Brain Sci. 2021;11(7):874. https://doi.org/10.21203/rs.3.rs-125420/v1.

9. Battaglini D, Anania P, Rocco PRM, et al. Escalate and de-escalate therapies for intracranial pressure control in traumatic brain injury. Front Neurol. 2020;11:564751. https://doi.org/10.3389/fneur.2020.564751.
10. Rasulo FA, Bertuetti R, Robba C, et al. The accuracy of transcranial Doppler in excluding intracranial hypertension following acute brain injury: a multicenter prospective pilot study. Crit Care. 2017;21(1):44. https://doi.org/10.1186/s13054-017-1632-2.
11. Wood MD, Boyd JG, Wood N, et al. The use of near-infrared spectroscopy and/or transcranial Doppler as non-invasive markers of cerebral perfusion in adult sepsis patients with delirium: a systematic review. J Intensive Care Med. 2021;37(3):408–22. https://doi.org/10.1177/0885066621997090.
12. Lau VI, Arntfield RT. Point-of-care transcranial Doppler by intensivists. Crit Ultrasound J. 2017;9(1):21. https://doi.org/10.1186/s13089-017-0077-9.
13. Cardim D, Robba C, Bohdanowicz M, et al. Non-invasive monitoring of intracranial pressure using transcranial Doppler ultrasonography: is it possible? Neurocrit Care. 2016;25(3):473–91. https://doi.org/10.1007/s12028-016-0258-6.
14. Brasil S, Renck AC, Taccone FS, et al. Obesity and its implications on cerebral circulation and intracranial compliance in severe COVID-19. Obes Sci Pract. 2021;7(6):751–9. https://doi.org/10.1002/osp4.534.
15. Asgari S, Bergsneider M, Hamilton R, Vespa P, Hu X. Consistent changes in intracranial pressure waveform morphology induced by acute hypercapnic cerebral vasodilatation. Neurocrit Care. 2011;15(1):55–62. https://doi.org/10.1007/s12028-010-9463-x.
16. Batra A, Clark JR, LaHaye K, et al. Transcranial Doppler ultrasound evidence of active cerebral embolization in COVID-19. J Stroke Cerebrovasc Dis. 2021;30(3):105542. https://doi.org/10.1016/j.jstrokecerebrovasdis.2020.105542.
17. Salazar-Orellana JLI, García-Grimshaw M, Valdés-Ferrer SI, et al. Detection of pulmonary shunts by transcranial Doppler in hospitalized non-mechanically ventilated Coronavirus disease-19 patients. Rev Invest Clin. 2021;73(2):61. https://doi.org/10.24875/RIC.20000569.
18. Ziai WC, Cho S-M, Johansen MC, Ergin B, Bahouth MN. Transcranial Doppler in acute COVID-19 infection. Stroke. 2021;52:2422–6. https://doi.org/10.1161/STROKEAHA.120.032150.
19. Reynolds AS, Lee AG, Renz J, et al. Pulmonary vascular dilatation detected by automated transcranial Doppler in COVID-19 pneumonia. Am J Respir Crit Care Med. 2020;202(7):1037–9. https://doi.org/10.1164/rccm.202006-2219LE.
20. Hakim SM, Abdellatif AA, Ali MI, Ammar MA. Reliability of transcranial sonography for assessment of brain midline shift in adult neuro-

critical patients: a systematic review and meta-analysis. Minerva Anestesiol. 2021;87(4):467–75. https://doi.org/10.23736/S0375-9393.20.14624-8.
21. Liao C-C, Chen Y-F, Xiao F. Brain midline shift measurement and its automation: a review of techniques and algorithms. Int J Biomed Imaging. 2018;2018:1–13. https://doi.org/10.1155/2018/4303161.
22. Cho S-M, Premraj L, Fanning J, et al. Ischemic and hemorrhagic stroke among critically ill patients with Coronavirus Disease 2019: An International Multicenter Coronavirus Disease 2019 Critical Care Consortium Study. Crit Care Med. 2021;49:e1223. https://doi.org/10.1097/CCM.0000000000005209.
23. Sekhon MS, Griesdale DE, Robba C, et al. Optic nerve sheath diameter on computed tomography is correlated with simultaneously measured intracranial pressure in patients with severe traumatic brain injury. Intensive Care Med. 2014;40(9):1267–74. https://doi.org/10.1007/s00134-014-3392-7.
24. Robba C, Cardim D, Tajsic T, et al. Ultrasound non-invasive measurement of intracranial pressure in neurointensive care: a prospective observational study. PLoS Med. 2017;14(7):e1002356. https://doi.org/10.1371/journal.pmed.1002356.
25. Robba C, Messina A, Battaglini D, et al. Early effects of passive leg-raising test, fluid challenge, and norepinephrine on cerebral autoregulation and oxygenation in COVID-19 critically ill patients. Front Neurol. 2021;12:674466. https://doi.org/10.3389/fneur.2021.674466.
26. Robba C, Ball L, Battaglini D, et al. Early effects of ventilatory rescue therapies on systemic and cerebral oxygenation in mechanically ventilated COVID-19 patients with acute respiratory distress syndrome: a prospective observational study. Crit Care. 2021;25(1):111. https://doi.org/10.1186/s13054-021-03537-1.
27. Chen J, Gombart Z, Rogers S, Gardiner S, Cecil S, Bullock R. Pupillary reactivity as an early indicator of increased intracranial pressure: the introduction of the neurological pupil index. Surg Neurol Int. 2011;2(1):82. https://doi.org/10.4103/2152-7806.82248.
28. Oddo M, Sandroni C, Citerio G, et al. Quantitative versus standard pupillary light reflex for early prognostication in comatose cardiac arrest patients: an international prospective multicenter double-blinded study. Intensive Care Med. 2018;44(12):2102–11. https://doi.org/10.1007/s00134-018-5448-6.
29. Suys T, Bouzat P, Marques-Vidal P, et al. Automated quantitative pupillometry for the prognostication of coma after cardiac arrest. Neurocrit Care. 2014;21(2):300–8. https://doi.org/10.1007/s12028-014-9981-z.
30. Favre E, Bernini A, Morelli P, et al. Neuromonitoring of delirium with quantitative pupillometry in sedated mechanically ventilated critically ill

patients. Crit Care. 2020;24(1):66. https://doi.org/10.1186/s13054-020-2796-8.
31. Sewell L, Abbas A, Kane N. Introduction to interpretation of the EEG in intensive care. BJA Educ. 2019;19(3):74–82. https://doi.org/10.1016/j.bjae.2018.11.002.
32. Kubota T, Gajera PK, Kuroda N. Meta-analysis of EEG findings in patients with COVID-19. Epilepsy Behav. 2021;115:107682. https://doi.org/10.1016/j.yebeh.2020.107682.

11 Management of Neurological Complications

Jaeho Hwang, Bo Soo Kim,
Ali Shabahang Saber Tehrani,
and Sung-Min Cho

11.1 Introduction

Critically ill patients with COVID-19 pneumonia in the intensive care unit (ICU) may develop neurological complications of their central nervous system (CNS) or peripheral nervous system (PNS) that may arise directly from the COVID-19 virus, indirectly as a complication of the COVID-19-related hospitalization, or by mechanisms that have not yet been elucidated. These include encephalopathy, delirium, ischemic stroke, intracranial hemorrhage, peripheral nerve injury, and critical illness myopathy. As

J. Hwang · A. S. S. Tehrani
Department of Neurology, Johns Hopkins University, Baltimore, MD, USA

B. S. Kim
Department of Medicine, Johns Hopkins University, Baltimore, MD, USA

S.-M. Cho (✉)
Neuroscience Critical Care Division, Departments of Neurology, Neurosurgery, Anaesthesiology and Critical Care Medicine, Johns Hopkins University School of Medicine, Baltimore, MD, USA
e-mail: csungmi1@jhmi.edu

D. Battaglini, P. Pelosi (eds.), *COVID-19 Critical and Intensive Care Medicine Essentials*, https://doi.org/10.1007/978-3-030-94992-1_11

the evidence of neurological complications in COVID-19 patients accumulate, we aim to provide a concise review on optimal management strategies of these complications. For the purpose of our review, we are excluding patients in the ICU who develop new neurological symptoms and are found to have otherwise asymptomatic SARS-CoV-2 PCR positivity.

11.2 Encephalopathy/Delirium

Encephalopathy and delirium are frequently observed complications in critically ill COVID-19 infected patients, and may be the primary presenting symptom or complication of a prolonged ICU admission [1–5]. The underlying causes may be a primary CNS process or secondary to dysfunction of other organs, such as the heart, lungs, liver, or kidneys. Patients should actively be screened for any changes in consciousness or mental status by the primary medical team performing serial neurological exams and making use of screening tools such as the Confusion Assessment Method Intensive Care Unit (CAM-ICU) instrument or the Intensive Care Delirium Screening Checklist (ICDSC) due to its impact on mortality and long-term cognitive outcome [3, 6–10].

Diagnostic workup to consider is the same as that of non-COVID ICU patients, including the review of medications that may be contributing; laboratory blood and urine tests to rule out hypoxic, toxic, metabolic, or infectious causes; neuroimaging such as computed tomography (CT) and/or magnetic resonance imaging (MRI) to rule out acute or subacute conditions such as ischemic stroke, hypoxic ischemic brain injury, or intracranial hemorrhage; blood vessel imaging such as CT angiography (CTA), magnetic resonance angiography (MRA) or transcranial doppler (TCD) to rule out stenoses, occlusions, or low-flow states if vascular event is suspected; electroencephalography (EEG) to identify patterns such as nonconvulsive seizures, diffuse slowing, or triphasic waves; and lumbar puncture (LP) with cerebrospinal fluid (CSF) analysis to rule out CNS infections such as meningitis or CNS inflammation such as encephalitis.

If any of these tests reveal CNS disease as a cause of encephalopathy, patients should receive the appropriate treatment specific to the underlying cause. However, if these tests are unremarkable or nondiagnostic, diagnoses of exclusion may include unspecified encephalopathy, ICU delirium, or psychiatric conditions. In these cases, management may include adequate pain control with analgesics, minimizing the number and dose of sedatives, promoting a normal sleep–wake cycle, and consideration of antipsychotics to manage delirium [3, 11, 12].

11.3 Effect of Prophylactic Anticoagulation on Neurological Conditions

As COVID-19 increases hypercoagulability, patients admitted to the ICU are generally given high-intensity prophylactic anticoagulation (AC) against venous thromboembolism (VTE) that consists of either subcutaneous enoxaparin or heparin. Exceptions for this include patients with contraindications, such as active hemorrhage, platelet count less than 50,000, thrombolysis within the past 24 h, or other conditions leading to high risk of bleeding. In such cases, multidisciplinary discussions weighing the risks and benefits of high-intensity prophylactic AC are required. The high-intensity prophylactic AC therapy consists of higher doses and/or frequency of enoxaparin and heparin compared to those given to non-ICU COVID-19 patients, with further dose adjustments depending on serial laboratory measurements of anti-Xa levels and/or creatinine levels. For example, for an average male of 90 kg and normal renal function, the starting doses of subcutaneous enoxaparin or heparin would be 30 mg every 12 h or 7500 units every 8 h respectively, rather than 40 mg daily or 5000 units every 8 h. There are randomized controlled trials at the time of this review that will answer this important question in the near future.

11.4 Ischemic Stroke

The association between COVID-19 and ischemic stroke has been controversial and not clearly determined [13–16]. Regardless, patients should be examined regularly for acute development of any focal neurological deficits. In patients with any concerns of an ischemic stroke, they should immediately undergo a head CT with consideration of CTA of the head and neck and CT-perfusion (CTP) [17]. If evidence of ischemic stroke is present, the remainder of the standard workup for ischemic stroke should be completed, including a MRI of the brain, transthoracic echocardiogram (TTE) with bubble study, electrocardiogram (EKG), and laboratory tests such as hemoglobin A1c, lipid panel, and thyroid-stimulating hormone (TSH) to determine the etiology of the stroke. If these studies are unrevealing, further hypercoagulable lab tests may be sent, including lupus anticoagulant, anti-cardiolipin antibodies, anti-phospholipid antibodies, protein C/S, antithrombin III (AT-III), prothrombin mutation, factor V Leiden mutation, homocysteine, hemoglobin electrophoresis, and syphilis serology, as well as those associated with COVID-19 such as D-dimer, fibrinogen, factor VIII, activated partial thromboplastin time (aPTT), prothrombin time/international normalized ratio (PT/INR), and von Willebrand factor (vWF).

Depending on the etiology of the stroke, the acute treatment will differ, following the preexisting guidelines for ischemic strokes in non-COVID patients, which may involve tissue plasminogen activator (tPA), intra-arterial thrombectomy, management of increased intracranial pressure from cerebral edema, permissive hypertension, statin, single or dual antiplatelet therapy (DAPT) with aspirin and/or clopidogrel, and/or AC [18]. However, if all other etiologies of stroke have been ruled out, and the patient's COVID-19 status appears to be the only pertinent finding, we recommend acute treatment with a daily single antiplatelet agent and statin, given the lack of current studies that indicate the superiority of DAPT over aspirin alone. The potential exception for this may be a situation in which the patient is concurrently found to have additional thromboses in other body parts, such as pulmonary embolism (PE), deep vein thrombosis (DVT), or infarcts of other organs, which would also warrant systemic AC. In these cases, the risks and benefits of combining antiplatelet therapy with systemic AC must be discussed with the involved health-care providers from other departments, and the treatment may be tailored on an individual basis. Additional procedures, such as the closure of patent foramen ovale (PFO), carotid endarterectomy (CEA), and/or carotid artery stent should also be considered based on any positive imaging findings mentioned above.

While stroke secondary to COVID-19 may be considered as a provoked stroke, the length of chronic treatment with antiplatelet therapy may differ for patients based on case-by-case discussions weighing the risks and benefits in context of their baseline medical history and risk factors, and may also be affected by the plan for long-term AC after discharge.

11.5 Intracranial Hemorrhage

On the opposite end of the spectrum, intracranial hemorrhages may also occur as a complication of COVID-19's disease course. Similar to ischemic stroke, a direct causal relationship between COVID-19 and intracranial hemorrhage has not been established. The diagnosis is made by head CT that is obtained if there is any concern for new focal neurological deficits. Etiologies may include unintended complications of systemic AC used for concurrent PEs or during extracorporeal membrane oxygenation (ECMO) support, or hemorrhagic conversions of ischemic strokes. Reversal of systemic AC is recommended for life-threatening intracranial hemorrhage [19]. Depending on the severity and location of the hemorrhage, blood product transfusions, neurosurgical interventions, management of increased intracranial pressure, adjustments in mechanical ventilation settings, and/or further imaging such as CTA may also be indicated. Subsequently, serial stability head CTs, neurological exams, and coagulopathy labs are necessary to monitor the progression of the hemorrhage. Multidisciplinary discussions weighing the risks and benefits of continued AC will be required prior to restarting it.

11.6 Peripheral Nerve and Muscle Injury

In addition to affecting the CNS, patients with COVID-19 in the ICU setting can also develop injury to the PNS or muscles, usually as unintended consequences of their treatment process. For example, the current guidelines for treatment of COVID-19 acute respiratory distress syndrome (ARDS) includes prone positioning for several hours per day, during which patients are mostly immobilized, and may at least in part be contributing to the development of peripheral neuropathies and/or plexopathies, usually of the upper limbs [20–23]. In addition, patients on ECMO support may also develop PNS injury either directly from ECMO cannulation or indirectly from complications of cannulation, such as an expanding hematoma. Another related condition more generalized to patients in the ICU setting is critical illness neuropathy and/or myopathy [24, 25]. In ICU patients who develop neuromuscular weakness, the diagnostic workup and treatment are the same as for those without COVID-19. In the event of diffuse generalized weakness or focal weakness with concern of a PNS lesion, the evaluation includes minimizing sedation, review of medications that may be contributing, standard laboratory tests, electrodiagnostic studies such as electromyography, nerve conduction studies, repetitive nerve stimulation, direct muscle stimulation, and muscle biopsy. The treatment is generally conservative, including frequent repositioning, continued treatment of the underlying primary illness, which in these cases is COVID-19, and aggressive rehabilitation. However, procedures by surgeons or interventional radiologists may be required in cases of traumatic PNS injury or expanding hematomas.

11.7 Special Consideration: Severe ARDS and ECMO

A situation more specific for critically ill COVID-19 patients is one in which the patients require ECMO support due to refractory severe ARDS. COVID-19 is known to cause ARDS that may require ICU admission for management of hypoxic respiratory failure and ECMO support in severe cases [26–30]. In addition to the ECMO support itself, patients who are cannulated for ECMO concurrently and routinely receive systemic AC. Independent of COVID-19, ECMO support has been shown to be associated with various neurological complications, including hypoxic-ischemic brain injury, ischemic stroke, intracranial hemorrhage, and seizures [31–33]. The management of these conditions are generally the same as for those without ECMO.

First, since ECMO patients are given paralytics and sedatives, they often do not have reliable neurological exams, and thus, the true onset of any exam changes or imaging findings may be difficult to determine. Given that a standardized neuromonitoring protocol can increase the detection of brain injury, a protocolized sedation cessation with serial neurological exams is recommended [34]. Second, the equipment used for ECMO support preclude patients from undergoing MRIs, and thus other modalities, such as CT, TCD, cerebral near-infrared spectroscopy, EEG, and/or somatosensory evoked potentials (SSEP) must be relied upon more frequently for the purpose of neurological monitoring and neuroprognostication [34, 35]. Third, the ECMO circuits may alter the pharmacokinetics and pharmacodynamics of medications, including those of anti-seizure drugs, potentially increasing the risk of seizures in high-risk patients. In these situations, patients would benefit from frequent lab checks of the drugs' serum levels or concentration, and continuous EEG monitoring to rule out nonconvulsive seizures if they continue to have impaired consciousness despite discontinuation of sedating medications [36]. Fourth, upon initiation of ECMO, rapid $PaCO_2$ corrections of large magnitude can occur, which have been independently associated with higher incidences of neurological complications, including seizures, ischemic stroke, intracranial hemorrhage, and brain death [37]. Thus, frequent arterial blood gas monitoring and the use of modest sweep gas flow rates particularly during the first 24 h is highly recommended [37]. Fifth, as mentioned in the discussion of intracranial hemorrhage above, patients on ECMO support who develop intracranial hemorrhage will require a multidisciplinary approach regarding the reversal and resumption of systemic AC.

11.8 Conclusions

Critically ill patients with COVID-19 pneumonia commonly develop neurological complications including encephalopathy, delirium, ischemic stroke, intracranial hemorrhage, peripheral nerve injury, and critical illness myopathy. The management strategy such complications is similar to those without COVID-19 disease in ICU. Sedatives and paralytics in COVID-19 ICU patients are major confounding factors. Early detection of acute brain injury through a standardized neuromonitoring protocol as well as a protocolized sedation cessation with serial neurological exams may lead to timely neurological care of critically ill COVID-19 patients.

References

1. Ellul MA, Benjamin L, Singh B, Lant S, Michael BD, Easton A, et al. Neurological associations of COVID-19. Lancet Neurol. 2020;19:767–83.
2. Hassett CE, Gedansky A, Migdady I, Bhimraj A, Uchino K, Cho SM. Neurologic complications of COVID-19. Cleve Clin J Med. 2020;87:729–34.
3. Kotfis K, Roberson SW, Wilson JE, Dabrowski W, Pun BT, Ely EW. COVID-19: ICU delirium management during SARS-CoV-2 pandemic. Crit Care. 2020;24:176.
4. Romero-Sanchez CM, Diaz-Maroto I, Fernandez-Diaz E, Sanchez-Larsen A, Layos-Romero A, Garcia-Garcia J, et al. Neurologic manifestations in hospitalized patients with COVID-19—the ALBACOVID registry. Neurology. 2020;95:e1060–70.
5. Nersesjan V, Amiri M, Lebech AM, Roed C, Mens H, Russell L, et al. Central and peripheral nervous system complications of COVID-19: a prospective tertiary center cohort with 3-month follow up. J Neurol. 2021;268(9):3086–104.
6. Ely EW, Inouye SK, Bernard GR, Gordon S, Francis J, May L, et al. Delirium in mechanically ventilated patients: validity and reliability of the confusion assessment method for the intensive care unit (CAM-ICU). JAMA. 2001;286:2703.
7. Luetz A, Heymann A, Radtke FM, Chenitir C, Neuhaus U, Nachtigall I, et al. Different assessment tools for intensive care unit delirium: which score to use? Crit Care Med. 2010;38:409.
8. Plaschke K, von Haken R, Scholz M, Engelhardt R, Brobeil A, Martin E, et al. Comparison of the confusion assessment method for the intensive care unit (CAM-ICU) with the Intensive Care Delirium Screening Checklist (ICDSC) for delirium in critical care patients gives high agreement rate(s). Intensive Care Med. 2008;34:431.
9. Bergeron N, Dubois MJ, Dumont M, Dial S, Skrobik Y. Intensive Care Delirium Screening Checklist: evaluation of a new screening tool. Intensive Care Med. 2001;27:859.

10. Cavallazzi R, Saad M, Marik PE. Delirium in the ICU: an overview. Ann Intensive Care. 2012;2:49.
11. Barr J, Fraser GL, Puntillo K, Ely EW, Gelinas C, Dasta JF, et al. Clinical practice guidelines for the management of pain, agitation, and delirium in adult patients in the intensive care unit. Crit Care Med. 2013;41:263–306.
12. Vincent JL, Shehabi Y, Walsh TS, Pandharipande PP, Ball JA, Spronk P, et al. Comfort and patient-centred care without excessive sedation: the eCASH concept. Intensive Care Med. 2016;42:962–71.
13. Bekelis K, Missios S, Ahmad J, Labropoulos N, Schirmer CM, Calnan DR, et al. Ischemic stroke occurs less frequently in patients with COVID-19: a multicenter cross-sectional study. Stroke. 2020;51:3570–6.
14. Oxley TJ, Mocco J, Majidi S, Kellner CP, Shoirah H, Singh P, et al. Large-vessel stroke as a presenting feature of Covid-19 in the young. N Engl J Med. 2020;382:e360.
15. Hoyer C, Ebert A, Huttner HB, Puetz V, Kallmunzer B, Barlinn K, et al. Acute stroke in times of the COVID-19 pandemic: a multicenter study. Stroke. 2020;51:2224–7.
16. Iadecola C, Anrather J, Kamel H. Effects of COVID-19 on the nervous system. Cell. 2020;183:16–27.
17. Albers GW, Marks MP, Kemp S, et al. Thrombectomy for stroke at 6 to 16 hours with selection by perfusion imaging. N Engl J Med. 2018;378:708–18.
18. Powers WJ, Rabinstein AA, Ackerson T, Adeoye OM, Bambakidis NC, Becker K, et al. Guidelines for the early management of patients with acute ischemic stroke: a guideline for healthcare professionals from the American Heart Association/American Stroke Association. Stroke. 2018;2018(49):e46–e110.
19. Frontera JA, Lewin JJ, Rabinstein AA, Aisiku IP, Alexandrov AW, Cook AM, et al. Guideline for reversal of antithrombotics in intracranial hemorrhage: a statement for healthcare professionals from the Neurocritical Care Society and Society of Critical Care Medicine. Neurocrit Care. 2016;24:6–46.
20. Weiss TT, Cerda F, Scott JB, Kaur R, Sungurlu S, Mirza SH, et al. Prone positioning for patients intubated for severe acute respiratory distress syndrome (ARDS) secondary to COVID-19: a retrospective observational cohort study. Br J Anaesth. 2021;126:48.
21. Shelhamer MC, Wesson PD, Solari IL, Jensen DL, Steele WA, Dimitrov VG, et al. Prone positioning in moderate to severe acute respiratory distress syndrome due to COVID-19: a cohort study and analysis of physiology. J Intensive Care Med. 2021;36:241.
22. Malik GR, Wolfe AR, Soriano R, Rydberg L, Wolfe LF, Deshmukh S, et al. Injury-prone: peripheral nerve injuries associated with prone positioning for COVID-19-related acute respiratory distress syndrome. Br J Anaesth. 2020;125:e478.
23. Fernandez CE, Franz CK, Ko JH, Walter JM, Koralnik IJ, Ahlawat S, et al. Imaging review of peripheral nerve injuries in patients with COVID-19. Radiology. 2021;298:E117–30.

24. Guidon AC, Amato AA. COVID-19 and neuromuscular disorders. Neurology. 2020;94:959–69.
25. Madia F, Merico B, Primiano G, Cutuli SL, De Pascale G, Servidei S. Acute myopathic quadriplegia in patients with COVID-19 in the intensive care unit. Neurology. 2020;95:492.
26. Wang D, Hu B, Hu C, Zhu F, Liu X, Zhang J, et al. Clinical characteristics of 138 hospitalized patients with 2019 novel Coronavirus-infected pneumonia in Wuhan, China. JAMA. 2020;323:1061–9.
27. Cummings MJ, Baldwin MR, Abrams D, Jacobson SD, Meyer BJ, Balough EM, et al. Epidemiology, clinical course, and outcomes of critically ill adults with COVID-19 in New York City: a prospective cohort study. Lancet. 2020;395:1763–70.
28. Grasseli G, Tonetti T, Protti A, Langer T, Girardis M, Bellani G, et al. Pathophysiology of COVID-19-associated acute respiratory distress syndrome: a multicentre prospective observational study. Lancet Respir Med. 2020;8:1201–8.
29. Schmidt M, Hajage D, Lebreton G, Monsel A, Voiriot G, Levy D, et al. Extracorporeal membrane oxygenation for severe acute respiratory distress syndrome associated with COVID-19: a retrospective cohort study. Lancet Respir Med. 2020;8:1121–31.
30. Barbaro RP, MacLaren G, Boonstra PS, Iwashyna TJ, Slutsky AS, Fan E, et al. Extracorporeal membrane oxygenation support in COVID-19: an international cohort study of the Extracorporeal Life Support Organization registry. Lancet. 2020;396:1071–8.
31. Cho SM, Canner J, Caturegli G, Choi C, Etchill E, Giuliano K, et al. Risk factors of ischemic and hemorrhagic strokes during venovenous extracorporeal membrane oxygenation: analysis of data from the extracorporeal life support organization registry. Crit Care Med. 2021;49:91–101.
32. Cho SM, Farrokh S, Whitman G, Bleck TP, Geocadin RG. Neurocritical care for extracorporeal membrane oxygenation patients. Crit Care Med. 2019;47:1773–81.
33. Mateen FJ, Muralidharan R, Shinohara RT, Parisi JE, Schears GJ, Wijdicks EFM. Neurological injury in adults treated with extracorporeal membrane oxygenation. Arch Neurol. 2011;68:1543–9.
34. Cho SM, Ziai W, Mayasi Y, Gusdon AM, Creed J, Sharrock M, et al. Noninvasive neurological monitoring in extracorporeal membrane oxygenation. ASAIO J. 2020;66:388–93.
35. Hunt MF, Clark KT, Whitman G, Choi CW, Geocadin RG, Cho SM, et al. The use of cerebral NIRS monitoring to identify acute brain injury in patients with VA-ECMO. J Intensive Care Med. 2020;36(12):1403–9.
36. Hunt MF, Clark KT, Grant MC, Choi CW, Whitman G, Cho SM, et al. Therapeutic drug monitoring of valproic acid in extracorporeal membrane oxygenation. Perfusion. 2020;36(8):868–72.
37. Cavayas YA, Munshi L, Del Sorbo L, Fan E. The early change in $PaCO_2$ after extracorporeal membrane oxygenation initiation is associated with neurological complications. Am J Respir Crit Care Med. 2020;201:1525–35.

Part IV

Cardiovascular Manifestations of COVID-19

12 Brief Pathophysiology

Roberta Della Bona, Claudia Canale, and Stefano Benenati

Coronavirus disease 2019 (COVID-19) due to severe acute respiratory syndrome coronavirus-2 (SARS-CoV-2) is primarily a respiratory illness with a highly variable clinical scenario, ranging from mild paucisymptomatic status up to severe respiratory distress needing intensive care [1].

Infection has been associated with multiple direct and indirect cardiovascular (CV) manifestations which, especially in the most severe forms, can further complicate the clinical picture [2].

CV system is evoked at multiple levels in COVID-19

- Patients with CV risk factors, in particular hypertension, and diabetes as well as patients with preexisting CV conditions have been identified as particularly vulnerable populations with increased morbidity and mortality when suffering from COVID-19 [3];

R. Della Bona (✉)
Cardiology Unit, Cardiothoracic and Vascular Department, IRCCS Ospedale Policlinico San Martino, Genoa, Italy

C. Canale · S. Benenati
Chair of Cardiovascular Disease, Department of Internal Medicine and Specialties (DIMI), University of Genoa, Genoa, Italy

D. Battaglini, P. Pelosi (eds.), *COVID-19 Critical and Intensive Care Medicine Essentials*, https://doi.org/10.1007/978-3-030-94992-1_12

- COVID-19 itself can promote the development of CV disorders such as acute myocardial injury, myocarditis, cardiac arrest, stress-induced cardiomyopathy, arrhythmias, venous thromboembolism, cardiogenic shock, and heart failure (HF) [4, 5]. The occurrence of these CV disorders is higher in severe COVID-19 and is associated to increased systemic complications and mortality rates [6];
- Drugs used to treat CV conditions could interfere with the progression or prevention of COVID-19 and, vice versa, drugs used to treat patients with COVID-19 could induce cardiotoxicity [7].

The available data indicate the presence of a bidirectional interplay between COVID-19 and the CV system. The underlying mechanisms, not yet completely elucidated, lie in different stages of the infection, including viral entry into the host cells, subsequent immune response, and organ injury (Fig. 12.1).

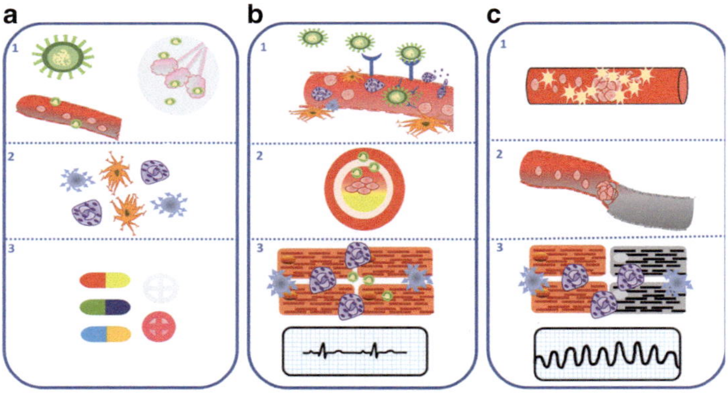

Fig. 12.1 Bidirectional interplay between COVID-19 and the CV system. Panel (**a**) Mechanisms involved in cardiovascular damage: (1) viral entry into the host cells; (2) inflammatory/immune response; (3) medications use to treat COVID-19. Panel (**b**) Targets organ injury: (1). endothelium, pericytes; (2) atherosclerotic plaques; (3) myocardiocytes, heart conduction system. Panel (**c**) Cardiovascular manifestations of SARS-CoV2 infection: (1) myocardial injury, acute coronary syndrome; (2) thromboembolism; (3) myocarditis, arrhythmias

SARS-CoV2 enters the cell through the angiotensin-converting enzyme-2 (ACE2) receptor that plays a central function in the virus's pathogenesis. The binding to ACE2 occurs through the viral spike (S)-protein, which is afterword cleaved by the transmembrane serine protease TMPRSS2 allowing the fusion of the viral membrane with the cellular one, the entry of the virus into the cytoplasm and its subsequent replication [8]. ACE2 is a membrane receptor protein that is highly expressed in the lung, heart, gut, and kidneys, and has many physiological functions. Mainly, it is involved in maintaining the surfactant production in the lungs and is a key counterregulator of the renin–angiotensin–aldosterone system (RAAS) by degrading angiotensin-2 into the peptide angiotensin 1–7. By counteracting the binding of angiotensin-2 to its receptor, ACE2 prevents the deleterious effects of its activation, including vasoconstriction, proinflammatory, profibrotic, prothrombotic, and arrhythmogenic effects [9].

The loss of ACE2 has been documented to have a negative impact on the CV system. Pathogenic *noxae* can lead to the cleavage of the extracellular portion of ACE2, thus rendering the rest of the protein ineffective and resulting in elevated plasma levels of ACE2. Plasma ACE2 has been shown to be increased in CV conditions, such as hypertension, HF, coronary artery disease, and atrial fibrillation [10]. Moreover, experimental data suggest that RAAS blockers, such as ACE-inhibitors and angiotensin receptors antagonists, drugs used to treat CV conditions, may increase the expression of ACE2 and its plasma levels [11].

The finding, from the early stages of the pandemic, that CV risk factors and preexisting CVD are the most common comorbidities in severe COVID-19 patients, suggested a role of ACE2 in the underling pathophysiological mechanisms and raised concerns that RAAS blockers could facilitate viral cell entry or worsen the infection [11]. Actually, human data on potential modification of ACE2 expression with RAAS blockers are limited and controversial, and clinical studies denied any clinical relevance of the upregulation of ACE2 on infection course [10]. Observational studies confirmed that COVID-19 patients with preexisting CVD are prone to more severe systemic and cardiac complications, supporting the hypothesis of a potential role of increased ACE2 expression in worse infection course in these patients, while no evidence supports that they are more susceptible to contracting SARS-CoV-2 infection [12]. Besides, it has been also proposed that SARS-CoV-2 might downregulate ACE2, with the result of promoting all the drawbacks of an undiscriminated RAAS-system activation. This hypothesis, originating from previous studies on SARS-CoV [13], remains, however, speculative.

The wide expression of ACE2 in different organs and cells (among others, pericytes, endothelium, and cardiomyocytes) may be predictive of several extrapulmonary manifestation of the infection.

Pathological evaluation of different affected organs in COVID-19 has shown microvascular inflammation, together with microvascular thrombi. Vascular smooth muscle membrane cells express both ACE2 receptors and TMPRSS2 protease and recent studies have shown the presence of viral particles within the endothelial cells and diffuse endothelial inflammation [14]. This suggest that SARS-CoV-2 infection can induce endotheliitis in several organs as a result of the host inflammatory response and the direct consequence of viral involvement. Endotheliitis may explain the systemically impaired microcirculatory function and its clinical sequelae in patients with COVID-19 such as organ ischemia, a procoagulant state, and thromboembolic phenomena [15]. Also in the heart, the recent demonstration of the presence of ACE2 on cardiac pericytes, with higher expression in patients with HF, suggested a potential direct role of SARS-COV-2 in microvascular coronary dysfunction eventually leading to myocardial injury [16].

Acute myocardial injury, defined as an increase in cardiac biomarkers, is the most described cardiac abnormality in COVID-19, reported in 8–12% of patients, and it has been associated with increased mortality [17]. Multiple potential mechanisms for cardiac injury have been considered, including myocardial ischemia related to coronary plaque rupture or supply/demand mismatch, stress cardiomyopathy, vasculitis phenomenon or direct myocarditis, and secondary effects of hyperinflammatory response.

Inflammation plays a crucial role in the progression of disease and organs damage in COVID-19, and it can be implicated in all the pathophysiological phenomena involved in myocardial damage. The interaction between SARS-CoV-2 and the host's immune system can trigger an inappropriate overproduction of pro-inflammatory cytokines, including colony stimulating factors, interleukin (IL)-1β, IL-6, tumor necrosis factor, and various chemokines such as IFNγ-induced protein 10, IP-10, which in turn induce systemic inflammation (the so-called cytokine release syndrome—CRS) and, in the most severe cases, a systemic inflammatory response syndrome (SIRS). The large amount of cytokines and chemokines leads to the activation of monocytes and macrophages and a massive infiltration of multiple organs and tissue [18].

Widespread inflammation and CRS can lead to changes in vascular tone, cause endothelium damage, increase platelet aggregation, activate the tissue-factor pathway, and increase thrombin production through the release of IL-6, triggering destabilization/rupture of preexisting atherosclerotic plaques and leading to acute coronary syndrome [19]. In the CRS, the positive feedback loop of immune activation can lead to myocardial damage, stress cardiomyopathy, and HF. Pathological findings showed that in patients dying with COVID-19, there is frequently present a myocardial interstitial macrophage infiltration that may largely result from the elevated systemic levels of proinflammatory cytokines [20]. Although cardiac inflammation has been documented in patients with COVID-19, and a recent study showed that myocardial cells express ACE2 which could mediate SARS-CoV-2 entry into cardiomyocytes [21], there is no robust histopathological evidence of intracellular viral material, thus the myocarditis due to direct myocardial infection as cause of myocardial injury remains to be demonstrated [22].

On the other hand, right ventricular (RV) strain clearly contributes to myocardial injury in these patients. Several causes contribute to RV overload and dysfunction including pulmonary parenchymal damage and subsequent fibrosis, hypoxia (a trigger for both demand myocardial ischemia and pulmonary vasoconstriction), widespread small pulmonary vessels microthrombosis and/or overt pulmonary thromboembolism, inflammation and cytokine storm, hyperstimulation of the RAAS pathway, and mechanical ventilation and/or positive end-expiratory pressure.

Due to chambers interdependence, RV remodeling may elicit a left ventricular dysfunction, leading to a vicious circle which finally results in a reduced cardiac output, HF, cardiogenic shock, and heightened mortality risk [23].

Acute myocardial injury along with hypoxia, fever, SIRS, electrolyte imbalances, sepsis, hypo- or hypervolemia, can also trigger cardiac arrhythmias, which are frequently reported in COVID-19 patients. Moreover, drugs used against COVID-19 can have proarrhythmic effects. For instance, aminoquinolines (chloroquine and hydroxychloroquine) and azithromycin (a macrolide-type antibiotic) are known to delay repolarization and prolong the QTc interval, triggering afterdepolarization and ventricular arrhythmias such as torsade de point, whereas lopinavir, a protease inhibitor administered in combination with ritonavir to obviate its degradation by the hepatic cytochromes, may prolong the PR and QRS intervals and cause atrioventricular blocks.

Several pathophysiological mechanisms, many still under investigation, account for the bidirectional interplay between COVID-19 and the CV system, and generally not a single but the interplay of multiple mechanisms can explain the complex scenario of the CV manifestations.

Further understanding of the pathophysiological mechanisms is crucial for the development of effective treatments to counteract the pathological effects of SARS-CoV-2 and its spread.

References

1. Chen N, Zhou M, Dong X, et al. Epidemiological and clinical characteristics of 99 cases of 2019 novel coronavirus pneumonia in Wuhan, China: a descriptive study. Lancet. 2020;395:507–13.
2. Tahir F, Bin Arif T, Ahmed J, Malik F, Khalid M. Cardiac manifestations of coronavirus disease 2019 (COVID-19): a comprehensive review. Cureus. 2020;12:e8021.
3. Pellicori P, Doolub G, Wong CM, et al. COVID-19 and its cardiovascular effects: a systematic review of prevalence studies. Cochrane Database Syst Rev. 2021;3:CD013879.
4. Madjid M, Safavi-Naeini P, Solomon SD, Vardeny O. Potential effects of coronaviruses on the cardiovascular system: a review. JAMA Cardiol. 2020;5:831–40.

5. Puntmann VO, Carerj ML, Wieters I, et al. Outcomes of cardiovascular magnetic resonance imaging in patients recently recovered from coronavirus disease 2019 (COVID-19). JAMA Cardiol. 2020;5:1265–73.
6. Guo T, Fan Y, Chen M, et al. Cardiovascular implications of fatal outcomes of patients with coronavirus disease 2019 (COVID-19). JAMA Cardiol. 2020;5:811–8.
7. Driggin E, Madhavan MV, Bikdeli B, et al. Cardiovascular considerations for patients, health care workers, and health systems during the COVID-19 pandemic. J Am Coll Cardiol. 2020;75:2352–71.
8. Nishiga M, Wang DW, Han Y, Lewis DB, Wu JC. COVID-19 and cardiovascular disease: from basic mechanisms to clinical perspectives. Nat Rev Cardiol. 2020;17:543–58.
9. Donoghue M, Hsieh F, Baronas E, et al. A novel angiotensin-converting enzyme-related carboxypeptidase (ACE2) converts angiotensin I to angiotensin 1–9. Circ Res. 2000;87:E1–9.
10. Gressens SB, Leftheriotis G, Dussaule JC, Flamant M, Levy BI, Vidal-Petiot E. Controversial roles of the renin angiotensin system and its modulators during the COVID-19 pandemic. Front Physiol. 2021;12:624052.
11. Ferrario CM, Jessup J, Chappell MC, et al. Effect of angiotensin-converting enzyme inhibition and angiotensin II receptor blockers on cardiac angiotensin-converting enzyme 2. Circulation. 2005;111:2605–10.
12. Fathi M, Vakili K, Sayehmiri F, et al. The prognostic value of comorbidity for the severity of COVID-19: a systematic review and meta-analysis study. PLoS One. 2021;16:e0246190.
13. Oudit GY, Kassiri Z, Jiang C, et al. SARS-coronavirus modulation of myocardial ACE2 expression and inflammation in patients with SARS. Eur J Clin Invest. 2009;39:618–25.
14. Varga Z, Flammer AJ, Steiger P, et al. Endothelial cell infection and endotheliitis in COVID-19. Lancet. 2020;395:1417–8.
15. Ackermann M, Verleden SE, Kuehnel M, et al. Pulmonary vascular endothelialitis, thrombosis, and angiogenesis in Covid-19. N Engl J Med. 2020;383:120–8.
16. Chen L, Li X, Chen M, Feng Y, Xiong C. The ACE2 expression in human heart indicates new potential mechanism of heart injury among patients infected with SARS-CoV-2. Cardiovasc Res. 2020;116:1097–100.
17. Lippi G, Lavie CJ, Sanchis-Gomar F. Cardiac troponin I in patients with coronavirus disease 2019 (COVID-19): evidence from a meta-analysis. Prog Cardiovasc Dis. 2020;63:390–1.
18. Lau SKP, Lau CCY, Chan KH, et al. Delayed induction of proinflammatory cytokines and suppression of innate antiviral response by the novel Middle East respiratory syndrome coronavirus: implications for pathogenesis and treatment. J Gen Virol. 2013;94:2679–90.
19. Petrovic V, Radenkovic D, Radenkovic G, Djordjevic V, Banach M. Pathophysiology of cardiovascular complications in COVID-19. Front Physiol. 2020;11:575600.

20. Basso C, Leone O, Rizzo S, et al. Pathological features of COVID-19-associated myocardial injury: a multicentre cardiovascular pathology study. Eur Heart J. 2020;41:3827–35.
21. Nicin L, Abplanalp WT, Mellentin H, et al. Cell type-specific expression of the putative SARS-CoV-2 receptor ACE2 in human hearts. Eur Heart J. 2020;41:1804–6.
22. Mele D, Flamigni F, Rapezzi C, Ferrari R. Myocarditis in COVID-19 patients: current problems. Intern Emerg Med. 2021;16(5):1123–9.
23. Pellikka PA, Naqvi TZ. The right ventricle: a target in COVID-19 cardiac insult. J Am Coll Cardiol. 2020;76:1978–81.

13 Biomarkers, Electrocardiography, and Echocardiography

Vered Gil Ad and Andrea Carlo Merlo

Similarly to severe acute respiratory syndrome (SARS) and Middle East respiratory syndrome (MERS), [1] coronavirus disease 2019 (COVID-19) is associated with a significant burden of cardiovascular (CV) complications ranging from isolated myocardial injury (elevation of cardiac troponin [cTn]) to acute heart failure, cardiac arrhythmias, venous thromboembolism, acute coronary syndromes, myocarditis, cardiogenic shock, and cardiac arrest [2, 3].

The assessment of cardiac biomarkers, electrocardiogram (ECG), and—in selected patients—transthoracic echocardiogram (TTE) or other cardiac imaging methods has a pivotal role in risk stratification, early detection of CV complications, and treatment management [4].

V. Gil Ad (✉)
Cardiology Unit, Cardiothoracic and Vascular Department, IRCCS Ospedale Policlinico San Martino, Genoa, Italy

A. C. Merlo
Cardiovascular Disease, Department of Internal Medicine and Specialties (Di.M.I.), University of Genova, Genova, Italy

D. Battaglini, P. Pelosi (eds.), *COVID-19 Critical and Intensive Care Medicine Essentials*, https://doi.org/10.1007/978-3-030-94992-1_13

13.1 Biomarkers

Increased levels of cardiac biomarkers—for example, cTn, creatine-kinase MB, myoglobin, D-dimer, brain natriuretic peptide (BNP) and its N-terminal pro-hormone (NT-proBNP)—are a common finding in hospitalized COVID-19 patients [2–6].

13.2 Cardiac Troponin

Myocardial injury—defined as a rise of cTn above the 99th percentile of the upper limit of normal (ULN)—has been widely reported in COVID-19 patients [2–6].

Myocardial injury may either signify CV involvement and complications or—more often—represent an epiphenomenon of systemic disease, related to severe inflammation and hypoxia [2, 5].

The important prognostic value of myocardial injury in COVID-19 has been demonstrated by several studies reporting a statistically significant association between cTn elevation and admission to an intensive care unit (ICU) as well as in-hospital death [6–8]. In a large multicenter Italian study, elevated cTn levels on admission were found in up to 45% of hospitalized COVID-19 patients and were independently associated with higher in-hospital mortality [8]. Moreover, myocardial injury correlated with a greater risk of CV and non-CV complications, including heart failure, sepsis, acute kidney failure, multiorgan failure, pulmonary embolism, delirium, and major bleeding. When myocardial injury was accompanied by CV comorbidities, highest mortality rates were observed [6–8].

Despite its evident prognostic significance, there is ongoing debate whether cTn should be routinely tested in COVID-19 patients [4]. Specifically, several other clinical and laboratory variables were demonstrated strong predictors of mortality in these patients (e.g., older age, higher Sequential Organ Failure Assessment score, D-dimer levels, interleukin 6, and lymphocyte count), and it is uncertain whether cTn would provide any incremental prognostic value. Furthermore, routine cTn measurements may trigger inappropriate diagnostic and therapeutic interventions.

In our opinion, cTn measurement on hospital admission is reasonable and may contribute to patient stratification and identification of subjects at higher risk of complications. Undoubtedly, a careful and accurate assessment is needed to avoid useless diagnostic exams and treatments. Mild increases in cTn levels (e.g., <fivefold the ULN), particularly in elderly subjects and in patients with respiratory disease, generally do not necessitate specific cardiologic workup unless symptoms or ECG strongly suggests CV involvement. Contrariwise, a rise of cTn >fivefold the ULN and an increasing cTn trend are powerful predictors of CV complications and are associated with worse prognosis. Therefore, in these patients prompt evaluation of symptoms, physical examination, and a 12-lead ECG are recommended. CV imaging—including TTE, cardiac computed tomography, and cardiac magnetic resonance, may help unfold CV involvement, yet, owing to contagion risk for operators and other patients, it should be reserved to patients whose treatment it is likely to impact.

Recommendations for CV diagnostic workup are shown in Flowchart 13.1.

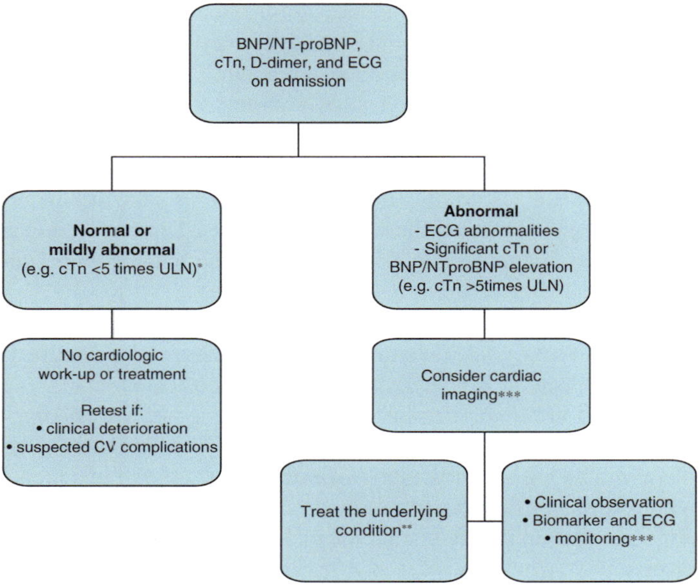

Flowchart 13.1 Recommendations for CV diagnostic workup. *BNP* brain natriureticpeptide, *cTn* cardiac troponin, *CV* cardiovascular, *ECG* electrocardiogram, *NT* N-terminal, *TTE* transthoracic echocardiography, *ULN* upper level of normal. *Mild abnormalities may not require further diagnostic investigations. **Only if potentially changing patient management. ***Frequency of controls based on clinical status, avoiding futility

13.3 Natriuretic Peptides

BNP and NT-proBNP are quantitative biomarkers of cardiac wall stress, typically increased in patients with congestive heart failure. High BNP/NT-proBNP plasma levels are common in patients with severe inflammatory and respiratory illnesses, and were demonstrated predictors of unfavorable outcome in patients with acute respiratory distress syndrome [9, 10].

In COVID-19 patients, a recent meta-analysis including thirteen observational studies and a total of 2,248 patients found a significant association between higher NT-proBNP levels on hospital admission and both disease severity and in-hospital mortality [11]. Nevertheless, limited evidence exists so far to define BNP/NT-proBNP as an independent prognostic marker in COVID-19 [11, 12].

13.4 D-Dimer

D-Dimers are generated by cleavage of fibrin monomers by prothrombin and indicate the presence of thrombin formation. Elevated D-dimer levels are often seen in patients with acute infection or inflammation and are associated with coagulation abnormalities and risk of thromboembolic events [13]. In COVID-19, elevated D-dimer levels were observed in almost 50% of hospitalized patients, particularly in patients admitted to ICUs and in those who died more than 80%, while very high levels (>1 μg/mL) were associated with an 18-fold increased risk of death [14, 15]. Although coagulation abnormalities in COVID-19 do not meet all criteria of disseminated intravascular coagulation established by the International Society on Thrombosis and Haemostasis [16], they most likely contribute to the development of the numerous CV complications of COVID-19.

13.5 Electrocardiography

ECG abnormalities are common in COVID-19 patients, and were found in up to 93% of critically ill patients [17]. A large spectrum of ECG alterations was described, including tachyarrhythmias and bradyarrhythmias, axis deviation, bundle branch blocks, pathologic Q waves, and repolarization abnormalities [17, 18].

Atrial arrhythmias mainly atrial fibrillation and atrial flutter, repolarization abnormalities QT-interval prolongation, ST-segment elevation or depression, and T-wave inversion, signs of right ventricular (RV) strain, and conduction disorders are associated with worse prognosis and increased mortality [19, 20].

While the most common ECG alterations are nonspecific and may be attributed to systemic disease and hypoxia, others may suggest CV complications and warrant further investigation. ST-segment elevation or depression and T-wave inversion may suggest acute coronary syndromes or myocarditis, and require prompt cardiologic evaluation. Notably, about 30% of critically ill patients develop ECG signs of acute RV pressure overload, presenting S1Q3T3 pattern, incomplete or complete right bundle branch block or ST abnormalities in leads V1–V4. These ECG signs are often associated with TTE evidence of RV dilatation and dysfunction [17].

ECG monitoring and the identification of risk factors of QT prolongation represent key points in preventing malignant arrhythmias during COVID-19, especially when potentially pro-arrhythmic drugs are administered. A summary of the main arrhythmogenic interactions between common drugs utilized for COVID-19 treatment is reported in Table 13.1 [21].

Table 13.1 Main cardiac effects and arrhythmic interactions of COVID-19 drugs

COVID-19 drugs	Cardiovascular effects	Pro-arrhythmic interactions
Azithromycin	• QT-interval prolongation	• Amiodarone • Amisulpride • Chloroquine • Citalopram • Clozapine • Disopyramide • Dofetilide • Dronedarone • Droperidol • Escitalopram • Haloperidol • Hydroxychloroquine • Ibutilide • Ivabradine • Moxifloxacin • Procainamide • Quinidine • Sotalol • Ziprasidone

Table 13.1 (continued)

COVID-19 drugs	Cardiovascular effects	Pro-arrhythmic interactions
Chloroquine/ hydroxychloroquine	• Cardiotoxicity • QT-interval prolongation	• Alfuzosin • Amiodarone • Amisulpride • Amitriptyline • Azithromycin • Buprenorphine • Chlorpromazine • Ciprofloxacin • Citalopram • Clarithromycin • Clomipramine • Clozapine • Desipramine • Disopyramide • Dofetilide • Dronedarone • Droperidol • Erythromycin • Escitalopram • Flecainide • Fluconazole • Fluoxetine • Haloperidol • Halothane • Hydroxyzine • Ibutilide • Imipramine • Ivabradine • Ketoconazole • Levofloxacin • Lithium • Mirtazapine • Moxifloxacin • Norfloxacin • Nortriptyline • Ofloxacin • Ondansetron • Posaconazole • Procainamide • Promazine

(continued)

Table 13.1 (continued)

COVID-19 drugs	Cardiovascular effects	Pro-arrhythmic interactions
		• Propafenone • Quetiapine • Quinidine • Ranolazine • Remdesivir • Risperidone • Sertraline • Sevoflurane • Sotalol • Tacrolimus • Tamoxifen • Telithromycin • Tramadol • Trazodone • Trimipramine • Venlafaxine • Voriconazole • Ziprasidone
Dexamethasone	• Arrhythmias • Bradycardia • Heart failure • Hypertension • Thromboembolism	• Amiodarone • Ranolazine
Remdesivir	• Bradycardia • Hypotension[a] • QT-interval prolongation[a]	None known
Tocilizumab	• Hypertension	None known

[a]These suspected effects have not been definitely proven yet

Measurement of baseline corrected QT interval and an electrolyte panel are recommended in all patients before starting treatment. Risk factors for malignant arrhythmias include congenital long QT syndrome, female sex, age > 65 years, structural heart disease, renal or liver impairment, hypocalcemia, hypokalemia, hypomagnesemia, and bradycardia [19, 21].

The proposed approach to arrhythmic risk assessment and management of QT-prolonging drugs are reported in Flowchart 13.2.

13.6 Echocardiography

TTE provides essential information about patient's heart and hemodynamic state when CV complications are suspected. Nonetheless, in COVID-19 important limitations exist owing to contagion risk for healthcare providers. Therefore, the European Association of Cardiovascular Imaging and the American Society of Echocardiography have recommended performing TTE in COVID-19 patients only if it is likely to impact patient management [22, 23]. In addition, in order to limit interpersonal contact, bedside, problem-tailored, and time-limited TTE is preferable [22, 23]. Transesophageal echocardiography, which carries a particularly high contagion risk due to aerosolization, should be performed only if providing significant incremental value [22, 23].

COVID-19 patients with myocardial injury show higher prevalence of TTE abnormalities than those without, and the combination of myocardial injury and TTE abnormalities significantly increases the risk for in-hospital mortality [5, 24, 25].

The most common TTE findings in COVID-19 include RV dilatation and dysfunction, left ventricular diastolic impairment, and mild pericardial effusion [24–26].

RV dilatation and dysfunction were reported in up to 40% of patients and reduced RV function parameters including tricuspid annular plane systolic excursion, pulmonary artery acceleration time, Tei index, and myocardial systolic excursion velocity [S'] were associated with in-hospital death [24, 25]. Notably, they were mostly mildly abnormal also in patients with pulmonary embolism [24], implying that in patients with high clinical suspicion chest computed tomography is recommended. Left ventricular systolic dysfunction was less common, although reported in up to 10% of patients [24–26]. Differentiation between coronary and noncoronary distribution of regional wall motion abnormalities on TTE may help underline CV conditions and guide management strategies.

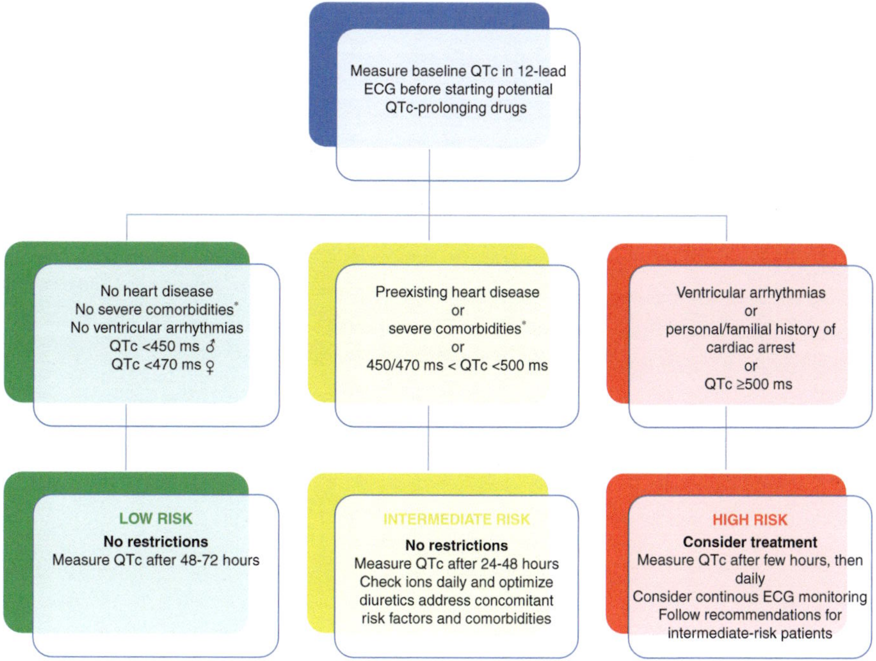

Flowchart 13.2 Arrhythmic risk and management of QTc-prolonging drugs. *ECG* electrocardiogram. *Comorbidities: chronic treatment with drugs that prolong QT interval, renal dysfunction, liver dysfunction, acute ischemic heart disease

References

1. Badawi A, Ryoo SG. Prevalence of comorbidities in the Middle East respiratory syndrome coronavirus (MERS-CoV): a systematic review and meta-analysis. Int J Infect Dis. 2016;49:129–33.
2. Clerkin KJ, Fried JA, Raikhelkar J, et al. COVID-19 and cardiovascular disease. Circulation. 2020;141(20):1648–55.
3. Pellicori P, Doolub G, Wong CM, et al. COVID-19 and its cardiovascular effects: a systematic review of prevalence studies. Cochrane Database Syst Rev. 2021;3(3):CD013879.
4. The European Society for Cardiology. ESC Guidance for the Diagnosis and Management of CV Disease during the COVID-19 Pandemic. https://www.escardio.org/Education/COVID-19-and-Cardiology/ESC-COVID-19-Guidance.
5. Giustino G, Croft LB, Stefanini GG, et al. Characterization of myocardial injury in patients with COVID-19. J Am Coll Cardiol. 2020;76(18):2043–55.
6. Parohan M, Yaghoubi S, Seraji A. Cardiac injury is associated with severe outcome and death in patients with coronavirus disease 2019 (COVID-19) infection: a systematic review and meta-analysis of observational studies. Eur Heart J Acute Cardiovasc Care. 2020;9(6):665–77.
7. Shi S, Qin M, Shen B, et al. Association of cardiac injury with mortality in hospitalized patients with COVID-19 in Wuhan, China. JAMA Cardiol. 2020;5(7):802–10.
8. Lombardi CM, Carubelli V, Iorio A, et al. Association of troponin levels with mortality in Italian patients hospitalized with coronavirus disease 2019: results of a multicenter study. JAMA Cardiol. 2020;5(11):1274–80.
9. Lai CC, Sung MI, Ho CH, et al. The prognostic value of N-terminal proB-type natriuretic peptide in patients with acute respiratory distress syndrome. Sci Rep. 2017;7:44784.
10. Mitaka C, Hirata Y, Nagura T, et al. Increased plasma concentrations of brain natriuretic peptide in patients with acute lung injury. J Crit Care. 1997;12:66–71.
11. Sorrentino S, Cacia M, Leo I, et al. B-type natriuretic peptide as biomarker of COVID-19 disease severity—a meta-analysis. J Clin Med. 2020;9(9):2957.
12. Gao L, Jiang D, Wen XS, et al. Prognostic value of NT-proBNP in patients with severe COVID-19. Respir Res. 2020;21(1):83.
13. Halaby R, Popma CJ, Cohen A, et al. D-Dimer elevation and adverse outcomes. J Thromb Thrombolysis. 2015;39(1):55–9.
14. Rostami M, Mansouritorghabeh H. D-Dimer level in COVID-19 infection: a systematic review. Expert Rev Hematol. 2020;13(11):1265–75.
15. Zhou F, et al. Clinical course and risk factors for mortality of adult inpatients with COVID-19 in Wuhan, China: a retrospective cohort study. Lancet. 2020;395:1054–62.

16. Taylor FB Jr, et al. Towards definition, clinical and laboratory criteria, and a scoring system for disseminated intravascular coagulation. Thromb Haemost. 2001;86:1327–30.
17. Bertini M, Ferrari R, Guardigli G, et al. Electrocardiographic features of 431 consecutive, critically ill COVID-19 patients: an insight into the mechanisms of cardiac involvement. Europace. 2020;22(12):1848–54.
18. Haseeb S, Gul EE, Çinier G, et al. Value of electrocardiography in coronavirus disease 2019 (COVID-19). J Electrocardiol. 2020;62:39–45.
19. Poterucha TJ, Elias P, Jain SS, et al. Admission cardiac diagnostic testing with electrocardiography and troponin measurement prognosticates increased 30-day mortality in COVID-19. J Am Heart Assoc. 2021;10(1):e018476.
20. Elias P, Poterucha TJ, Jain SS, et al. The prognostic value of electrocardiogram at presentation to emergency department in patients with COVID-19. Mayo Clin Proc. 2020;95(10):2099–109.
21. Bhatla A, Mayer MM, Adusumalli S, et al. COVID-19 and cardiac arrhythmias. Heart Rhythm. 2020;17(9):1439–44.
22. Skulstad H, Cosyns B, Popescu BA, et al. COVID-19 pandemic and cardiac imaging: EACVI recommendations on precautions, indications, prioritization, and protection for patients and healthcare personnel. Eur Heart J Cardiovasc Imaging. 2020;21(6):592–8.
23. Kirkpatrick JN, Mitchell C, Taub C, Kort S, Hung J, Swaminathan M. ASE statement on protection of patients and echocardiography service providers during the 2019 novel coronavirus outbreak: endorsed by the American College of Cardiology. J Am Soc Echocardiogr. 2020;33(6):648–53.
24. Szekely Y, Lichter Y, Taieb P, et al. Spectrum of cardiac manifestations in COVID-19: a systematic echocardiographic study. Circulation. 2020;142(4):342–53.
25. Li Y, Li H, Li M, et al. The prevalence, risk factors and outcome of cardiac dysfunction in hospitalized patients with COVID-19. Intensive Care Med. 2020;46(11):2096–8.
26. Gilad V, De Marzo V, Guglielmi G, et al. Cardiac point-of-care ultrasound in hospitalized coronavirus disease-2019 patients: findings and association with outcome. J Cardiovasc Med. 2021;23(1):e3–7.

14 Clinical Characteristics

Vered Gil Ad and Vincenzo De Marzo

In COVID-19 patients, CV manifestations include venous and pulmonary thromboembolism, acute heart failure, cardiac arrhythmias, arterial thrombotic events, acute coronary syndromes, myocarditis, cardiogenic shock, and cardiac arrest.

14.1 Venous Thromboembolism and Pulmonary Embolism

Since the first months of pandemic, thrombotic complications were described in hospitalized COVID-19 patients [1–3] and subsequently microvascular thrombosis were reported in postmortem studies [4, 5]. In recent two systematic reviews and meta-analysis, the overall incidence of VTE among inpatients with COVID-19 was estimated between 14 to 17%, and there was a fourfold higher incidence rate in patients admitted to intensive care units (ICUs) [5, 6]. Acute pulmonary

V. Gil Ad (✉)
Cardiology Unit, Cardiothoracic and Vascular Department, IRCCS Ospedale Policlinico San Martino, Genoa, Italy

V. De Marzo
Cardiovascular Disease, Department of Internal Medicine, University of Genova, Genova, Italy

D. Battaglini, P. Pelosi (eds.), *COVID-19 Critical and Intensive Care Medicine Essentials*, https://doi.org/10.1007/978-3-030-94992-1_14

embolism (PE), however, has been probably underdiagnosed as symptoms largely overlap with pulmonary and systemic disease. Unexpected respiratory worsening, unexplained tachycardia or fall in blood pressure, electrocardiogram (ECG) changes, and signs of deep vein thrombosis of the extremities should trigger a suspicion of PE.

The specificity of D-dimer tests may be lower in patients with COVID-19 compared to other clinical settings. Notwithstanding, it is still advised to follow general diagnostic algorithms for PE starting with pretest probability and D-dimer [7]. However, CT pulmonary angiography remains the gold standard for diagnosis of PE.

14.2 Heart Failure and Cardiogenic Shock

Acute heart failure (HF) and exacerbation of chronic HF are common complications of COVID-19 and were reported in up to 20–30% of hospitalized patients, showing high mortality rates, especially in patients with severe comorbidities [8, 9].

Trigger mechanisms include increased cardiac workload, hypoxemia, hypervolemia, myocardial injury, arrhythmias, myocarditis, stress-induced cardiomyopathy, acute kidney injury, and systemic inflammatory activation ("cytokine storm") [7, 8].

Clinical signs include cardiomegaly, pulmonary vascular congestion or peripheral oedema cardiac biomarkers increase. ECG and echocardiography may reveal underlying mechanisms and complication (right or left ventricle involvement and dysfunction) and guide therapy.

A small number of patients with COVID-19 may develop cardiogenic shock (CS). CS is typically characterized by impaired end-organ perfusion frequently triggered by concomitant sepsis and is associated with high mortality rates [10].

14.3 Acute Myocarditis

Diagnosis of myocarditis is suspected in the presence of clinical features (chest pain, dyspnea, fever), electrocardiogram alterations (ST-segment elevation, T-wave inversion), laboratory testing (an increase of cardiac biomarkers), and imaging findings (myocardial regional or global dysfunction on echocardiography), yet definite diagnosis requires the execution of cardiac magnetic resonance (CMR) and or endomyocardial biopsy (EMB) [11].

In patients with COVID-19, however, there are consistent limitations to diagnostic assessments, mainly related to the infectious risk for operators (e.g., echocardiography, EMB) and clinical instability (e.g., CMR). As a result, data regarding prevalence, clinical characteristics and prognosis is amply lacking, and nearly all the information comes from case reports or small series [12–14]. In reported cases, inflammatory indices and cardiac troponin were commonly increased (the last without the typical "rise and fall" curve), several ECG alterations were found (most common diffuse ST elevation following T waves inversion), and in up to 50% of cases left ventricular (LV) dysfunction was documented, most often mildly (LV ejection fraction 40–55%). In all cases undergoing CMR, diffuse intense myocardial oedema was reported while late gadolinium enhancement (LGE) images were unremarkable. EBM and autopsy data were obtained only in a small number of patients, with the most common finding of interstitial macrophage infiltration and few cases of lymphocytic infiltrates [11]. The presence of virus particles was also reported in few cases; however, these particles may originated from interstitial cells or macrophages invading the myocardial tissue. The prognosis reported appears favorable, yet data available is insufficient and myocarditis in the COVID-19 settings are extensively under diagnosed.

14.4 Acute Coronary Syndromes and Takotsubo Syndrome

As with other infectious diseases, including SARS and influenza, COVID-19 can trigger acute coronary syndrome (ACS). The mechanisms underlying COVID-19-induced ACS may involve plaque rupture, coronary spasm or microthrombi triggered by systemic inflammation and cytokine storm [15–17]. However, many cases are not related to coronary complications and may be attributed to an imbalance between heightened cardiac workload and reduced oxygen supply secondary to systemic conditions (type-2 myocardial infarction). Furthermore, there are increasing reports of stress-like cardiomyopathy, also known as Takotsubo syndrome (TTS), in patients with COVID-19, probably triggered by emotional or physical stress [18, 19].

Differential diagnosis is challenging and symptoms (mainly persistent angina) and ECG pattern are the key elements. Furthermore, synchronized cardiac computed tomography may contribute to risk assessment, enabling infection risk containment to operators and other patients.

There is growing evidence from autopsy studies of microthrombi in myocardial capillaries, arterioles, and small muscular arteries rather than epicardial arteries [20]. Furthermore, COVID-19 patients have microthrombi with significantly greater fibrin and terminal complement C5b-9 immunostaining and lower arteriolar ACE-2 endothelial expression [21].

Despite the prothrombotic status, there have been no reports of excess myocardial infarctions during the first months of the pandemic, probably due to decreased admission of non-COVID-19 patients due to a fear of contagion.

14.5 Cardiac Arrhythmias and Cardiac Arrest

Cardiac arrhythmias constitute a major concern in COVID-19. Atrial fibrillation (AF) and flutter (AFL) are the most common, being detected in up to 22% of hospitalized patients [22]. Higher rates of AF/AFL were associated with male gender, older age, and azithromycin treatment. Patients with AF/AFL showed a threefold increase in mortality, with no significant differences between newly diagnosed and chronic persistent patterns [23].

Ventricular arrhythmias are less frequent, although reported in about 6% of patients, and may result from electrolyte imbalances, severe bradycardia and the usage of specific drugs—all possible causes of QT-interval prolongation, a condition that may induce the onset of torsade de pointes [24]. A clear association was demonstrated between QT-interval prolongation and the use of hydroxychloroquine/chloroquine, azithromycin, and antiviral drugs such as lopinavir/ritonavir, especially in patients with pre-existing hepatic or renal disease [22, 24]. Thus, ECG monitoring is advisable in all patients treated with antivirals or other well-known QT-prolonging drugs.

However, COVID-19 patients with cardiac arrest rarely showed shockable rhythms (reported in only 5.9% of cases) [25].

Finally, pathological variations in heart rate with or without conduction abnormalities may also represent side-effects of antiviral therapy. Concerning this topic, a recent real-word study showed a high incidence of bradycardia and severe bradycardia in patients treated with remdesivir [26].

14.6 Multisystem Inflammatory Disorder in Children (MIS-C)

Children with COVID-19 are often asymptomatic or present mild respiratory symptoms. However, few cases of children with hyperinflammatory syndrome referred to as multisystem inflammatory disorder in children (MIS-C) were reported, and by the end of June 2020, approximately 1000 MIS-C cases had been documented globally [27]. MIS-C can develop in previously healthy children with no known comorbidities and usually presents within 4 weeks following SARS-CoV-2 infection.

MIS-C patients typically present with a multiorgan involvement, and common clinical manifestations include persistent fever and dermatological, mucocutaneous and gastrointestinal manifestations [28]. Cardiac abnormalities are almost ubiquitous [28], including reduced LV systolic function (described in 31–100% of patients) and dilatation of coronary arteries (described in the majority of patients), similar to Kawasaki disease (KD).

Unlike KD, MIS-C tends to affect older children and present greater multiorgan involvement, particularly of the gastrointestinal and CV systems. A significant proportion of MIS-C patients are admitted to the ICU, often requiring vasopressor support or even venoarterial extracorporeal membrane oxygenation because of CS and or severe vasoplegia.

Underlying mechanisms are still unknown, and the prevailing hypothesis is a postinfectious phenomenon mediated by antibody and immune complex [27, 28].

14.7 Long COVID-19

"Long COVID-19" describes a syndrome characterized by persistent symptoms and or delayed or long-term complications beyond 4 weeks from the acute disease [29].

There are increasing reports of persistent symptoms in most patients recovered from acute COVID-19, and up to 80% of patients discharged from the hospital report at least one symptom, even several months after. Dyspnea and fatigue are the prevalent symptoms, followed by joint pain, chest pain (20% of patients), and palpitation (9% of patients) [29, 30].

Preliminary data with CMR suggest that ongoing myocardial inflammation may be present at rates as high as 60% 2 months after a diagnosis of COVID-19 [31]. Moreover, autonomic dysfunction resulting in postural orthostatic tachycardia syndrome and inappropriate sinus tachycardia has previously been reported as a result of adrenergic modulation [32]. At last, a preliminary study of 200 patients who undergone cardiopulmonary exercise testing at 3 months from hospital discharge demonstrated abnormal peak oxygen uptake in about 50% of them [33]. However, more studies are needed to elucidate the underlying mechanism and the subsequent treatment.

References

1. Piazza G, Campia U, Hurwitz S. Registry of arterial and venous thromboembolic complications in patients with COVID-19. J Am Coll Cardiol. 2020;76(18):2060–72.
2. Schulman S, Hu Y, Konstantinides S. Venous thromboembolism in COVID-19. Thromb Haemost. 2020;120:1642–53.
3. Ackermann M, Verleden SE, Kuehnel M. Pulmonary vascular endothelialitis, thrombosis, and angiogenesis in Covid-19. N Engl J Med. 2020;383:120–8.

4. Wichmann D, Sperhake JP, Lütgehetmann M. Autopsy findings and venous thromboembolism in patients with COVID-19: a prospective cohort study. Ann Intern Med. 2020;173:268–77.
5. Jiménez D, García-Sanchez A, Rali P. Incidence of venous thromboembolism and bleeding among hospitalized patients with COVID-19: a systematic review and meta-analysis. Chest. 2020;209:94–8.
6. Nopp S, Moik F, Jilma B, Pabinger I, Ay C. Risk of venous thromboembolism in patients with COVID-19: a systematic review and meta-analysis. Res Pract Thromb Haemost. 2020;6:1178–91.
7. The European Society for Cardiology. ESC guidance for the diagnosis and management of CV disease during the COVID-19 pandemic: part 2-care pathways, treatment, and follow-up. Eur Heart J. 2022;43(11):1059–103.
8. Zhou F, Yu T, Du R, et al. Clinical course and risk factors for mortality of adult inpatients with COVID-19 in Wuhan, China: a retrospective cohort study. Lancet. 2020;395(10229):1054–62.
9. Yang J, Zheng Y, Gou X, et al. Prevalence of comorbidities and its effects in patients infected with SARS-CoV-2: a systematic review and meta-analysis. Int J Infect Dis. 2020;94:91–5.
10. Ranard LS, Fried JA, Abdalla M, Anstey DE, et al. Approach to acute cardiovascular complications in COVID-19 infection. Circ Heart Fail. 2020;13:e007220.
11. Caforio ALP, Pankuweit S, Arbustini E, et al. Current state of knowledge on aetiology, diagnosis, management, and therapy of myocarditis: a position statement of the European Society of Cardiology Working Group on myocardial and pericardial diseases. Eur Heart J. 2013;34:2636–48.
12. Sawalha K, Abozenah M, Kadado AJ, et al. Systematic review of COVID-19 related myocarditis: insights on management and outcome. Cardiovasc Revasc Med. 2020;23:107–13.
13. Kariyanna PT, Sutarjono B, Grewal E, et al. A systematic review of COVID-19 and myocarditis. Am J Med Case Rep. 2020;8:299–305.
14. Ho JS, Sia CH, Chan MY, Lin W, Wong RC. Coronavirus-induced myocarditis: a meta-summary of cases. Heart Lung. 2020;49:681–5.
15. Schiavone M, Gobbi C, Biondi-Zoccai G, et al. Acute coronary syndromes and Covid-19: exploring the uncertainties. J Clin Med. 2020;9(6):1683.
16. Rivero F, Antuña P, Cuesta J, et al. Severe coronary spasm in a COVID-19 patient. Catheter Cardiovasc Interv. 2020;97(5):E670–2. https://doi.org/10.1002/ccd.29056.
17. Nakao M, Matsuda J, Iwai M, et al. Coronary spasm and optical coherence tomography defined plaque erosion causing ST-segment-elevation acute myocardial infarction in a patient with COVID-19 pneumonia. J Cardiol Cases. 2020;23(2):87–9.
18. Jabri A, Kalra A, Kumar A, et al. Incidence of stress cardiomyopathy during the coronavirus disease 2019 pandemic. JAMA Netw Open. 2020;3(7):e2014780.

19. Okura H. Update of Takotsubo syndrome in the era of COVID-19. J Cardiol. 2021;77(4):361–9.
20. Bois MC, Boire NA, Layman AJ, et al. COVID-19-associated nonocclusive fibrin microthrombi in the heart. Circulation. 2021;143(3):230–43.
21. Pellegrini D, Kawakami R, Guagliumi G, et al. Microthrombi as a major cause of cardiac injury in COVID-19: a pathologic study. Circulation. 2021;143(10):1031–42.
22. Bertini M, Ferrari R, Guardigli G, et al. Electrocardiographic features of 431 consecutive, critically ill COVID-19 patients: an insight into the mechanisms of cardiac involvement. Europace. 2020;22(12):1848–54.
23. Yarmohammadi H, Morrow JP, Dizon J, et al. Frequency of atrial arrhythmia in hospitalized patients with COVID-19. Am J Cardiol. 2021;147:52–7.
24. Bhatla A, Mayer MM, Adusumalli S, et al. COVID-19 and cardiac arrhythmias. Heart Rhythm. 2020;17(9):1439–44.
25. Shao F, Xu S, Ma X, et al. In-hospital cardiac arrest outcomes among patients with COVID-19 pneumonia in Wuhan, China. Resuscitation. 2020;151:18–23.
26. Touafchia A, Bagheri H, Carrié D, et al. Serious bradycardia and remdesivir for coronavirus 2019 (COVID-19): a new safety. Clin Microbiol Infect. 2021;27(5):791.
27. Levin M. Childhood multisystem inflammatory syndrome—a new challenge in the pandemic. N Engl J Med. 2020;383(4):393–5. https://doi.org/10.1056/NEJMe2023158.
28. Rafferty MS, Burrows H, Joseph JP, et al. Multisystem inflammatory syndrome in children (MIS-C) and the coronavirus pandemic: current knowledge and implications for public health. J Infect Public Health. 2021;14(4):484–94.
29. Nalbandian A, Sehgal K, Gupta A, et al. Post-acute COVID-19 syndrome. Nat Med. 2021;27(4):601–15.
30. Carfì A, Bernabei R, Landi F, Group ftGAC-P-ACS. Persistent symptoms in patients after acute COVID-19. JAMA. 2020;324:603–5.
31. Puntmann VO, Carerj ML, Wieters I, et al. Outcomes of cardiovascular magnetic resonance imaging in patients recently recovered from coronavirus disease 2019 (COVID-19). JAMA Cardiol. 2020;5(11):1265–73.
32. Lazzerini PE, Laghi-Pasini F, Boutjdir M, Capecchi PL. Cardioimmunology of arrhythmias: the role of autoimmune and inflammatory cardiac channelopathies. Nat Rev Immunol. 2019;19:63–4.
33. Clavario P, De Marzo V, Lotti R, et al. Cardiopulmonary exercise testing in COVID-19 patients at 3 months follow-up. Int J Cardiol. 2021;340:113–8.

15 Management

Roberta Della Bona, Fabio Pescetelli, and Alberto Valbusa

15.1 CV Comorbidities

Patients with CV risk factors or preexisting CV disease are prone to worse infection course [1]. For this vulnerable population, strict measures (such as self-isolation, social distancing, use of face masks and vaccines) must be applied to prevent exposure and infection.

Patients with CV morbidities should be urged to adhere to prescribed medication and monitoring regimens (e.g., blood pressure, blood glucose monitoring). About medication, experimental

R. Della Bona (✉) · A. Valbusa
Cardiology Unit, Cardiothoracic and Vascular Department, IRCCS Ospedale Policlinico San Martino, Genoa, Italy

F. Pescetelli
Chair of Cardiovascular Diseases, Department of Internal Medicine and Specialties (DIMI), University of Genoa, Genoa, Italy

D. Battaglini, P. Pelosi (eds.), *COVID-19 Critical and Intensive Care Medicine Essentials*, https://doi.org/10.1007/978-3-030-94992-1_15

data suggest that expression of ACE2 (membrane receptor and entry point for SARS-CoV-2) may be increased by renin–angiotensin–aldosterone system (RAAS) blockers, raising concerns that these drugs may facilitate viral cell entry or worsen the infection [2].

The available human data on potential modification of ACE2 expression with RAAS blockers are limited and controversial, and clinical studies denied any clinical relevance of the upregulation of ACE2 on infection course [2]. In experimental models these drugs showed a potentially protective influence and clinical studies demonstrated that in hospitalized patients their use was associated with lower risk of COVID-19 infection and its serious complication including deaths [3, 4]. To date, as recommended by scientific societies, RAAS blockers therapy should not be discontinued in the patient that develops COVID-19 [5].

15.2 Venous and Pulmonary Thromboembolism

Due to an impairment of the coagulation cascade, COVID-19 is associated with high rates of venous thromboembolism (VTE). The incidence and the severity of clinical manifestations vary according to the setting of care and antithrombotic treatment should be tailored, focusing on the estimated risk of bleeding and thrombosis [6].

Since thrombotic complications are associated with higher rate in-hospital mortality, current practice guidelines propose pharmacological thromboprophylaxis in all hospitalized COVID-19 patients in absence of contraindications [7–11]. The best strategy for this purpose has been investigated in several trials [12]. Heparins have proven effective for both prophylaxis and treatment of VTE in hospitalized patients, probably due to the heparin's unique pharmacology demonstrating a reduction in both inflammation and coagulation markers in COVID-19 [12]. Low-molecular-weight heparin (LMWH) is recommended for prophylaxis over unfractionated heparin (UFH) to decrease the number of injections and risk of healthcare worker exposure, reserving the use of UFH for patients with severe renal insufficiency and the use of fondaparinux for patients with a history of heparin-induced thrombocytopenia. Most guidelines recommend standard doses of anticoagulant prophylaxis while some of them give an option for using therapeutic anticoagulation in the highest risk patients [10]. Direct-acting oral anticoagulants (DOACs) are not recommended for VTE prophylaxis, due to the potential interactions with antiviral or immunosuppressive therapy [7]. "Routine" post–hospital discharge prophylaxis is not recommended but guidelines suggest individualized patient decision making based on residual VTE risk especially for patients who were hospitalized in the intensive care units (ICUs) [9]. When indicated, either enoxaparin or DOACs for a duration of 14–45 days postdischarge can be administered [9].

In patients with proved VTE, conventional therapy should be promptly started according to current guidelines [13], including systemic thrombolysis in case of hemodynamic instability [14]. Parenteral anticoagulation is preferred in ICUs or for patients with impending clinical deterioration, while oral treatment with DOACs (assuming no drug interactions) can be started in stable patients or after transition in outpatients setting [6, 12].

15.2.1 Acute Coronary Syndromes (ACS)

Most of patients with COVID-19 may have troponin elevation with or without associated electrocardiographic changes. Mild elevations in cardiac troponin are in general well explained by preexisting cardiac disease and/or the acute injury/stress related to COVID-19 and do not require workup for type 1 myocardial infarction (MI) [15, 16]. Marked elevations in cardiac troponin may are associated with myocarditis, Takotsubo syndrome, type 2 MI triggered by severe respiratory failure, systemic hypoxemia or shock [17]. These patients might be conservatively treated with anti-ischemic drugs and therapy targeting underlying acute conditions [18].

Patients with undoubted ST-segment elevation myocardial infarction (STEMI) or very high-risk non-ST elevation myocardial infarction (NSTEMI) should receive reperfusion therapy as soon as possible according to current guidelines and primary percutaneous coronary intervention remain the standard of care [17, 19, 20].

Patients with low risk-NSTEMI should be evaluated with non-invasive test, preferably a coronary computerized tomography angiography [16, 17] according to which a conservative or a selective invasive approach can be adopted [18].

About medication, while low dose of aspirin can be safely used [15], clopidogrel and ticagrelor have specific interactions with lopinavir–ritonavir due to their potent CYP3A4 inhibition, which results in a weaker effect of clopidogrel and an increased effect of ticagrelor [9]; prasugrel should be used if no contraindications are present [21]. Beta-blockers should be given with caution in patients on chloroquine or hydroxychloroquine due to CYP2D6 inhibition and the potential role of hydroxychloroquine in reducing heart rate. RAAS blockers can be safely started and should not be discontinued especially in patients with left ventricular dysfunction [15, 21].

15.2.2 Myocarditis

There are currently no specific treatments for COVID-19 related myocarditis and treatment should be based on treatment of ventricular dysfunction and clinical status [22] and in according to current guideline recommendations for heart failure [23, 24]. Data of efficacy of antiviral agents in the setting of COVID-19 myocarditis are lacking. Some antiviral agents such as remdesivir, hydroxychloroquine, and lopinavir–ritonavir, showed indeed little or no effect on overall mortality, need of ventilation and duration of hospital stay [25, 26]. Some authors suggested to use high-dose steroids and intravenous immunoglobulins (IVIG) driven by the evidence of a diffuse nonspecific immune activation in late stage of COVID-19. However, the use of high-dose steroids in COVID-19 showed conflicting results [27–30]. IVIG seem to be associated with improved ventricular function and increased survival in acute fulminant myocarditis, but more data are needed in COVID-19 patients [31, 32]. In patients with hemodynamic deterioration and end-organ dysfunction, use of inotropes and/or vasopressors and mechanical circulatory support (extracorporeal membrane oxygenation, ventricular assist device, or intra-aortic balloon pump) should be considered [33].

15.2.3 Cardiac Arrhythmias

Arrhythmias can arise in association with heart failure, myocarditis and it is important to investigate and correct secondary causes such as fever, hypoxia, and metabolic or electrolyte imbalances [34].

To treat bradyarrhythmia, use of isoprenaline, atropine, and temporary pacing prior to permanent pacemaker should be considered due to the possible transient nature of bradycardia and risk of device infection [34].

In patients with atrial fibrillation electrical cardioversion should be the first choice in case of hemodynamic instability. Amiodarone should be used with caution in patients receiving lopinavir–ritonavir (due its metabolism via CYP-3A4) and/or hydroxychloroquine and/or azithromycin (risk of QT interval increase) [35]. To rate control, calcium channel blockers may be preferred over beta-blockers, and among latter metoprolol or esmolol should be preferred due to their selective action toward heart receptors [36]. Digoxin should be used with caution due to the risk of toxicity if associated with antiviral agents.

For patients with sustained ventricular arrhythmias and hemodynamic instability, prompt defibrillation is recommended [37], and in case of polymorphic ventricular tachycardia or ventricular fibrillation, infusion of magnesium, potassium, and isoprenaline or overdrive pacing, with discontinuation of drugs that prolong the QT interval, is recommended [34].

References

1. Pellicori P, et al. COVID-19 and its cardiovascular effects: a systematic review of prevalence studies. Cochrane Database Syst Rev. 2021;3(3):CD013879.

2. Gressens SB, et al. Controversial roles of the renin angiotensin system and its modulators during the COVID-19 pandemic. Front Physiol. 2021;12:624052.
3. Bean DM, et al. Angiotensin-converting enzyme inhibitors and angiotensin II receptor blockers are not associated with severe COVID-19 infection in a multi-site UK acute hospital trust. Eur J Heart Fail. 2020;22(6):967–74.
4. Li J, et al. Association of renin–angiotensin system inhibitors with severity or risk of death in patients with hypertension hospitalized for coronavirus disease 2019 (COVID-19) infection in Wuhan, China. JAMA Cardiol. 2020;5(7):825–30.
5. Bozkurt B, Kovacs R, Harrington B. Joint HFSA/ACC/AHA statement addresses concerns re: using RAAS antagonists in COVID-19. J Card Fail. 2020;26(5):370.
6. Robba C, et al. Coagulative disorders in critically ill COVID-19 patients with acute distress respiratory syndrome: a critical review. J Clin Med. 2021;10(1):140.
7. Marietta M, et al. COVID-19 and haemostasis: a position paper from Italian Society on Thrombosis and Haemostasis (SISET). Blood Transfus. 2020;18(3):167–9.
8. Zhai Z, et al. Prevention and treatment of venous thromboembolism associated with coronavirus disease 2019 infection: a consensus statement before guidelines. Thromb Haemost. 2020;120(6):937–48.
9. Bikdeli B, et al. COVID-19 and thrombotic or thromboembolic disease: implications for prevention, antithrombotic therapy, and follow-up: JACC state-of-the-art review. J Am Coll Cardiol. 2020;75(23):2950–73.
10. Spyropoulos AC, et al. Scientific and standardization committee communication: clinical guidance on the diagnosis, prevention, and treatment of venous thromboembolism in hospitalized patients with COVID-19. J Thromb Haemost. 2020;18(8):1859–65.
11. Barnes GD, et al. Thromboembolism and anticoagulant therapy during the COVID-19 pandemic: interim clinical guidance from the anticoagulation forum. J Thromb Thrombolysis. 2020;50(1):72–81.
12. Ali MAM, Spinler SA. COVID-19 and thrombosis: from bench to bedside. Trends Cardiovasc Med. 2021;31(3):143–60.
13. Konstantinides SV, et al. 2019 ESC Guidelines for the diagnosis and management of acute pulmonary embolism developed in collaboration with the European Respiratory Society (ERS). Eur Heart J. 2020;41(4):543–603.
14. Della Bona R, et al. Systemic fibrinolysis for acute pulmonary embolism complicating acute respiratory distress syndrome in severe COVID-19: a case series. Eur Heart J Cardiovasc Pharmacother. 2021;7(1):78–80.
15. Schiavone M, et al. Acute coronary syndromes and Covid-19: exploring the uncertainties. J Clin Med. 2020;9(6):1683.

16. Cameli M, et al. COVID-19 and acute coronary syndromes: current data and future implications. Front Cardiovasc Med. 2020;7:593496.
17. Chieffo A, et al. EAPCI position statement on invasive Management of Acute Coronary Syndromes during the COVID-19 pandemic. Eur Heart J. 2020;41(19):1839–51.
18. Collet JP, et al. 2020 ESC Guidelines for the management of acute coronary syndromes in patients presenting without persistent ST-segment elevation. Eur Heart J. 2021;42(14):1289–367.
19. Ibanez B, et al. 2017 ESC Guidelines for the management of acute myocardial infarction in patients presenting with ST-segment elevation: the task force for the management of acute myocardial infarction in patients presenting with ST-segment elevation of the European Society of Cardiology (ESC). Eur Heart J. 2018;39(2):119–77.
20. Mahmud E, et al. Management of acute myocardial infarction during the COVID-19 pandemic: a position statement from the Society for Cardiovascular Angiography and Interventions (SCAI), the American College of Cardiology (ACC), and the American College of Emergency Physicians (ACEP). J Am Coll Cardiol. 2020;76(11):1375–84.
21. Driggin E, et al. Cardiovascular considerations for patients, health care workers, and health systems during the COVID-19 pandemic. J Am Coll Cardiol. 2020;75(18):2352–71.
22. Mele D, et al. Myocarditis in COVID-19 patients: current problems. Intern Emerg Med. 2021;16(5):1123–9.
23. Caforio AL, et al. Current state of knowledge on aetiology, diagnosis, management, and therapy of myocarditis: a position statement of the European Society of Cardiology Working Group on Myocardial and Pericardial Diseases. Eur Heart J. 2013;34(33):2636–48.
24. McDonagh TA, et al. 2021 ESC Guidelines for the diagnosis and treatment of acute and chronic heart failure. Eur Heart J. 2021;42(36):3599–726.
25. WHO Solidarity Trial Consortium. Repurposed antiviral drugs for Covid-19—interim WHO solidarity trial results. N Engl J Med. 2021;384(6):497–511.
26. Young B, Tan TT, Leo YS. The place for remdesivir in COVID-19 treatment. Lancet Infect Dis. 2021;21(1):20–1.
27. Russell CD, Millar JE, Baillie JK. Clinical evidence does not support corticosteroid treatment for 2019-nCoV lung injury. Lancet. 2020;395(10223):473–5.
28. Shi S, et al. Association of cardiac injury with mortality in hospitalized patients with COVID-19 in Wuhan, China. JAMA Cardiol. 2020;5(7):802–10.
29. Mehta P, et al. COVID-19: consider cytokine storm syndromes and immunosuppression. Lancet. 2020;395(10229):1033–4.

30. Wang D, et al. Clinical characteristics of 138 hospitalized patients with 2019 novel coronavirus-infected pneumonia in Wuhan, China. JAMA. 2020;323(11):1061–9.
31. Huang X, et al. Intravenous immunoglobulin therapy for acute myocarditis in children and adults. Int Heart J. 2019;60(2):359–65.
32. Zeng W, et al. Characterization of SARS-CoV-2-specific antibodies in COVID-19 patients reveals highly potent neutralizing IgA. Signal Transduct Target Ther. 2021;6(1):35.
33. Kociol RD, et al. Recognition and initial management of fulminant myocarditis: a scientific statement from the American Heart Association. Circulation. 2020;141(6):e69–92.
34. Dherange P, et al. Arrhythmias and COVID-19: a review. JACC Clin Electrophysiol. 2020;6(9):1193–204.
35. Hindricks G, et al. 2020 ESC Guidelines for the diagnosis and management of atrial fibrillation developed in collaboration with the European Association for Cardio-Thoracic Surgery (EACTS): the task force for the diagnosis and management of atrial fibrillation of the European Society of Cardiology (ESC) developed with the special contribution of the European heart rhythm association (EHRA) of the ESC. Eur Heart J. 2021;42(5):373–498.
36. Desai AD, et al. Management of arrhythmias associated with COVID-19. Curr Cardiol Rep. 2020;23(1):2.
37. Karamchandani K, et al. Cardiac arrhythmias in critically ill patients with COVID-19: a brief review. J Cardiothorac Vasc Anesth. 2020;35 (12):3789–96.

Part V

Renal Manifestations of COVID-19

16 Brief Pathophysiology

Silvia De Rosa, Gianluca Villa,
Zaccaria Ricci, and Stefano Romagnoli

16.1 Introduction

The severe acute respiratory syndrome due to coronavirus-2 infection (SARS-CoV-2) was first described in humans in December 2019 in Wuhan, China [1]. SARS-CoV-2 is the third coronavirus that has emerged in the last 20 years, and its pandemic infection was declared on March 11, 2020, by the World Health Organization [1]. The potential impact of SARS-CoV-2

S. De Rosa (✉)
International Renal Research Institute of Vicenza (IRRIV), Vicenza, Italy

Department of Anesthesia and Intensive Care, San Bortolo Hospital, Vicenza, Italy

G. Villa · S. Romagnoli
Department of Health Science, University of Florence, Florence, Italy

Department of Anesthesiology and Intensive Care, Azienda Ospedaliero-Universitaria Careggi, Florence, Italy
e-mail: gianluca.villa@unifi.it

Z. Ricci
Department of Health Science, University of Florence, Florence, Italy

Pediatric Intensive Care Unit, Department of Emergency and Intensive Care, Azienda Ospedaliero Universitaria Meyer, Florence, Italy

D. Battaglini, P. Pelosi (eds.), *COVID-19 Critical and Intensive Care Medicine Essentials*, https://doi.org/10.1007/978-3-030-94992-1_16

disease (COVID-19) on the kidney is still undetermined. Emerging evidence indicates that renal involvement is frequently observed in COVID-19 patients, with peculiar characteristics among those with chronic kidney disease, end-stage renal disease, and kidney transplant recipients [2]. Patients diagnosed with acute kidney injury (AKI) present a more severe clinical picture, worst illness severity scores, persistent lymphopenia, and require invasive mechanical ventilation and vasoactive support during hospitalization. These characteristics ultimately suggest AKI as a marker of COVID-19 severity [3].

16.2 SARS-CoV-2 and COVID-19 Pathophysiology

SARS-CoV-2 has a spherical virion with spike proteins (S). The spike protein represents its high virality, as the RNA virus enters cells through the binding between the S protein and its host receptor. The virus effectively binds angiotensin-converting enzyme 2 (ACE2) receptor, and is expressed ubiquitously in many tissues (e.g., bronchia and lung parenchyma, heart, kidneys, and gastrointestinal tract [4–6]. In particular, some studies have shown that ACE2 is highly expressed in type II alveolar epithelial cells (AECII), suggesting them as potential virus reservoirs. Other studies have shown that AECII has several genes related to the viral process (e.g., replication, life cycle, and assembly), thus promoting the lung viral tropism [6] (Fig. 16.1). The cellular transmembrane protease serine 2 (TMPRSS2) allows the virus to enter host cells through endocytosis [4]. At this point, the virus exploits the cellular transcriptional mechanism to replicate and alter host cells and tissues' behavior, making them unable to perform their normal function.

Two different phases characterize the SARS-CoV-2-induced immune response. In the former, the patients' adaptive immune response prevents the disease progression and attempt to eliminate the virus during the early stages of incubation [7]. The second phase consists of an uncontrolled inflammatory response characterized by a cytokine storm that can favor apoptosis or

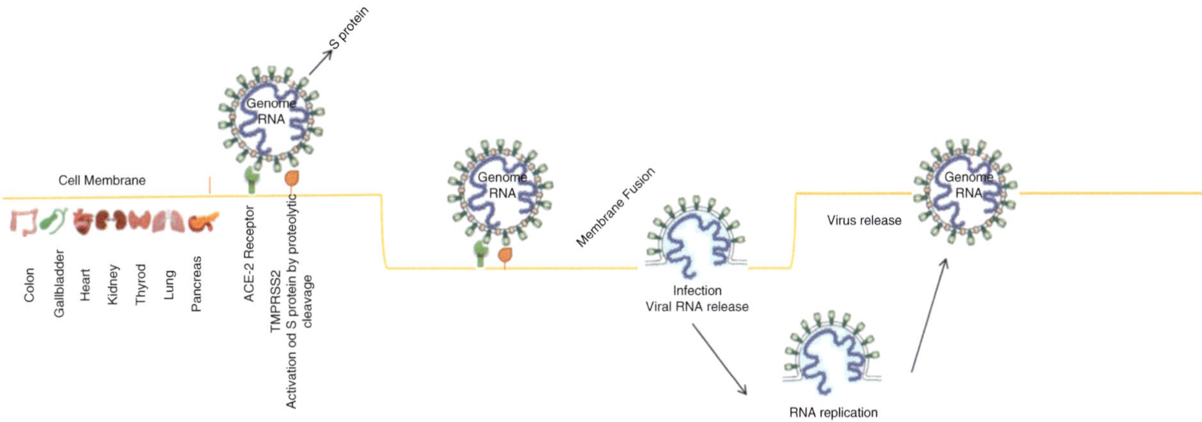

Fig. 16.1 The entry of SARS-CoV-2 into cells. ACE2, expressed on the cell surface, is recognized by the SARS-CoV-2 spike protein. This triggers the viral peak glycoprotein by means of a host serine protease (TMPRSS2), which allows for internalization by endocytosis. Once inside the cells, SARS-CoV-2 replicates using the cellular transcriptional mechanism. *ACE2* angiotensin-converting enzyme 2, *SARS-CoV-2*, severe acute respiratory syndrome Coronavirus 2, *TMPRSS2* transmembrane serine protease 2

necrosis of T lymphocytes, leading to their reduction. It is hypothesized that uncontrolled inflammation while promoting ARDS alters viral clearance by inducing T cell depletion [8].

16.3 ACE-2 Receptors and Direct Tubular Damage Hypothesis

The etiopathogenetic mechanisms of renal involvement are currently not completely clarified. As previously mentioned, in the renal cells where ACE2 expression is the highest [9], the disease can be caused by the binding of SARS-CoV-2 to the ACE2 receptor. The proximal tubules epithelia, parietal epithelial cells, and in some cases, the podocyte membrane expresses ACE2 [4, 10]. The preference of SARS-CoV-2 toward the kidneys is likely due to a low pH environment. Acidosis seems to facilitate the virus inclusion into the cells via endocytosis after the binding between ACE2 receptor and SARS-CoV-2 during viremia [11, 12].

Recent observational studies have reported elevated urinary proteins in 40–60% of SARS-CoV-2 patients [13]. Both proteinuria and AKI are associated with increased mortality rates [13]. Mainly, podocytes are involved in filtration and synthesizing aspects of the glomerular filtration barrier that prevent serum protein filtration [14]. In patients with SARS-CoV-2 infection, light and electron microscopies have observed process effacement on podocytes' foot and glomerular basal membrane detachment, signifying viral-related cell destruction [15]. These findings could explain the etiology of proteinuria found in SARS-CoV-2 patients.

Severe acute tubular necrosis associated with lymphocytic infiltration was found in the postmortem renal tissue; immunohistochemistry analyses have also detected SARS-CoV-2 nucleocapsid protein (NP) in renal tubules [16]. The viral infection could probably induce tubular damage-inducing the deposition of the membrane attack complex (MAC) complex (the final phase of the complement cascade) on the tubules and promote the infiltration of CD68+ macrophages into the tubulointerstitial space [16]. Su et al. examined renal tissue from 26 COVID-19 patients, 9 of whom had clinical evidence of renal damage. The loss of the edge of the brush and vacuolar degeneration were evident in the proximal tubules, along with diffuse erythrocyte aggregation, endothelial damage, and capillary obstruction without fibrin thrombi or erythrocyte and platelet fragmentation in the peritubular and glomerular capillaries [15].

Electron microscopy has demonstrated SARS-CoV-2 clusters in the tubular epithelium and podocytes [15]. Nevertheless, this finding may not be specific, and the presence of viral proteins may not represent direct virus-mediated damage but instead indicate clathrin-coated vesicles [17, 18]. In an autopsy study, Menter et al. [19] examined renal tissue of 18 patients deceased for COVID-19; in these, the authors demonstrated acute tubule damage with dilated clearings and flattened epithelium and interstitial edema as the most frequent findings. Moreover, three patients also showed small fibrin thrombi in the glomerular capillaries, consistent with disseminated intravascular coagulation (DIC). In a similar autoptic study on COVID-19 patients, Puelles et al. [20] showed SARS-CoV-2 RNA and proteins in the kidney, particularly in the glomerular cells, in half of the cases. The authors have not observed inflammatory vascular changes or interstitial nephritis. However, it seems that neutrophil extracellular traps (NET) had a pathophysiological role as microcirculation disturbance in the kidneys of severe COVID-19 patients.

Activation of neutrophil granulocytes in the blood and an increased formation of NETs can entirely or partially occlude capillaries and lead to tissue damage [21]. This pathophysiological role of dysfunctional neutrophil granulocytes or a dysregulated immune response in COVID-19 infection may explain why patients with diabetes mellitus and impaired immune competence have an increased risk for mortality [22].

Renal biopsies would help to understand better the histological pattern lesions (tubular, glomerular, and vascular) and the main pathogenetic mechanisms leading to AKI. Unfortunately, the unstable patients' clinical conditions and the correlated risk of bleeding rarely allow this maneuver.

Interestingly, kidney biopsies in two African American patients with high-risk APOL1 genotype and SARS-CoV-2 infection showed collapsing focal segmental glomerulosclerosis in the absence of detection of virus RNA in the renal tissue; this may suggest that the cytokine storm increased APOL1 expression, leading to podocyte damage [23, 24]. Notably, in patients with dysfunctional APOL1 protein, the collapsing glomerulopathy can be precipitated by direct SARS-CoV-2 insult and/or by immunologic responses to the virus in which leads to the segmental and global collapse of the glomerular capillaries, marked hypertrophy and hyperplasia of podocytes, and severe tubulointerstitial disease [25–27].

16.4 Indirect Causes of AKI

Several studies in the literature have found acute tubule epithelial damages in the absence of characteristic virus particles; this may indirectly cause AKI in COVID-19 patients. Superimposed bacterial sepsis, cytokine storm syndrome, hemodynamic instability with hypotensiona and hypoperfusion, rhabdomyolysis, and renal tissue hypoxia are other indirect mechanisms that potentially induce tubular damage in these patients [13, 28] (Fig. 16.2). Moreover, other iatrogenic factors may have a causative relationship with AKI development, such as the use of nephrotoxic drugs, mechanical ventilation, and sustained fluid restriction. Among nephrotoxic drugs, radiographic contrast media (often used to investigate thromboembolic events, such as pulmonary embolism), antibiotics, and antiviral therapies are the most commonly associated with AKI. Unfortunately, these factors have been poorly investigated in COVID-19 patients. Fluid restriction and hypovolemia associated with prolonged fever, tachypnea, and gastrointestinal disturbances could also cause prerenal AK [8]. However, to the best of our knowledge, no studies have reported specific data on the volume status at the time of hospital admission. We can only assume the role of these factors in the onset of AKI [29].

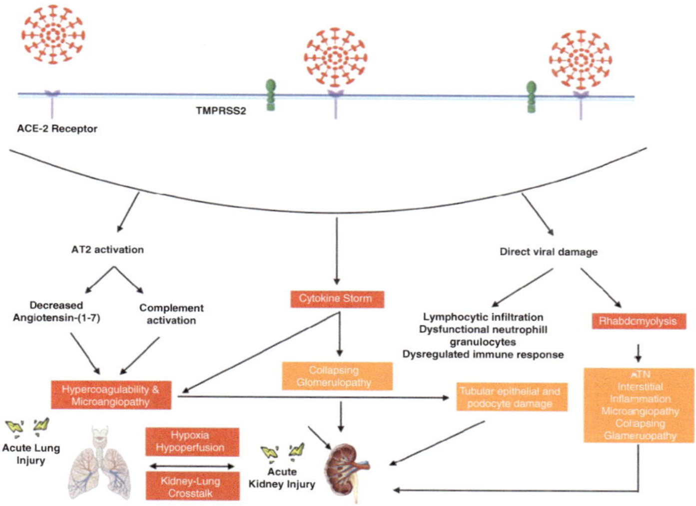

Fig. 16.2 Pathophysiological mechanisms leading to kidney damage in COVID-19

16.4.1 Kidney–Lung Cross Talk

The acute and combined injuries of both kidney and lung represent a complex clinical problem that drastically decreases patient survival.

Most of critically ill patients with COVID-19 require ventilatory support. In a recent study, 45% of COVID-19 patients admitted to the intensive care unit for respiratory support developed an AKI (Fig. 16.2), and 20% of the total ICU cohort required renal replacement therapy acutely for an average duration of 12.5 days [30].

Several clinical and experimental studies have revealed the harmful effects of acute respiratory failure on renal function. In critically ill patients with COVID-19, respiratory failure can trigger AKI due to hypoxia, hypercapnia, acute lung injury, systemic inflammation, and even mechanical ventilation [31]. Most of the mechanisms identified to date are related to mechanical ventilation rather than acute respiratory failure. As we know, changes in intrathoracic pressure associated with mechanical ventilation affect systemic and renal hemodynamics, leading to a decrease in glomerular filtration rate, free water clearance, urinary sodium excretion, and creatinine clearance [32]. Also, mechanical ventilation can further lead to apoptosis of renal epithelial cells [33].

16.4.2 Cytokine Storm

A growing body of clinical data suggests that a cytokine storm is associated with the severity of COVID-19. After its inclusion into the respiratory epithelial cells, SARS-CoV-2 provokes an immune response with inflammatory cytokine production associated with weak interferon (IFN) response. The pro-inflammatory immune responses of pathogenic Th1 cells and intermediate CD14+ CD16+ monocytes are mediated by membrane-bound immune receptors and downstream signaling pathways. Macrophages and neutrophils lung tissue infiltration usually follow this phase, resulting in a cytokine storm [34]. This persistent cytokine response leads to immune-related damage of both lung and kidney tissues [35] (Fig. 16.2). Diao et al. supported the idea that innate immune cells were responsible for indirect cytotoxic damage to renal tubules [16]. Cytokine storm has even been suggested to cause collapsing glomerulopathy due to elevated pro-inflammatory cytokines resulting in immune-directed injury to the glomeruli.

16.4.3 Hypoperfusion

Septic shock is observed in up to 70% of patients who did not survive to COVID-19 [15]; it can cause hypoxia and ischemia to the kidneys due to the impairment of local microcirculation (Fig. 16.2). Acute tubular injury can be seen for SARS-CoV-2 cell infiltration or tissue hypoperfusion. Behind the occurrence of septic shock, other events may increase ischemic events, such as the high circulating levels of AGII. AGII can induce vasoconstriction of renal vessels that further reduce renal blood flow, leading to ischemia [36, 37].

16.4.4 Hypercoagulability

The pathogenesis of hypercoagulability in COVID-19 is still being defined. All three components of Virchow's triad appear to be involved, including endothelial injury (direct invasion of endothelial cells), stasis (immobilization), and hypercoagulable state (elevated circulating prothrombotic factors) [38]. AGII levels will be increased in SARS-CoV-2 infection, resulting in the release of multiple inflammatory mediators, most of which are prothrombotic and predisposed to macro and microthrombosis development [39]. The pathological hallmark is diffuse, small-vessel platelet–fibrin thrombi and intravascular megakaryocytes in all major organs, including kidneys [40] (Fig. 16.2). Microscopic findings demonstrated inflammatory capillary injury, capillary congestion with luminal fibrin deposition, and angiogenesis. The kidneys' autopsy showed diffuse tubular injury, interstitial edema, and fibrin thrombi in the glomerular capillaries [19]. Autopsy findings have revealed that D-dimer was markedly elevated in 73% of SARS-CoV-2 patients [15]. Mainly, elevated D-dimer levels have been observed to correlate with illness severity and 28 day mortality [41].

16.4.5 Rhabdomyolysis

Many viral, bacterial, fungal, and protozoal infections have been associated with rhabdomyolysis. Influenza A is the most commonly implicated, but the exact mechanism of muscle damage in viral infections has not been wholly established [42].

Autopsy findings of renal tissue from patients with SARS-CoV-2 revealed the presence of hemosiderin granules in the tubular epithelium and pigmented casts under light microscopy, suggesting rhabdomyolysis as a potential etiology of acute renal failure [15]. The first incidence of coronavirus-related rhabdomyolysis has been reported in a case series of SARS-CoV patients who all developed AKI with peak creatine kinase levels between 7000 and 330,000 IU/L. It is currently unclear whether rhabdomyolysis in SARS-CoV-2 patients is related to direct viral invasion as skeletal muscle lacks ACE2 receptors. The overactive immune system in SARS-CoV-2 patients may be responsible for developing rhabdomyolysis and AKI as part of multiorgan dysfunction secondary to the cytokine storm [43] (Fig. 16.2). In SARS-CoV-2-infected patients, elevated serum creatine kinase and myoglobin values were found along with a marked increase in inflammatory markers. No evidence can currently define the presence of skeletal muscle thrombosis. Still, we can assume that microthrombosis can occur at the skeletal muscle level, causing tissue hypoperfusion similar to the lungs and kidneys [15].

16.5 Conclusions

The pathophysiology and mechanisms of AKI in COVID-19 patients have not been fully elucidated and appear multifactorial. The significant value of recognizing and understanding the pathophysiology of AKI is significant for improving outcomes in SARS-CoV2 patients. A deeper understanding of the etiology of AKI will allow for a timely diagnosis and improvement in the management of patients with SARS-CoV-2.

References

1. McMichael TM, Currie DW, Clark S, Pogosjans S, Kay M, Schwartz NG, Public Health–Seattle and King County, EvergreenHealth, and CDC COVID-19 Investigation Team, et al. Epidemiology of Covid-19 in a long-term care facility in King County, Washington. N Engl J Med. 2020;382(21):2005–11.
2. Perico L, Benigni A, Remuzzi G. Should COVID-19 concern nephrologists? Why and to what extent? The emerging impasse of angiotensin blockade. Nephron. 2020;144(5):213–21.

3. Fung M, Babik JM. COVID-19 in immunocompromised hosts: what we know so far. Clin Infect Dis. 2020;1:ciaa863. https://doi.org/10.1093/cid/ciaa863.
4. Hoffmann M, Kleine-Weber H, Schroeder S, Krüger N, Herrler T, Erichsen S, et al. SARS-CoV-2 cell entry depends on ACE2 and TMPRSS2 and is blocked by a clinically proven protease inhibitor. Cell. 2020;181:271–80.
5. Li W, Moore MJ, Vasilieva N, Sui J, Wong SK, Berne MA, et al. Angiotensin-converting enzyme 2 is a functional receptor for the SARS coronavirus. Nature. 2003;426(6965):450–4.
6. Zhang H, Penninger JM, Li Y, Zhong N, Slutsky AS. Angiotensin-converting enzyme 2 (ACE2) as a SARS-CoV-2 receptor: molecular mechanisms and potential therapeutic target. Intensive Care Med. 2020;46:586–90.
7. Shi Y, Wang Y, Shao C, Huang J, Gan J, Huang X, et al. COVID-19 infection: the perspectives on immune responses. Cell Death Differ. 2020;27:1451–4.
8. Huang C, Wang Y, Li X, Ren L, Zhao J, Hu Y, et al. Clinical features of patients infected with 2019 novel coronavirus in Wuhan, China. Lancet. 2020;395:497–506.
9. Du M, Cai G, Chen F, Christiani DC, Zhang Z, Wang M. Multiomics evaluation of gastrointestinal and other clinical characteristics of COVID-19. Gastroenterology. 2020;158(8):2298–301.
10. Letko M, Marzi A, Munster V. Functional assessment of cell entry and receptor usage for SARS-CoV-2 and other lineage B betacoronaviruses. Nat Microbiol. 2020;5:562–9.
11. Allison SJ. SARS-CoV-2 infection of kidney organoids prevented with soluble human ACE2. Nat Rev Nephrol. 2020;16(6):316.
12. Zumla A, Chan JF, Azhar EI, Hui DS, Yuen KY. Coronaviruses—drug discovery and therapeutic options. Nat Rev Drug Discov. 2016;15(5):327–47.
13. Cheng Y, Luo R, Wang K, Zhang M, Wang Z, Dong L, et al. Kidney disease is associated with in-hospital death of patients with COVID-19. Kidney Int. 2020;97(5):829–38.
14. Menzel S, Moeller MJ. Role of the podocyte in proteinuria. Pediatr Nephrol. 2011;26(10):1775–80.
15. Su H, Yang M, Wan C, Yi LX, Tang F, Zhu HY, et al. Renal histopathological analysis of 26 post-mortem findings of patients with COVID-19 in China. Kidney Int. 2020;98(1):219–27.
16. Diao B, Wang C, Wang R, Feng Z, Tan Y, Wang H, et al. Human kidney is a target for novel severe acute respiratory syndrome coronavirus 2 (SARS-CoV-2) infection. In: medRxiv, vol. 4; 2020. p. 1120. https://doi.org/10.1101/2020.03.04.20031120.

17. Calomeni E, Satoskar A, Ayoub I, Brodsky S, Rovin BH, Nadasdy T. Multivesicular bodies mimicking SARS-CoV-2 in patients without COVID-19. Kidney Int. 2020;98(1):233–4.
18. Miller SE, Brealey JK. Visualization of putative coronavirus in kidney. Kidney Int. 2020;98(1):231–2.
19. Menter T, Haslbauer JD, Nienhold R, Savic S, Hopfer H, Deigendesch N, et al. Postmortem examination of COVID-19 patients reveals diffuse alveolar damage with severe capillary congestion and variegated findings in lungs and other organs suggesting vascular dysfunction. Histopathology. 2020;77(2):198–209.
20. Puelles VG, Lütgehetmann M, Lindenmeyer MT, Sperhake JP, Wong MN, Allweiss L, et al. Multiorgan and renal tropism of SARS-CoV-2. N Engl J Med. 2020;383(6):590–2.
21. Leppkes M, Knopf J, Naschberger E, Lindemann A, Singh J, Herrmann I, et al. Vascular occlusion by neutrophil extracellular traps in COVID-19. EBioMedicine. 2020;58:102925. https://doi.org/10.1016/j.ebiom.2020.102925.
22. Schulte-Schrepping J, Reusch N, Paclik D, Baßler K, Schlickeiser S, Zhang B, Deutsche COVID-19 OMICS initiative (DeCOI), et al. Severe COVID-19 is marked by a dysregulated myeloid cell compartment. Cell. 2020;182(6):1419–40.
23. Kissling S, Rotman S, Gerber C, Halfon M, Lamoth F, Comte D, et al. Collapsing glomerulopathy in a COVID-19 patient. Kidney Int. 2020;98(1):228–31.
24. Larsen CP, Bourne TD, Wilson JD, Saqqa O, Sharshir MA. Collapsing glomerulopathy in a patient with COVID-19. Kidney Int Rep. 2020;5(6):935–9.
25. Lu T-C, He JC, Wang Z-H. HIV-1 Nef disrupts the podocyte actin cytoskeleton by interacting with diaphanous interacting protein. J Biol Chem. 2008;283(13):8173–82.
26. Nasr SH, Kopp JB. COVID-19—associated collapsing glomerulopathy: an emerging entity. Kidney Int Rep. 2020;22(1):1–9. https://doi.org/10.1016/j.ekir.2020.04.030.
27. Rosenberg AZ, Naicker S, Winkler CA, Kopp JB. HIV-associated nephropathies: epidemiology, pathology, mechanisms and treatment. Nat Rev Nephrol. 2015;11(3):150–60.
28. Naicker S, Yang CW, Hwang SJ, Liu BC, Chen JH, Jha V. The novel coronavirus 2019 epidemic and kidneys. Kidney Int. 2020;97:824–8.
29. Gabarre P, Dumas G, Dupont T, Darmon M, Azoulay E, Zafrani L. Acute kidney injury in critically ill patients with COVID-19. Intensive Care Med. 2020;46(7):1339–48.
30. Lowe R, Ferrari M, Nasim-Mohi M, Jackson A, Beecham R, Veighey K, University Hospital Southampton Critical Care Team and the REACT COVID Investigators, et al. Clinical characteristics and outcome of

critically ill COVID-19 patients with acute kidney injury: a single centre cohort study. BMC Nephrol. 2021;22(1):92.
31. Husain-Syed F, Slutsky AS, Ronco C. Lung–kidney cross-talk in the critically ill patient. Am J Respir Crit Care Med. 2016;194(4):402–14.
32. Kuiper JW, Groeneveld AB, Slutsky AS, Plötz FB. Mechanical ventilation and acute renal failure. Crit Care Med. 2005;33(6):1408–15.
33. Imai Y, Parodo J, Kajikawa O, de Perrot M, Fischer S, Edwards V, et al. Injurious mechanical ventilation and end-organ epithelial cell apoptosis and organ dysfunction in an experimental model of acute respiratory distress syndrome. JAMA. 2003;289(16):2104–12.
34. Hussman JP. Cellular and molecular pathways of COVID-19 and potential points of therapeutic intervention. Front Pharmacol. 2020;29(11):1169.
35. Ye Q, Wang B, Mao J. The pathogenesis and treatment of the 'Cytokine Storm' in COVID-19. J Infect. 2020;80(6):607–13.
36. Long DA, Price KL, Herrera-Acosta J, Johnson RJ. How does angiotensin II cause renal injury? Hypertension. 2004;43(4):722–3.
37. Zhou F, Yu T, Du R, Fan G, Liu Y, Liu Z, et al. Clinical course and risk factors for mortality of adult inpatients with COVID-19 in Wuhan, China: a retrospective cohort study. Lancet. 2020;395(10229):1054–62.
38. Singhania N, Bansal S, Nimmatoori DP, Ejaz AA, McCullough PA, Singhania G. Current overview on hypercoagulability in COVID-19. Am J Cardiovasc Drugs. 2020;20(5):393–403.
39. Senchenkova EY, Russell J, Esmon CT, Granger DN. Roles of coagulation and fibrinolysis in angiotensin II-enhanced microvascular thrombosis. Microcirculation. 2014;21(5):401–7.
40. Fox SE, Akmatbekov A, Harbert JL, Li G, Quincy Brown J, Vander Heide RS. Pulmonary and cardiac pathology in African American patients with COVID-19: an autopsy series from New Orleans. Lancet Respir Med. 2020;8(7):681–6.
41. Tang N, Bai H, Chen X, Gong J, Li D, Sun Z. Anticoagulant treatment is associated with decreased mortality in severe coronavirus disease 2019 patients with coagulopathy. J Thromb Haemost. 2020;18(5):1094–9.
42. Fadila MF, Wool KJ. Rhabdomyolysis secondary to influenza a infection: a case report and review of the literature. N Am J Med Sci. 2015;7(3):122–4.
43. Chong WH, Saha B. Severe acute respiratory syndrome coronavirus 2 (SARS-CoV-2) associated with rhabdomyolysis and acute kidney injury (AKI). Am J Med Sci. 2020;360(6):738–9.

17 Clinical Features and Biomarkers

Silvia De Rosa, Gianluca Villa,
Zaccaria Ricci, and Stefano Romagnoli

17.1 Introduction

Prevalence and long-term outcomes of acute kidney injury (AKI) in patients with Coronavirus Disease 19 (COVID-19) are not entirely known. Nevertheless, the incidence of AKI in those severe cases requiring hospitalization ranges from 2.9 to 50%, depending on definitions and clinical settings [1–5]. Several pathophysiological mechanisms leading to AKI have been recognized in COVID-19 disease. Beyond the direct renal cell invasion from the Severe Acute Respiratory Syndrome Virus-2 (SARS-CoV-2), restrictive fluid strategies, hypoxia, cytokine

S. De Rosa (✉)
International Renal Research Institute of Vicenza (IRRIV), Vicenza, Italy

Department of Anesthesia and Intensive Care, San Bortolo Hospital, Vicenza, Italy

G. Villa · S. Romagnoli
Department of Health Science, University of Florence, Florence, Italy

Department of Anesthesiology and Intensive Care, Azienda Ospedaliero-Universitaria Careggi, Florence, Italy
e-mail: gianluca.villa@unifi.it; stefano.romagnoli@unifi.it

Z. Ricci
Department of Health Science, University of Florence, Florence, Italy

Pediatric Intensive Care Unit, Department of Emergency and Intensive Care, Azienda Ospedaliero Universitaria Meyer, Florence, Italy

D. Battaglini, P. Pelosi (eds.), *COVID-19 Critical and Intensive Care Medicine Essentials*, https://doi.org/10.1007/978-3-030-94992-1_17

storm, nephrotoxic drugs, and bacterial superinfections may be identified as co-acting factors for the AKI development and worsening (see Chap. 20) (Fig. 17.1). When associated with COVID-19, AKI (AKI COVID-19) worsens the patient's outcomes, and affects health care staffing by increasing the requirement of personnel, equipment, and organizational resources.

17.2 COVID-19 and Acute Kidney Injury

During hospitalization, the development of kidney impairment seems to be an independent risk factor of complicated clinical course in COVID-19 patients [1, 6, 7]. As described elsewhere, acute tubular lesions and lymphocytic infiltrations are common histopathologic findings among patients with COVID-19 [8, 9]. Proximal tubular dysfunction, hypouricemia and uricosuria have been observed in specific subgroups of patients. Interestingly, these seem to correlate with the systemic disease severity and with the occurrence of acute respiratory decompensation [10]. Li et al. found that 34% of patients had proteinuria on the first day after the admission for COVID-19, while 63% developed proteinuria during the entire hospital stay [1, 11]. Proteinuria is often transient in nature, similar to what was observed during Middle Eastern Respiratory Syndrome (MERS)-CoV infection. Although the mechanism is not entirely understood, proteinuria can be the consequence of fever, systemic inflammation, or the effect of direct viral infection of the renal epithelium [8]. Hematuria is another common finding, being observed in 27–53% of the cases. Although studies on the exact mechanisms leading to hematuria are lacking in the literature, its occurrence is considered a multifactorial phenomenon [1, 8, 12]. Blood urea nitrogen (BUN) is elevated in 27% of COVID-19 patients, specifically among two-thirds of those who ultimately died [4]. Proteinuria, hematuria, and hyperazotemia are all associated with an increased risk of mortality in patients with COVID-19.

In addition, hypercoagulability is a prominent feature of many COVID-19 patients who experience thrombotic complications. Although the kidney presents a broad susceptibility to thrombotic

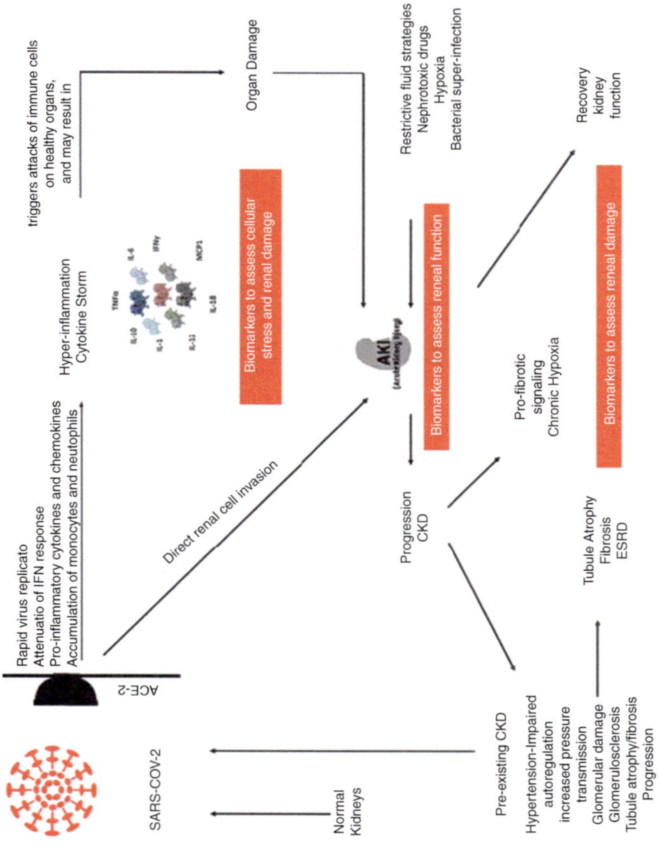

Fig. 17.1 Biomarkers, recovery or CKD progression

microangiopathy, most of the microangiopathic damage in COVID-19 has been documented in extra-renal organs. On the other hand, computerized tomography (CT) abdominal scan presents radiographic abnormalities of the kidneys with reduced density suggesting inflammation and edema, mainly [11].

17.3 COVID-19 and Chronic Kidney Disease

Chronic kidney disease (CKD) has been recognized among the main risk factors for death and other adverse long-term outcomes in COVID-19 [13]. The high incidence of clinical and subclinical AKI observed in hospitalized patients with COVID-19 is undoubtedly related to the high prevalence of preexisting CKD (Fig. 17.1). The superimposed systemic inflammation associated with COVID-19 to the already present CKD-related maladaptive inflammatory state might lead to the acute development of organ dysfunction, the worsening of systemic illness, and a higher mortality rate. Cheng et al. showed that AKI incidence was significantly higher in patients with elevated baseline serum creatinine (SCr) (11.9 vs. 4.0%, $p = 0.001$) [1]. In addition, after univariate Cox regression analysis, elevated baseline SCr has been associated with increased risk of in-hospital death by almost threefold (hazard ratio 2.99 [CI 95% 2.00–4.47], $p < 0.001$). Notably, CKD tripled the risk of patients developing severe symptoms [14]. Abrishami et al. described in a single-center study that patients with CKD are vulnerable to a more severe form of COVID-19. On admission, 58.1% of CKD patients had severe COVID-19. The mean duration of hospitalization in these patients was 11.65 ± 6.67 days, and more prolonged among those with stage V CKD (15.4 ± 6.4 days) and those who died (16.6 ± 8.38 days) [15].

Evidence concerning the management of CKD patients on dialysis therapy infected with SARS-CoV-2 is still scarce. It is still not clear if dialysis therapy is associated with a worse prognosis in patients infected with SARS-CoV-2, although infections, in general, can decompensate underlying CKD.

17.4 COVID-19 and Kidney Transplantation

If compared to the general population, kidney-transplant recipients seem particularly at high risk for severe forms of COVID-19, probably for the effect of long-term immunosuppressive therapy. Only a few studies, and mainly with a limited sample size, have reported conflicting results for the characteristics of COVID-19 in these patients. Akalin et al. identified 36 consecutive adult kidney-transplant recipients who tested positive for COVID-19, reporting less fever as an initial symptom, lower CD3, CD4, and CD8 cell counts, and more rapid clinical progression than persons with COVID-19 in the general population [16]. Considering very low CD3, CD4, and CD8 cell counts [17], the authors retain that it indirectly supports the need to decrease doses of immunosuppressive agents in patients with COVID-19, especially in those who have recently received antithymocyte globulin, which decreases all T-cell subsets for many weeks [16].

In addition, kidney-transplant recipients with COVID-19 showed a very high mortality rate at 3 weeks after symptoms initiation. Other reports of patients with kidney transplants have shown a high mortality rate among kidney transplant patients with percentages of 20% and 28% compared to the 1–5% mortality ratio among COVID-19 patients in the general population [18–20]. The literature lacks specific investigations on the prevalence and risk factors related to COVID-19 disease in the kidney transplant population.

17.5 Renal Biomarkers in AKI and COVID-19

The understanding of the AKI pathophysiology during COVID-19 is of paramount importance and certainly needs further research. Identifying patients susceptible to AKI development may allow the timely adoption of nephroprotective strategies and potentially lead to better outcomes. Hemodynamic optimization and prevention of nephrotoxic exposures are strategies generally suggested in patients at higher risk of developing AKI. Nevertheless, identifying these susceptible patients and specifically those who might benefit from renal replacement therapy (RRT), hemoperfusion, and sequential extracorporeal therapies is a process mainly based on clinical practice and physician perception. Indeed, AKI diagnosis and severity staging are nowadays mainly based on clinical parameters, such as urine production and serum creatinine. Studies aimed at identifying and validating novel biomarkers and recognizing patients at highier risk for AKI in COVID-19 are very much needed. Biomarkers detecting renal damage before or without a clinically evident loss of functional renal (i.e., subclinical AKI) may have a prominent role in modifying the clinical management of COVID-19 patients [20, 21]]. Several biomarkers of kidney damage have been identified. Although they differ in anatomical origin, physiological function, kinetics, and detection time after kidney damage, all of them are potentially applicable in the context of COVID-19. Among these, neutrophil gelatinase-associated lipocalin (NGAL) seems particularly relevant (Fig. 17.2).

NGAL is a 25 kDa glycoprotein secreted by neutrophils in response to infections [22, 23]. NGAL has been found in numerous tissues, including pulmonary, gastric, and renal [24], and its

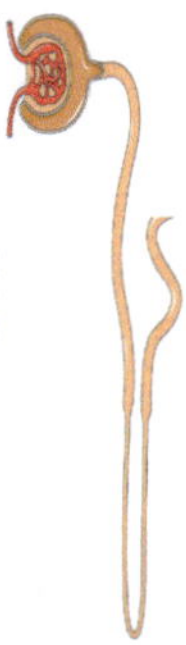

		Molecular weight	Fluids analysed	POC availability
Markers of function	sCr	113 Da	Blood	-
	CysC	13 Kda	Blood	-
Markers of stress	TIMP1-IGFBP7	21 KDa/29 Kda	Urine	+
Markers ok damage	NGAL	25 Kda	Urine	+
	KIM-1	104 Kda	Urine	-

Fig. 17.2 Clinical characteristics of the most relevant biomarkers of kidney insult. *POC* point-of-care

secretion has been related to various pathological conditions [25]. Several studies, conducted in different clinical settings, have investigated its potential role as an early biomarker of AKI [26]. These described the positive and negative predictive value of NGAL regarding the diagnosis and staging of AKI, the site of injury, the need for RRT, and renal recovery or progression to CKD [27]. Unfortunately, NGAL levels increase not only in AKI but also in the presence of other diseases such as sepsis [28] and diabetes mellitus [29], CKD [30], and in extracorporeal circulation [31]. The usefulness of urinary NGAL levels and the platelet/lymphocyte index as predictive markers of AKI in the context of COVID-19 is currently under study (Clinical Trial.Gov ID: NCT04603664).

Considering the effects that critical illness and prolonged hospitalization might have on muscle mass, serum creatinine has been frequently questioned as unspecific and insensitive in identifying kidney disfunction in COVID patients. For these reasons, new biomarkers aimed at identifying the loss of renal function in sarcopenic patients are critically important. Plasma cystatin C (pCys-C) is a marker of kdiney function. Secreted by glomeruli, it does not undergo tubular excretion or reabsorption. Different than serum creatinine, circulating levels of pCys-C are independent by muscle production [32–34]. Studies on COVID-19 patients are currently lacking even if this biomarker could be considered as a valid alternative to creatinine in sarcopenic critically ill patients.

Kidney damage and kidney dysfunction represent clinical conditions where kidney insults have already occurred. Thus, the physician can only limit the severity of organ dysfunction or prevent multiple organ dissemination. Identifying conditions of kidney stress may represent the only possibility we have to prevent the AKI occurrence in COVID-19 patients. In this context, biomarkers of cell cycle arrest (i.e., Tissue Inhibitor of Metalloproteinase 2 [TIMP2] and Insulin-like Growth Factor-binding Protein 7 [IGFBP7]) can be usefully adopted to identify stressful conditions. The former is a 21 kDa protein that suppresses endothelial cell proliferation in response to angiogenic factors and inhibits protease activity in tissues undergoing extracellular matrix remodeling [35]. On the other hand, IGFBP7 is a

29 kDa protein with numerous biological functions, including regulating the availability of insulin-like growth factors and their binding to receptors [36]. Both TIMP2 and IGFBP7 are involved in cell cycle arrest in the G1 phase, which occurs during the early stages of cellular stress [37]. Cell cycle arrest biomarkers have been the subject of numerous subsequent studies aimed at investigating their predictive role of AKI [38], but also of mortality [39], the need for RRT [39] and renal functional recovery [40]. In critically ill patients without COVID-19, the combination of TIMP2–IGFBP7 has been shown to predict AKI development. Whether these new biomarkers also predict AKI development in critically ill patients with COVID-19 is currently unknown. Ongoing observational study will perhaps bring further clarity to the use of biomarkers in COVID-19 patients (Clinical Trial.Gov ID: NCT04408248).

17.6 Conclusions

AKI appears to be an independent risk factor for negative outcomes in COVID-19. Although clinical evidence regarding the management of COVID-19 patients with CKD is unknown, it is still unclear whether RRT is associated with a worse prognosis in infected patients. Furthermore, the literature lacks specific investigations into the prevalence and risk factors related to COVID-19 disease in the kidney transplant population. The discovery and validation of novel biomarkers capable of identifying cellular stress, damage without renal dysfunction, and early renal dysfunction before the increase in sCr have been proposed to redefine the diagnostic and staging criteria for AKI. Furthermore, such biomarkers may contribute to construct a conceptual model of AKI that encompasses the entire spectrum of events and situations ranging from normal kidney, or already affected by CKD, to resolution of the clinical picture or irreversible organ death. For each phase of this model, biomarkers can help elucidate possible damage mechanisms and predict the clinical evolution of kidney damage. Today, with the increase in the number of available biomarkers, the studies in progress are increasing simultaneously.

These have so far demonstrated the superiority of clinical data integration models with biomarker levels in the management of patients at risk or with AKI. Further studies on new biomarkers in the COVID-19 scenario, alone or more likely combined in a panel, will provide valuable tools for its early diagnosis and AKI risk stratification and recovery assessment.

References

1. Cheng Y, Luo R, Wang K, Zhang M, Wang Z, Dong L, et al. Kidney disease is associated with in-hospital death of patients with COVID-19. Kidney Int. 2020;97:829–38.
2. Guan WJ, Ni ZY, Hu Y, Liang WH, Ou CQ, He JX, et al. China Medical Treatment Expert Group for COVID-19: clinical characteristics of coronavirus disease 2019 in China. N Engl J Med. 2020;382:1708–20.
3. Hirsch JS, Ng JH, Ross DW, Sharma P, Shah HH, Barnett RL, et al. Acute kidney injury in patients hospitalized with COVID-19. Kidney Int. 2020;98(1):209–18.
4. Naicker S, Yang CW, Hwang SJ, Liu BC, Chen JH, Jha V. The novel coronavirus 2019 epidemic and kidneys. Kidney Int. 2020;97(5):824–8.
5. Yang X, Yu Y, Xu J, Shu H, Xia J, Liu H, et al. Clinical course and outcomes of critically ill patients with SARS-CoV-2 pneumonia in Wuhan, China: a single-centered, retrospective, observational study. Lancet Respir Med. 2020;8:475–81.
6. Portolés J, Marques M, Sánchez PL, De Valdenebro M, Muñez E, Serrano ML, et al. Chronic kidney disease and acute kidney injury in the COVID-19 Spanish outbreak. Nephrol Dial Transplant. 2020;35(8):1353–61.
7. Uribarri A, Nuñez-Gil IJ, Aparisi A, Becerra-Muñoz VM, Feltes G, Trabattoni D, et al. Impact of renal function on admission in COVID-19 patients: an analysis of the international HOPE COVID-19 (Health Outcome Predictive Evaluation for COVID-19) Registry. J Nephrol. 2020;33:737–45.
8. Pei G, Zhang Z, Peng J, Liu L, Zhang C, Yu C, et al. Renal involvement and early prognosis in patients with COVID-19 pneumonia. J Am Soc Nephrol. 2020;31(6):1157–65.
9. Xia P, Wen Y, Duan Y, Su H, Cao W, Xiao M, et al. Clinicopathological features and outcomes of acute kidney injury in critically ill COVID-19 with prolonged disease course: a retrospective cohort. J Am Soc Nephrol. 2020;31(9):2205–21.
10. Werion A, Belkhir L, Perrot M, Schmit G, Aydin S, Chen Z, et al. SARS-CoV-2 causes a specific dysfunction of the kidney proximal tubule. Kidney Int. 2020;98(5):1296–307.

11. Li ZMW, Guo J, Yao J, Guo J, Liao X, Song S, et al. Caution on kidney dysfunction of COVID-19 patients. medRxiv. 2020. https://doi.org/10.2139/ssrn.3559601.
12. Cao M, Zhang D, Wang Y, Lu Y, Zhu X, Li Y, et al. Clinical features of patients infected with the 2019 novel coronavirus (COVID-19) in Shanghai, China. medRxiv. 2020;2020:20030395.
13. ERA-EDTA Council, ERACODA Working Group. Chronic kidney disease is a key risk factor for severe COVID-19: a call to action by the ERA-EDTA. Nephrol Dial Transplant. 2021;36:87–94.
14. Henry BM, Lippi G. Chronic kidney disease is associated with severe coronavirus disease 2019 (COVID-19) infection. Int Urol Nephrol. 2020;52(6):1193–4.
15. Abrishami A, Khalili N, Dalili N, Tabari R, Farjad R, Samavat S, et al. Clinical and radiologic characteristics of COVID-19 in patients with CKD. Iran J Kidney Dis. 2020;14(4):267–77.
16. Akalin E, Azzi Y, Bartash R, Seethamraju H, Parides M, Hemmige V, et al. COVID-19 and kidney transplantation. N Engl J Med. 2020;382(25):2475–7.
17. Diao B, Wang C, Tan Y, Chen X, Liu Y, Ning L, et al. Reduction and functional exhaustion of T cells in patients with coronavirus disease 2019 (COVID-19). Front Immunol. 2020;1(11):827.
18. Coates PT, Wong G, Drueke T, Rovin B, Ronco P, Associate Editors, for the Entire Editorial Team. Early experience with COVID-19 in kidney transplantation. Kidney Int. 2020;97(6):1074–5.
19. Columbia University Kidney Transplant Program. Early description of coronavirus 2019 disease in kidney transplant recipients in New York. J Am Soc Nephrol. 2020;31(6):1150–6.
20. Murray PT, Mehta RL, Shaw A, Ronco C, Endre Z, Kellum JA, Chawla LS, Cruz D, Ince C, Okusa MD, ADQI 10 Workgroup. Potential use of biomarkers in acute kidney injury: report and summary of recommendations from the 10th Acute Dialysis Quality Initiative consensus conference. Kidney Int. 2014;85(3):513–21.
21. Haase M, Devarajan P, Haase-Fielitz A, Bellomo R, Cruz DN, Wagener G, et al. The outcome of neutrophil gelatinase-associated lipocalin-positive subclinical acute kidney injury: a multicenter pooled analysis of prospective studies. J Am Coll Cardiol. 2011;57(17):1752–61.
22. Kjeldsen L, Johnsen AH, Sengeløv H, Borregaard N. Isolation and primary structure of NGAL, a novel protein associated with human neutrophil gelatinase. J Biol Chem. 1993;268(14):10425–32.
23. Xu SY, Carlson M, Engström A, Garcia R, Peterson CG, Venge P. Purification and characterization of a human neutrophil lipocalin (HNL) from the secondary granules of human neutrophils. Scand J Clin Lab Invest. 1994;54(5):365–76.
24. Cowland JB, Borregaard N. Molecular characterization and pattern of tissue expression of the gene for neutrophil gelatinase-associated lipocalin from humans. Genomics. 1997;45:17–23.

25. Xu S, Venge P. Lipocalins as biochemical markers of disease. Biochim Biophys Acta. 2000;1482:298–307.
26. Mårtensson J, Martling CR, Bell M. Novel biomarkers of acute kidney injury and failure: clinical applicability. Br J Anaesth. 2012a;109:843–50. https://doi.org/10.1093/bja/aes357.
27. Agarwal A, Dong Z, Harris R, Murray P, Parikh SM, Rosner MH, Acute Dialysis Quality Initiative XIII Working Group, et al. Cellular and molecular mechanisms of AKI. J Am Soc Nephrol. 2016;27(5):1288–99.
28. Bagshaw SM, Bennett M, Haase M, Haase-Fielitz A, Egi M, Morimatsu H, et al. Plasma and urine neutrophil gelatinase-associated lipocalin in septic versus non-septic acute kidney injury in critical illness. Intensive Care Med. 2010;36(3):452–61.
29. Nauta FL, Boertien WE, Bakker SJ, van Goor H, van Oeveren W, de Jong PE, Bilo H, Gansevoort RT. Glomerular and tubular damage markers are elevated in patients with diabetes. Diabetes Care. 2011;34(4):975–81.
30. Mcilroy DR, Wagener G, Lee HT. Kidney injury after cardiac surgery: the effect of baseline renal function on diagnostic performance. Clin J Am Soc Nephrol. 2010;5:211–9.
31. Cai L, Borowiec J, Xu S, Han W, Venge P. Assays of urine levels of HNL/NGAL in patients undergoing cardiac surgery and the impact of antibody configuration on their clinical performances. Clin Chim Acta. 2009;403(1–2):121–5.
32. De Rosa S, De SS, Ronco C. Creatinine-based definitions: from baseline creatinine to serum creatinine adjustment in intensive care. Crit Care. 2016;20:1–5.
33. Mårtensson J, Martling CR, Oldner A, Bell M. Impact of sepsis on levels of plasma cystatin C in AKI and non-AKI patients. Nephrol Dial Transplant. 2012b;27(2):576–81.
34. Vaidya VS, Waikar SS, Ferguson MA, Collings FB, Sunderland K, Gioules C, et al. Urinary biomarkers for sensitive and specific detection of acute kidney injury in humans. Clin Transl Sci. 2008;1(3):200–8.
35. Edelstein CL. Chapter six—Biomarkers in acute kidney injury. In: Edelstein CL, editor. Biomarkers of kidney disease. 2nd ed. Amsterdam: Academic Press; 2017. p. 241–315.
36. Evdokimova V, Tognon CE, Benatar T, Yang W, Krutikov K, Pollak M, et al. IGFBP7 binds to the IGF-1 receptor and blocks its activation by insulin-like growth factors. Sci Signal. 2012;5(255):ra92.
37. Ortega LM, Heung M. The use of cell cycle arrest biomarkers in the early detection of acute kidney injury. Is this the new renal troponin? Nefrologia. 2018;38:361–7.
38. Gocze I, Koch M, Renner P, Zeman F, Graf BM, Dahlke MH, Nerlich M, Schlitt HJ, Kellum JA, Bein T. Urinary biomarkers TIMP-2 and IGFBP7 early predict acute kidney injury after major surgery. PLoS One. 2015;10(3):e0120863.

39. Koyner JL, Shaw AD, Chawla LS, Hoste EA, Bihorac A, Kashani K, Haase M, Shi J, Kellum JA, Investigators S. Tissue inhibitor metalloproteinase-2 (TIMP-2)·IGF-binding protein-7 (IGFBP7) levels are associated with adverse long-term outcomes in patients with AKI. J Am Soc Nephrol. 2015;26(7):1747–54.
40. Meersch M, Schmidt C, Van Aken H, Martens S, Rossaint J, Singbartl K, Görlich D, Kellum JA, Zarbock A. Urinary TIMP-2 and IGFBP7 as early biomarkers of acute kidney injury and renal recovery following cardiac surgery. PLoS One. 2014;9(3):e93460.

18 COVID-19 and Renal Replacement Therapies

Stefano Romagnoli, Zaccaria Ricci, Gianluca Villa, and Silvia De Rosa

18.1 Introduction, Incidence, and Outcomes

Although *Severe Acute Respiratory Syndrome CoronaVirus* (SARS-CoV-2) infection primarily manifests as an acute pulmonary disease (*COronaVirus Disease 2019*; COVID-19) and respiratory failure with interstitial and alveolar pneumonia, it frequently affects multiple organs, including the kidneys, heart, gut, and nervous system. Acute kidney injury (AKI) is emerging as a common and important sequela of COVID-19, with rates as high as 33–43% among hospitalized patients [1]. In case of respiratory failure,

S. Romagnoli (✉) · G. Villa
Department of Health Science, University of Florence, Florence, Italy

Department of Anesthesiology and Intensive Care, Azienda Ospedaliero-Universitaria Careggi, Florence, Italy
e-mail: stefano.romagnoli@unifi.it; gianluca.villa@unifi.it

Z. Ricci
Pediatric Intensive Care Unit, Department of Emergency and Intensive Care, Azienda Ospedaliero Universitaria Meyer, Florence, Italy

S. De Rosa
International Renal Research Institute of Vicenza (IRRIV), Vicenza, Italy

Department of Anesthesia and Intensive Care, San Bortolo Hospital, Vicenza, Italy

D. Battaglini, P. Pelosi (eds.), *COVID-19 Critical and Intensive Care Medicine Essentials*, https://doi.org/10.1007/978-3-030-94992-1_18

AKI affects over 50% of patients admitted to the intensive care unit (ICU) [2]. Among critically ill patients, AKI frequently manifests as a severe oligo-anuric phenotype and imposes the use of renal replacement therapy (RRT) [3, 4]. In fact, RRT is frequently required to treat ICU patients with severe COVID-19 related AKI (C-19-AKI), and different modalities have been described in the literature (Continuous RRT-CRRT; Intermittent Hemodialysis—IHD; Peritoneal Dialysis—PD) [3]. Specifically, careful management of fluid balance and electrolyte disorders has been found to be beneficial in patients with severe C-19-AKI requiring RRT [5]. Not surprisingly, C-19-AKI requiring RRT is also associated with a particularly poor outcome. In fact, renal failure is now a well-established independent risk factor linked with increased in-hospital mortality [3, 4]. A recent study involving COVID-19 patients found that 63% of the patients exhibited proteinuria, 19% had an elevated plasma creatinine level, and 27% had an elevated urea nitrogen level [6]. During the first pandemic peak, 451 adult COVID-19 patients admitted to ICUs at the Karolinska University Hospital showed an overall incidence of AKI of 43.7% (9.5% had AKI grade I, 8.9% AKI grade II, and 25.3% experienced AKI grade III) [7]. Compared to non-AKI patients, AKI patients had a prolonged, doubled, length of stay, higher SAPS III scores, and 18.2% received CRRT while on ICU [7]. Even if the overall 30-day mortality for the COVID-19 cohort was 19.1% (and 23.1% at 60 days), mortality of AKI patients was much higher (42.6%) compared to patients with no-AKI (8.7%). As expected, mortality was proportional to the severity of AKI being 27.9% in grade I, 40.0% in grade II, and 49.1% in grade III [7]. Finally, 45.1% of those who received CRRT died up until the end of follow-up, showing that mortality in the CRRT group was significantly higher than in non-CRRT patients with a hazard ratio of 2.59 (confidence interval, CI 1.73–3.86, $P \leq 0.001$) [7]. Interestingly, predictors of hospital mortality for CRRT patients were a higher age at admission, being 55 (IQR 52–64) years in survivors vs. 63 (IQR 58–68) years in nonsurvivors, weight change during hospital stay, being −10.5 (−15.3 to 6.7)% in survivors and −1.2 (−4.1 to +0.7)% in nonsurvivors, and a higher baseline creatinine value [7]. These data show that older subjects with accumulation of fluid excess and preinfection renal disfunction showed the worse outcomes. Mortality appeared to be highly variable in different publications. In one Italian report of COVID-19 patients, it was 38.9% and 52.9% for AKI patients and for those who received CRRT, respectively [8]. In a second report, AKI incidence was 22.6% with a mortality of 63% [9]. In a cohort of nearly 4000 hospitalized patients in New York, 76% of the 976 ICU patients had AKI, 19% received RRT and in-hospital mortality in the AKI group was 50% [10]. The largest prospective study on RRT in C-19-AKI is the Study of the Treatment and Outcomes in Critically Ill Patients with COVID-19 (STOP-COVID), a multicenter cohort study at 67 geographically diverse hospitals across the USA [1]. A total of 3099 patients were included in the analysis and 637 of them patients (20.6%) developed AKI requiring RRT within 14 days following ICU admission. Patients with RRT were similar in age to patients without AKI-RRT and were more likely to have comorbidities (e.g., diabetes mellitus, hypertension, and chronic kidney disease—CKD), and to have greater severity of illness on arrival to the ICU, including higher rates of invasive mechanical ventilation and treatment with vasopressors. In the 637 AKI-RRT patients, the median time from ICU admission to RRT initiation was 4 days (IQR 2–7 days), and in 52.4% of the cases the modality was CRRT. The remaining modalities included intermittent hemodialysis in 30.0%, "hybrid" RRT (a CRRT conducted for <12 h/day) in 14.9%, and PD in 1.3%. CKD was associated with a higher risk of AKI-RRT (odds ratio, 5.63), and additional patient-specific risk factors for AKI-RRT included sex (men at higher risk), nonwhite race, hypertension, diabetes mellitus, higher body mass index, lower PaO_2: FiO_2 ratio on ICU admission, and D-dimer >2500 ng/mL on ICU admission. Among the 637 patients with AKI-RRT, 28-day mortality was 54.9%. Older age, receipt of two or more vasopressors at the time of RRT initiation, and severe oliguria (urine output <100 mL/day) at the time of RRT initiation were each associated with a higher risk of 28-day mortality, whereas CKD stage 4 or 5 was associated with a lower risk of 28-day mortality. Among the 216 patients discharged, 33.8% remained RRT dependent on discharge [1]. A recent large meta-analysis on AKI and RRT in COVID-19 patients analyzed 58 observational studies and 22,671 patients [11]. The pooled AKI incidence rate was 12.3% and 39% among the ICU patients. A total of 12 studies reported that AKI incidence among deceased patients was 42.0%. Furthermore, in 7 studies, among 1588 AKI patients, the proportions of stage 1, 2, and 3 AKI were 36.3%, 20.7%, and 43.0%, respectively. RRT was used to treat 939 out of 17,664 COVID-19 patients in 39 selected studies, for a pooled application rate of 5.4% and in the overall ICU patients RRT use was 16.3% [11].

18.2 Availability of Dialysis Machines and Resource Shortages

Figure 18.1 summarizes a hypothetical decisional flowchart from RRT indication to RRT application throughout the available modalities. In the face of unprecedented hospitalization and ICU admittance, the sudden dramatic increase in demand has presented a unique challenge to the healthcare systems. Considering the high number of severely ill patients and the unexpected need for multiple dialytic treatments, managing this new and complex syndrome has led to additional problems for patients requiring RRT. The healthcare systems, the hospitals, and the caregivers had to face and address such novel clinical and organizational issues without forewarning. Providing RRT is an expensive procedure that requires significant economic investments for the dialysis machines, consumables circuits and filters, dialysate solutions, and healthcare workers with appropriate advanced training. During the first pandemic peak in New York City, the number of patients with indications for RRT exceeded the availability of renal support resources [12]. As the dialysis needs began to challenge resources, the nephrologists, in New York City, recognized the need for a coordinated response for RRT across all New York Presbyterian Hospital-affiliated hospitals. A workgroup that included a lead nephrologist from all campuses was formed and the workgroup gathered via video calls daily to track needs and inventory, share dialytic resources, and develop standard protocols and innovative solutions. Due to the novelty of the SARS-CoV-2 pandemic and the severe C-19-AKI cases, different strategies for delivering RRT needed to be rapidly explored as

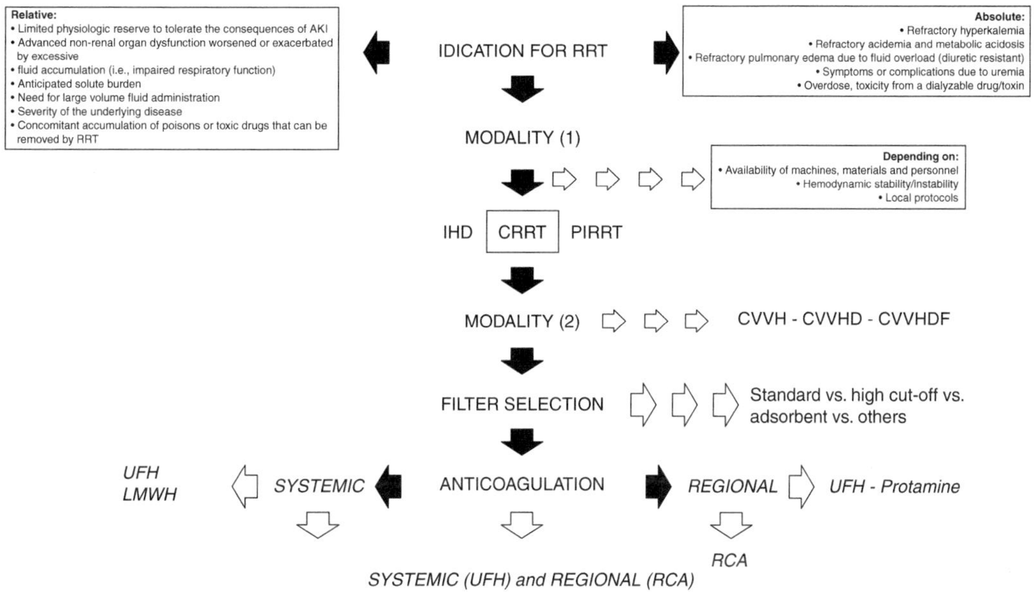

Fig. 18.1 Decisional flowchart in case of RRT indication. *CVVH*, continuous venovenous hemofiltration, *CVVHD* continuous venovenous hemodialysis, *CVVHDF* continuous venovenous hemodiafiltration, *IHD* intermittent hemodialysis, *LMWH* low-molecular-weight heparin, *PIRRT* prolonged intermittent renal replacement therapy, *RCA* regional citrate anticoagulation, *RRT* renal replacement therapy, *UFH* unfractioned heparin

many factors were clearly involved and played a critical role in the decisional process: IHD may be particularly challenging in hemodynamically unstable patients and CRRT is suggested as initial renal support modality in these patients by current guidelines [13] due to the benefit of a slow, continuous support in clearing solutes and managing fluid balance [14]. Nevertheless, in many centers, devices for CRRT have been used in a noncontinuous manner to treat more patients given the paucity of devices. The hybrid approach, called prolonged intermittent renal replacement therapy (PIRRT) or accelerated venovenous hemofiltration (AVVH), has been used in severe C-19-AKI [15, 16]. The shortage of dialysis machine was also described by Fisher and collaborators in London. Initially, the physicians increased the use of continuous venovenous hemodiafiltration (CVVHDF) applying strategies aimed at prolonging the life span of filters and circuits (e.g., higher dialysis flow, high blood flow rate, low filtration fraction, careful anticoagulation strategy). However, rapidly, the number of patients needing a dialytic treatment overwhelmed the ability to provide RRT due to lack of hemofiltration machines and a national issue with the delivery of hemofiltration-related consumables. Thus, PD and IHD started gaining novel indications and applications [3]. The constant support of a nephrology team in the ICUs helped in the management of noncontinuous RRT modalities [3]. CVVHDF with PrisMax machines (Baxter Healthcare, Deerfield, Illinois, USA) represented the standard treatment before the pandemic. Prismaflex CRRT machines (Baxter Healthcare, Deerfield, Illinois, USA) were acquired from nephrology services and Aquarius CRRT machines (Edwards Lifesciences AG, Irvine, CA, USA) from the pediatric ICU which increased device capacity from 33 to 46 (an increase of 39%). However, even after the upgrade in the RRT capacity, PD and IHD, still resulted necessary [3]. Given the paucity of devices and the challenges of IHD in hemodynamically unstable patients, several large academic centers shifted to protocols that allowed devices to be shared between patients resulting in the use of traditionally continuous therapies in a noncontinuous manner (PIRRT or sustained low efficiency dialysis, SLED) or accelerated venovenous hemofiltration [16].

18.3 RRT in C-19-AKI: Rational and (Standard) Modalities

Most single center studies have focused on single geographic regions and locally available resources, and, therefore, they provide incomplete descriptions of the modalities applied to C-19-AKI patients undergoing RRT. It is widely accepted that in severe AKI (especially oliguric/anuric AKI) RRT produces beneficial effects by reverting life-threatening alterations (e.g., fluid overload resistant to diuretics, electrolytes alterations, acidosis) and may prevent extrarenal injuries (e.g., respiratory failure, gut congestion, and bacterial translocation). In this light, RRT may have three different and contemporary beneficial mechanisms: (1) fluid overload management; (2) normalization of acid–base and electrolytes imbalance together with solute clearance; (3) immunomodulation. In a recent study by Fisher and collaborators on C-19-AKI patients, among the 82 patients who commenced RRT, all patients received CVVHDF except for one patient who received (acute) peritoneal dialysis (APD), which was started before ICU admission and eventually continued; 31.5% received also acute APD and 13.5% received IHD [3]. Interestingly, prior to the pandemic the typical CVVHDF prescription was 24–44 mL/kg/h effluent dose (by ideal body weight). The effluent dose was divided on a 1:1 basis between diffusion and convection, with one third of the replacement fluid given as predilution prior to the blood passing over the filter membrane, to minimize clotting and anticoagulation was with either heparin or epoprostenol. It was clear early in the pandemic that the filter life span was a challenge in C-19-AKI (see below). The average filter life span was 24.3 h, compared with an average filter lifespan of 31.6 h in 2019. To increase filter life span, the authors adjusted the ratio of dialysate to replacement fluid from 1:1 to 3:1 to reduce the effect of the filtration fraction effect. Because of the high incidence of filter clotting and evidence in the literature of a prothrombotic state in COVID-19 patients, systemic anticoagulation with heparin was commenced for all patients receiving CVVHDF targeting an activated partial thromboplastin time (aPTT) ratio of 2.0–2.5 unless contraindicated. APD was undertaken by a specialist team lead by a senior clinical nurse specialist, a consultant nephrologist, and a consultant in critical care in patients with a BMI <40 kg/m^2, no midline laparotomy scar and no known abdominal aortic aneurysm. In addition to APD, to further reduce demand for CVVHDF they also introduced IHD (82 hemodialysis sessions delivered to 15 patients). The hybrid techniques (i.e., PIRRT or SLED) were not employed as the longer dialysis sessions (usually 8 h) would have limited the possibility to treat more patients. IHD was dedicated to patients with stable or improving clinical trajectory, modest ventilatory requirements ($FiO_2 < 0.5$), and cardiovascular support with norepinephrine dose < 0.15 μg/kg/min. Patients received daily IHD for the first 3 days followed by three times weekly sessions once established [3]. In a recent observational single center study performed at the Medstar Georgetown University Hospital, the decision to start RRT and the choice between continuous venovenous hemofiltration (CVVH) and IHD was made by the treating intensivist in conjunction with a consulting nephrologist. A total of 43 patients (26%) required RRT. Seven received IHD in the ICU, and the remainder received CVVH. Details on specific machine settings have not been provided by the authors [17].

18.4 RRT in C-19-AKI: Rational and (Special) Modalities for Cytokines Clearance

Proinflammatory and anti-inflammatory cytokines (CKs) response may have a role in leading to cellular and organ injury in C-19-AKI and in COVID-19 in general [18]. CRRT has three forms of depurative mechanisms: diffusion, convection, and adsorption by the filtering membrane. By applying the second and third mechanisms, CRRT may remove pro- and anti-inflammatory CKs [19]. There has been growing evidence throughout the course of the pandemic that suggests that many (even if not all) patients with severe COVID-19 infection have an intense cytokine storm release [20]. In these patients, multiorgan failure is possibly associated with increased levels of interleukin (IL)-2, IL-6, IL-7, IL-8, IL-10, granulocyte-colony stimulating factor (G-CSF), interferon (INF)-

gamma and since high viral titer and an intense inflammatory CK response, has been associated with higher morbidity and mortality, treatments that counteract these CKs has been a hotbed for research and clinical trials [21]. Therapies aimed at modulating the inflammatory response (e.g., INF-gamma inhibitors, corticosteroids, intravenous immunoglobulin G, TNF blockers, chloroquine) have been postulated to be beneficial in the treatment of CK release; however, they have not yet shown significant efficacy. An alternative immunomodulating strategy in the treatment of sepsis syndrome is the use of CRRT. Although its use is still controversial and large studies are needed to clarify its effectiveness, CRRT can remove inflammatory mediators, thus limiting the CK storm and, therefore, ultimately reducing the damage done to multiple organs. Villa et al. described, in an observational study, the overtime variations of clinical and biochemical features of C-19-AKI patients treated with extracorporeal blood purification with a hemodiafilter characterized by enhanced CK adsorption properties. In 37 patients, the median baseline IL-6 was 1230 pg/mL (IQR 895) and decreased overtime ($p < 0.001$ Kruskal–Wallis test) during the first 72 h of the treatment, with the most significant decrease in the first 24 h ($P = 0.001$). The reduction in serum IL-6 concentrations correlated with the improvement in organ function, as measured in the decrease of SOFA score (rho = 0.48, $P = 0.0003$). Median baseline SOFA was 13 (IQR 6) and decreased significantly overtime ($P < 0.001$) during the first 72 h of the treatment, with the most significant decrease in the first 48 h (median 8 IQR 5, $P = 0.001$). Finally, compared to the expected mortality rates, as calculated by APACHE IV, the mean observed rates were 8.3% lower after treatment [21].

18.5 Anticoagulation Strategies, Thrombogenicity and Filter Clotting

Figures 18.2 and 18.3 is a schematic representation of anticoagulation procedures during CRRT with heparin and citrate respectively, while Fig. 18.4 shows a decisional flowchart that may help the clinician in choosing a coagulation strategy. Hypercoagulability

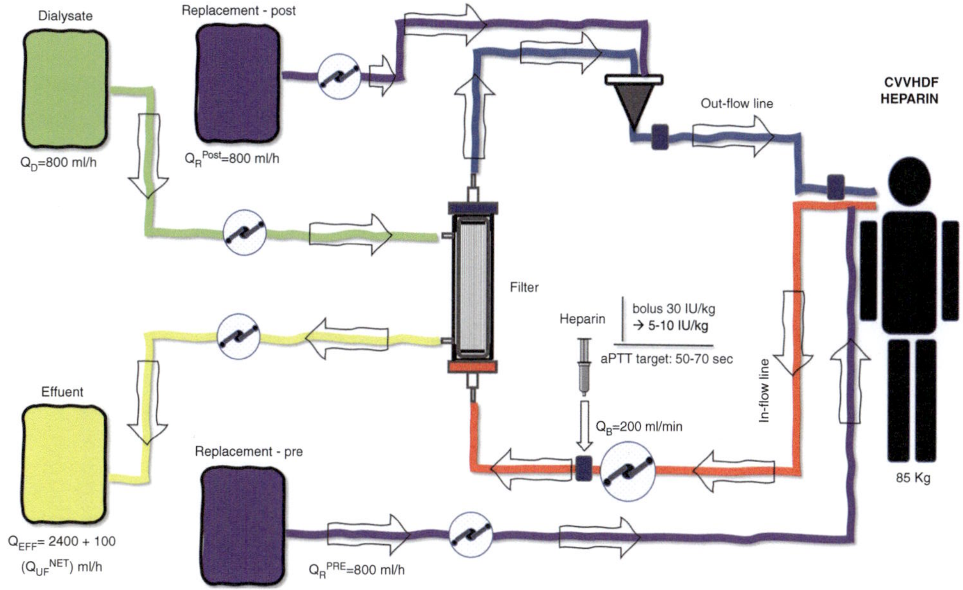

Fig. 18.2 Schematic representation of a CRRT circuit (CVVHDF) anticoagulated with heparin. *CVVHDF* continuous venovenous hemodiafiltration, Q_B blood flow, Q_D dialysate flow, Q_{EFF} effluent flow, Q_R^{POST} replacement in postdilution flow, Q_R^{PRE} replacement in predilution flow, Q_{UF}^{NET} net ultrafiltration flow

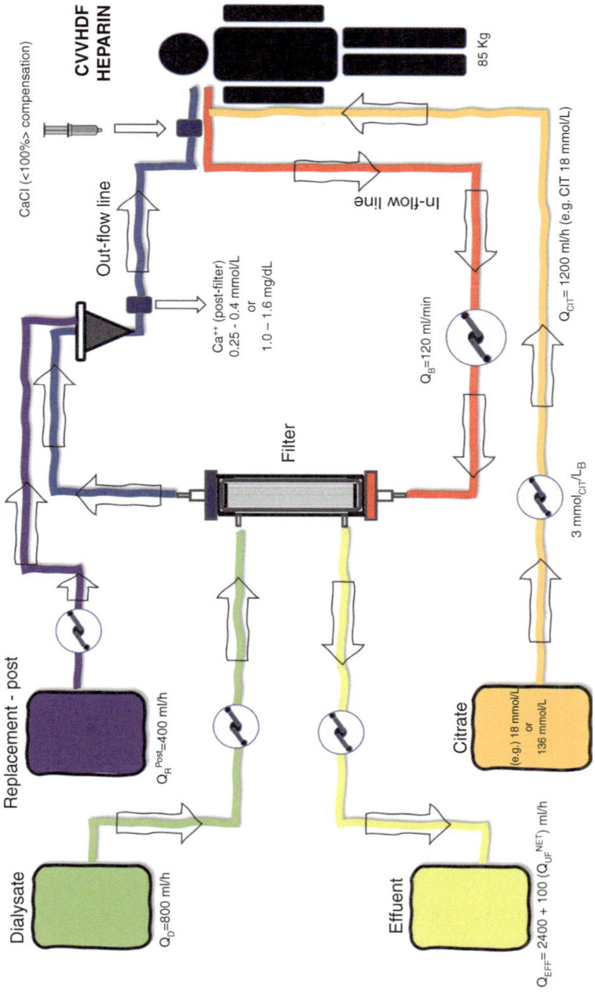

Fig. 18.3 Schematic representation of a CRRT circuit (CVVHDF) with regional citrate anticoagulation. *CVVHDF* continuous veno-venous hemodiafiltration, Q_B blood flow, *CIT* citrate, Q_{CIT} citrate flow, Q_D dialysate flow, Q_{EFF} effluent flow, Q_R^{POST} replacement in postdilution flow, Q_{UF}^{NET} net ultrafiltration flow

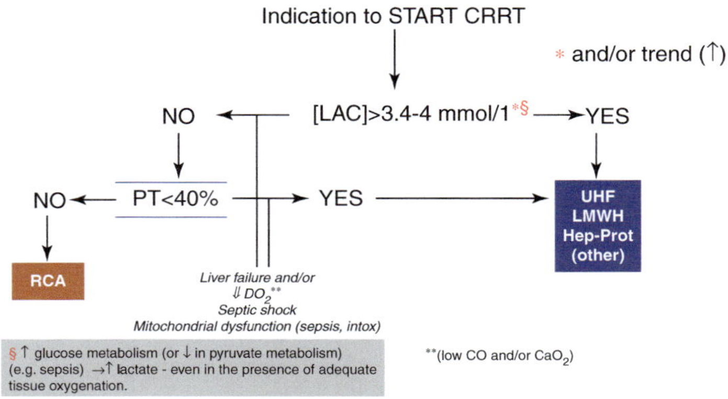

Fig. 18.4 Flowchart for anticoagulation strategy [26–28]. *CaO_2* arterial oxygen content, *CO* cardiac output, *CRRT* continuous renal replacement therapy, *DO_2* oxygen delivery, *Hep-Prot* heparin–protamine, *LAC* lactate, *LMWH* low-molecular-weight heparin, *PT* prothrombin time, *RCA* regional citrate anticoagulation, *UHF* unfractioned heparin

has been recognized as a salient feature of COVID-19 in the critically ill and due to this thrombogenicity, filter life may be shorter due to filter clotting [22]. A Dutch study specifically investigated filter life span in 22 C-19-AKI patients undergoing RRT. CVVH with regional citrate anticoagulation (RCA) was the standard treatment with filter change scheduled routinely every 72 h [23]. Alternatively, when patients received systemic anticoagulation with unfractioned heparin (UFH) for another indication, a target of aPTT of 50–70 s was maintained. Filter lifetime (53 filters) was 27 h (14–63), 35 (66%) of which were under RCA. Thirty filters (57%) failed prematurely, and the lifetime of these filters was 21 h (13–33). The authors did not find a correlation between filter life and type of anticoagulation attributing a premature filter failure to additional reasons that included inflammatory proteins, late response to alarms by the nursing staff due to personal protection equipment requirements or the decreased catheter performance due to prone positioning. Interestingly, in an American center, systemic anticoagulation was applied in all 16 ICUs, whereas RCA remained restricted to the surgical ICU, albeit with less frequent postfilter ionized calcium monitoring to reduce nurse exposure to infected patients [24]. In an observational study, this group described their experience with 502 CRRT circuits on different anticoagulation regimens in 80 patients who received CVVHD by using the NxStage System One, a portable hemodialysis system commercialized for home use in the USA. The different anticoagulation regimens were heparin (systemic UFH or low–molecular weight heparin [LMWH]) (n = 32), prefilter heparin (n = 8), argatroban (n = 2), RCA (citrate) (n = 3), citrate plus heparin (when patients received systemic heparin for medical indications) (n = 1), or no anticoagulation (none) (n = 34). Of the 502 circuits, 350 (70%) received anticoagulation, and 152 (30%) did not. Median clotting-free survival was 21 h for no anticoagulation and 25 h for anticoagulation with prefilter UFH, 40 h for citrate, 49 h for systemic UFH, 72 h for argatroban and 72 h for citrate plus heparin.

Another group described, in 65 patients, a protocol based on systemic UFH dosing by following anti-factor Xa levels (targeting 0.3–0.7 IU/mL) rather than PTT [25]. The median survival time of the first filter was very short, resulting in 6.5 [2.5, 33.5] h. A retrospective single-center study performed in the USA specifically investigated the role of anticoagulation in 52 C-19-AKI patients requiring RRT by SLED (blood flow rate 250 mL/min and standard dialysate flow rate 200 mL/min) for >8 h [25]. In this center, CVVHDF with CRRT machines was restricted to the neuro-intensive care unit and was not expanded during the pandemic due to logistics. Anticoagulation modalities included: none, RCA (22.4 mmol/h), prefilter UFH (200 U/h), minimally intensive UFH (12 U/kg/h), systemic low intensity UFH (initial bolus 60 U/kg followed by 12 U/kg/h), systemic high-intensity UFH (initial bolus 80 U/kg followed by 18 U/kg/h), and combined systemic high-intensity UFH plus RCA. The aPTT goal for heparin strategy was 39–69 s and anti-Xa 0.3–0.7 IU/mL. The changes in transmembrane pressure between the beginnings and ends of the SLED runs was investigated. The median (IQR) duration of SLED/session under each anticoagulation protocol was as follows: 4.1 h (2.5–11.3 h) without anticoagulation, 4.5 h (2.5–9.3 h) with RCA, 12.0 h (3.9–17.0 h) with prefilter UFH, 10.1 h (4.0–20.1 h) with minimally intensive UFH, 11.2 h (4.2–17.0 h) with systemic low-intensity UFH, 10.5 h (5.3–22.0 h) with systemic high-intensity UFH, and 12.3 h (7.2–24.5 h) with combined systemic high-intensity UFH plus RCA. These findings suggest that systemic heparin may be more effective than regional citrate in maintaining circuit lifes pan. Moreover, anticoagulation with pre-filter heparin and combined systemic high-intensity UFH and RCA were associated with numerically longer median duration of SLED sessions suggesting the beneficial synergistic effect of heparin and citrate.

18.6 Conclusions

AKI is a common complication among patients hospitalized with COVID-19, especially among those with more severe infections and C-19-AKI requiring RRT is associated with a particularly poor outcome. Understanding the pathophysiology of C-19-AKI is an actively evolving issue. In these critically ill patients, it is crucial to prevent and actively manage AKI and renal organ cross talk to decrease mortality. Studies comparing different RRT techniques are still running, and results aimed at selecting the most efficient are needed. To date, no data is available to compare different modalities in COVID-19 patients, and it remains an area of future research. In addition, the relationship between CK storm and tissue injury and organ failure and the potential role of extracorporeal CK clearance is still under investigation.

However, the dramatic increase in demand for RRT in the face of unprecedented hospitalization rates to accommodate the surge of patients has presented a unique challenge to the hospitals. Providing RRT both in the ICU and in hospital wards has represented an unforeseen logistic challenge that has required significant capital and human investments. The application of alternative organizational strategies was not related to any specific clinical requirement and included intermittent and hybrid techniques, allowing devices to be shared between patients. Likely due to these aspects, even if several studies have examined the incidence of AKI in hospitalized patients with COVID-19 and their outcomes, few of them have focused on RRT modalities and machine settings (anticoagulation strategies, pumps flow, solute clearance, etc.) and detailed information are rarely provided.

As an additional challenge, hypercoagulability seen in COVID-19 disease led to frequent clotting and consumption of CRRT filter-circuit packages that exceeded, again, any prevision. Even if few data are available, different strategies have been applied and the most extended filter lifespan seems RCA plus systemic UFH (for non-CRRT indications).

New and more extensive studies are needed to identify the best timing, modality, anticoagulation, and membranes in these difficult and dramatic conditions.

References

1. Gupta S, Coca SG, Chan L, Melamed ML, Brenner SK, Hayek SS, Sutherland A, Puri S, Srivastava A, Leonberg-Yoo A, Shehata AM, Flythe JE, Rashidi A, Schenck EJ, Goyal N, Hedayati SS, Dy R, Bansal A, Athavale A, Nguyen HB, Vijayan A, Charytan DM, Schulze CE, Joo MJ, Friedman AN, Zhang J, Sosa MA, Judd E, Velez JCQ, Mallappallil M, Redfern RE, Bansal AD, Neyra JA, Liu KD, Renaghan AD, Christov M, Molnar MZ, Sharma S, Kamal O, Boateng JO, Short SAP, Admon AJ, Sise ME, Wang W, Parikh CR, Leaf DE, the STOP-COVID Investigators. AKI treated with renal replacement therapy in critically ill patients with COVID-19. J Am Soc Nephrol. 2021;32(1):161–76. https://doi.org/10.1681/ASN.2020060897.
2. Nadim MK, Forni LG, Mehta RL, Connor MJ, Liu KD, Ostermann M, et al. COVID-19-associated acute kidney injury: consensus report of the 25th acute disease quality initiative (ADQI) workgroup. Nat Rev Nephrol. 2020;16:747–64.
3. Fisher R, Clarke J, Al-Arfi K, Saha R, Lioudaki E, Mehta R, Pahl C, Sharpe C, Bramham K, Hutchings S. Provision of acute renal replacement therapy, using three separate modalities, in critically ill patients during the COVID-19 pandemic. An after action review from a UK tertiary critical care centre. J Crit Care. 2021;62:190–6. https://doi.org/10.1016/j.jcrc.2020.12.023.
4. Zhang G, Hu C, Luo L, Fang F, Chen Y, Li J, Peng Z, et al. Clinical features and short-term outcomes of 221 patients with COVID-19 in Wuhan, China. J Clin Virol. 2020;127:104364.
5. Ronco C, Bagshaw SM, Bellomo R, Clark WR, Husain-Syed F, Kellum JA, et al. Extracorporeal blood purification and organ support in the critically ill patient during COVID-19 pandemic: expert review and recommendation. Blood Purif. 2021;50:17–27.

6. Li Z, Wu M, Yao J, et al. Caution on kidney dysfunctions of COVID-19 patients. medRxiv. 2020. https://doi.org/10.1101/2020.02.08.20021212.
7. Eriksson KE, Campoccia-Jalde F, Rysz S, Rimes-Stigare C. Continuous renal replacement therapy in intensive care patients with COVID-19; survival and renal recovery. J Crit Care. 2021;16(64):125–30. https://doi.org/10.1016/j.jcrc.2021.04.002.
8. Fominskiy EV, Scandroglio AM, Monti G, et al. Prevalence, characteristics, risk factors, and outcomes of invasively ventilated COVID-19 patients with acute kidney injury and renal replacement therapy. Blood Purif. 2020;50(1):102–9.
9. Russo E, Esposito P, Taramasso L, et al. Kidney disease and all-cause mortality in patients with COVID-19 hospitalized in Genoa, Northern Italy. J Nephrol. 2020;55:105924.
10. Chan L, Chaudhary K, Saha A, et al. Acute kidney injury in hospitalized patients with COVID-19. medRxiv. 2021;32(1):151–60. https://doi.org/10.1681/ASN.2020050615.
11. Yang X, Tian S, Guo H. Acute kidney injury and renal replacement therapy in COVID-19 patients: a systematic review and meta-analysis. Int Immunopharmacol. 2021;90:107159. https://doi.org/10.1016/j.intimp.2020.107159.
12. Goldfarb DS, Goldfarb DS, Benstein JA, Zhdanova O, Hammer E, Block CA, Caplin NJ, Thompson N, Charytan DM. Impending shortages of kidney replacement therapy for COVID-19 patients. Clin J Am Soc Nephrol. 2020;15(6):880–2. https://doi.org/10.2215/CJN.05180420.
13. Kidney Disease: Improving Global Outcomes (KDIGO) Acute Kidney Injury Work Group. KDIGO clinical practice guideline for acute kidney injury. Section 2: AKI definition. Kidney Int Suppl. 2012;2:19–36.
14. Tandukar S, Palevsky PM. Continuous renal replacement therapy: who, when, why, and how. Chest. 2019;155(3):626–38. https://doi.org/10.1016/j.chest.2018.09.004.
15. Akomeah J, Apostol A, Barnes E, et al. Optimizing kidney replacement therapy during the COVID-19 pandemic across a complex healthcare system. Front Med. 2020;7:892. https://doi.org/10.3389/fmed.2020.604182.
16. Stevens JS, Velez JCQ, Mohan S. Continuous renal replacement therapy and the COVID pandemic. Semin Dial. 2021;34(6):561–6. https://doi.org/10.1111/sdi.12962.
17. Burke E, Haber E, Pike CW, Sonti R. Outcomes of renal replacement therapy in the critically ill with COVID-19. Med Intensiva. 2021;45(6):325–31. https://doi.org/10.1016/j.medin.2021.02.004.
18. Fraser DD, Cepinskas G, Slessarev M, Martin C, Daley M, Miller MR, O'Gorman DB, Gill SE, Patterson EK, Dos Santos CC. Inflammation profiling of critically ill coronavirus disease 2019 patients. Crit Care Explor. 2020;2(6):e0144. https://doi.org/10.1097/CCE.0000000000000144.
19. Ronco C, Tetta C, Mariano F, et al. Interpreting the mechanisms of continuous renal replacement therapy in sepsis: the peak concentration

hypothesis. Artif Organs. 2003;27:792–801. https://doi.org/10.1046/j.1525-1594.2003.07289.x.
20. Zhu N, Zhang D, Wang W, et al. A novel coronavirus from patients with pneumonia in China, 2019. N Engl J Med. 2020;382:727–33. https://doi.org/10.1056/NEJMoa2001017.
21. Villa G, Romagnoli S, De Rosa S, Greco M, Resta M, Montin DP, Prato F, Patera F, Ferrari F, Rotondo G, Ronco C. Blood purification therapy with a hemodiafilter featuring enhanced adsorptive properties for cytokine removal in patients presenting COVID-19: a pilot study. Crit Care. 2020;24:605. https://doi.org/10.1186/s13054-020-03322-6.
22. Spiezia L, Boscolo A, Poletto F, et al. COVID-19-related severe hypercoagulability in patients admitted to intensive care unit for acute respiratory failure. Thromb Haemost. 2020;120(06):998–1000. https://doi.org/10.1055/s-0040-1710018.
23. Wilbers TJ, Koning MV. Renal replacement therapy in critically ill patients with COVID-19: a retrospective study investigating mortality, renal recovery and filter lifetime. J Crit Care. 2020;60:103–5. https://doi.org/10.1016/j.jcrc.2020.07.025.
24. Shankaranarayanan D, Muthukumar T, Barbar T, Bhasin A, Gerardine S, Lamba P, Leuprecht L, Neupane SP, Salinas T, Shimonov D, Varma E, Liu F. Anticoagulation strategies and filter life in COVID-19 patients receiving continuous renal replacement therapy: a single-center experience. Clin J Am Soc Nephrol. 2020;16(1):124–6. https://doi.org/10.2215/CJN.08430520.
25. Endres P, Rosovsky R, Zhao S, et al. Filter clotting with continuous renal replacement therapy in COVID-19. J Thromb Thrombolysis. 2020;51(4):966–70. https://doi.org/10.1007/s11239-020-02301-6.
26. Bianchi NA, Altarelli M, Eckert P, Schneider AG. Complications of regional citrate anticoagulation for continuous renal replacement therapy: an observational study. Blood Purif. 2020;49(5):567–75. https://doi.org/10.1159/000506253.
27. Schneider AG, Journois D, Rimmelé T. Complications of regional citrate anticoagulation: accumulation or overload? Crit Care. 2017;21:281.
28. Zhang W, Bai M, Yu Y, Li L, Zhao L, Sun S, Chen X. Safety and efficacy of regional citrate anticoagulation for continuous renal replacement therapy in liver failure patients: a systematic review and meta-analysis. Crit Care. 2019;23(1):22. https://doi.org/10.1186/s13054-019-2317-9.

Part VI

Haemostasis and Coagulation in COVID-19

Pathophysiology of Coagulopathy in COVID-19

19

Michael Mazzeffi and Jonathan Chow

19.1 Introduction

Severe acute respiratory syndrome coronavirus-2 (SARS-CoV-2) infection is now well established to cause a myriad of coagulation changes. Specifically, SARS-CoV-2 disrupts normal endothelial cell function leading to endotheliosis. The fibrinolytic system is activated, and in cases of severe disease, becomes exhausted leading to hypercoagulability and macro and microthrombosis. In this chapter, we review the mechanisms of coronavirus diasease-2019 (COVID-19) related coagulopathy.

19.2 Link Between Acute Inflammation and Coagulation Activation in Viral Infection

The acute inflammatory response to viral infection is intended to clear virus from the body and heal injured cells. Viruses can cause direct cellular damage, but excessive host immune response also contributes. Multiple cells respond to viral infection through pattern

M. Mazzeffi (✉) · J. Chow
Department of Anesthesiology and Critical Care Medicine, George Washington University School of Medicine and Health Sciences, Washington, DC, USA

D. Battaglini, P. Pelosi (eds.), *COVID-19 Critical and Intensive Care Medicine Essentials*, https://doi.org/10.1007/978-3-030-94992-1_19

recognition receptors (PRRs) [1]. PRRs on cell surfaces or in endosomes recognize pathogen associated molecular patterns (PAMPs) [1]. Toll-like receptors (TLRs) are an important part of the innate immune response to viral infection. TLR-4 binds to the SARS-CoV-2 S protein [2]. Both interleukin-6 (IL-6) and tumor necrosis factor-α (TNF-α) are produced downstream from TLR-4, leading to activation of other immune cells. Cell surface activation of TLRs 1, 4, and 6 increases pro-inflammatory cytokine production and endosomal activation increases interferon production [3]. Type I interferons activate dendritic cells, monocytes, and lymphocytes (B cells, T cells, and natural killer cells). Infected respiratory epithelial cells secrete chemokines which recruit neutrophils and lymphocytes to the lung [1]. Some respiratory viruses, including SARS-CoV-2, also infect endothelial cells. Respiratory viruses that infect endothelial cells, including Hantavirus and respiratory syncytial virus (RSV), cause more severe lung injury, extensive pulmonary edema, and in some cases coagulation derangements [1]. Activation of the lectin and classical complement pathways by SARS-CoV-2 leads to platelet activation and von Willebrand factor (VWF) release, which creates a prothrombotic state [4].

Pro-inflammatory cytokines including IL-1, IL-6, IL-12, and TNF-α, activate the coagulation system by enhancing tissue factor expression on endothelial cells and monocytes [5–7]. Pro-inflammatory cytokines increase the release of VWF from endothelial cells, which increases platelet adhesion to collagen [6]. Activation of protein C decreases because of reduced thrombomodulin expression on endothelial cells [8, 9]. Plasminogen activator inhibitor-1 (PAI-1) is upregulated, which reduces fibrinolysis and propagates a procoagulant state in some viral infections [10]. Table 19.1 summarizes important coagulation changes that contribute to a prothrombotic state in severe COVID-19.

19.3 Critical Role of Endothelial Cell Infection in COVID-19

Multiple studies have demonstrated that SARS-CoV-2 infects endothelial cells. The angiotensin converting enzyme 2 (ACE2) receptor is widely expressed on endothelial surfaces, and this is

Table 19.1 Mechanisms of coagulopathy in severe COVID-19

Factor	Normal function	Change in COVID-19
Endothelium	– Expresses thrombomodulin and heparin-like molecules on surface – Minimal tissue factor expressed under normal conditions – Releases prostacyclin to maintain normal vascular homeostasis	– Surface thrombomodulin is reduced – Surface tissue factor is increased – Prostacyclin synthesis is reduced
Fibrinogen	– Substrate for thrombin – Creates fibrin mesh which leads to secondary hemostasis	– Fibrinogen concentration increased in response to IL-6
Factor VIII	– Stored in endothelium, circulates bound to VWF – Participates in intrinsic tenase complex – Helps bring factor IXa into contact with factor X cleavage site	– Activity is increased to 300–400% in severe disease
von Willebrand factor	– Binds platelets to collagen at an injury site	– Increased release of VWF from endothelium and reduced ADAMTS13 activity, which leads to "TTP like" syndrome in some patients

(continued)

Table 19.1 (continued)

Factor	Normal function	Change in COVID-19
Plasminogen activator inhibitor-1 (PAI-1)	– Inhibits conversion of plasminogen to plasmin	– PAI-1 levels increase compared to controls, which leads to impaired fibrinolysis or fibrinolysis shutdown
Antithrombin	– Counteracts effects of thrombin (factor IIa) and factor Xa	– In cases of severe disease antithrombin becomes exhausted in the setting of excessive thrombin generation
Protein C	– When activated cleaves factors Va and VIIIa	– In cases of severe disease where factor VIII is extremely elevated becomes exhausted, also has reduced activation because of thrombomodulin deficiency

ADAMTS13 a disintegrin and metalloproteinase with a thrombospondin-like *motif* member 13, *IL* interleukin, *TTP* thrombotic thrombocytopenic purpura, *VWF* von Willebrand factor

the receptor by which SARS-CoV-2 gains cell entry [11, 12]. Some authors have suggested that above all else, COVID-19 is primarily an endothelial cell disease [13]. Endothelial cells have a critical role in normal vascular homeostasis, maintaining vascular integrity and the normal procoagulant–anticoagulant balance. Under resting conditions, endothelial cells promote vasodilation, fibrinolysis, and anticoagulation, and have anti-oxidant properties [13]. Expression of thrombomodulin and heparin-like molecules along with release of prostacyclin prevents coagulation in circulating blood. When endothelial cells are infected by SARS-CoV-2, their barrier function becomes impaired, and they propagate coagulation through increased tissue factor expression, reduced thrombomodulin expression, and increased release of PAI-1 [14, 15]. These changes contribute to microvascular and macrovascular thrombosis in the pulmonary vasculature and in other organs.

19.4 Release of Extracellular Vesicle Tissue Factor, Procoagulant Enzymes, and Fibrinogen

In a cohort of 100 patients with COVID-19, extracellular vesicle tissue factor levels were two to three times higher than in controls [16]. In this study, extracellular vesicle tissue factor levels were also strongly associated with mortality [16]. The authors speculated that the source of extracellular vesicle tissue factor was monocytes, endothelial cells, and perhaps perivascular cells. Elevated tissue factor levels were correlated with reduced antithrombin activity, reduced factor II activity, reduced a disintegrin and metalloproteinase with a thrombospondin type I motif, member 13 (ADAMTS13) activity, and increased VWF antigen levels [16].

Patients with COVID-19 have severely increased factor VIII activity and plasma fibrinogen concentration. Factor VIII is released from endothelial cells during inflammation, and in patients with severe COVID-19, factor VIII activity can increase up to 300–400% [17]. Fibrinogen is synthesized in hepatocytes at a rate of around 2–5 g per day and is released during inflammation. Fibrinogen's release is mainly regulated by IL-6, which is capable of increasing plasma fibrinogen concentration tenfold [18].

19.5 Excess Thrombin Generation

High levels of expressed tissue factor on endothelial cells and monocytes, as well as increased circulating tissue factor increases thrombin generation. In a cohort study of 20 COVID-19 patients with acute respiratory distress syndrome (ARDS), the authors found increased markers of thrombin activity (e.g., prothrombin fragments 1 + 2) [19]. Furthermore, the authors found that markers of thrombin activity continued to rise over time in non-survivors, while they decreased in survivors [19].

In a second study that compared 46 COVID-19 patients with 53 septic patients, the authors found that endogenous thrombin potential and peak thrombin generation were increased in COVID-19 patients compared to septic patients and healthy controls [20].

19.6 Depletion of Endogenous Anticoagulants

Figure 19.1 shows the important role that anticoagulants have in reversing the prothrombotic changes that occur in ARDS. Patients with severe COVID-19 have low-normal or reduced endogenous anticoagulant activity including antithrombin and protein C [17]. In a study of 49 hospitalized patients with COVD-19, antithrombin levels were significantly lower in non-survivors, when compared to survivors (72% vs. 95%, $p = 0.001$) [21]. A second study of 102 hospitalized patients with COVID-19 found lower antithrombin levels were associated with increased mortality [22]. In many cases, antithrombin levels are initially normal, but decrease as disease severity progresses and endogenous anticoagulants are depleted. A small retrospective study suggested that treatment with fresh frozen plasma restores antithrombin activity and may improve outcome [23].

Protein C is activated by thrombin–thrombomodulin complex and cleaves both factor V and factor VIII. Cleavage of factor V leads to a significant decrease in thrombin generation, as factor V massively augments thrombin generation by bringing factor Xa into close proximity with prothrombin's cleavage site in the prothrombinase complex. In patients with severe COVID-19, protein C activity is low normal or decreased [17]. Protein S, which is a cofactor for protein C, may also have decreased activity in patients with severe COVID-19, but data is relatively sparse [24]. Activated protein C could present an interesting therapeutic option for COVID-19 patients with hypercoagulability, but it was withdrawn from the market by its manufacturer due to multiple randomized controlled studies showing a lack of efficacy in patients with bacterial sepsis [25].

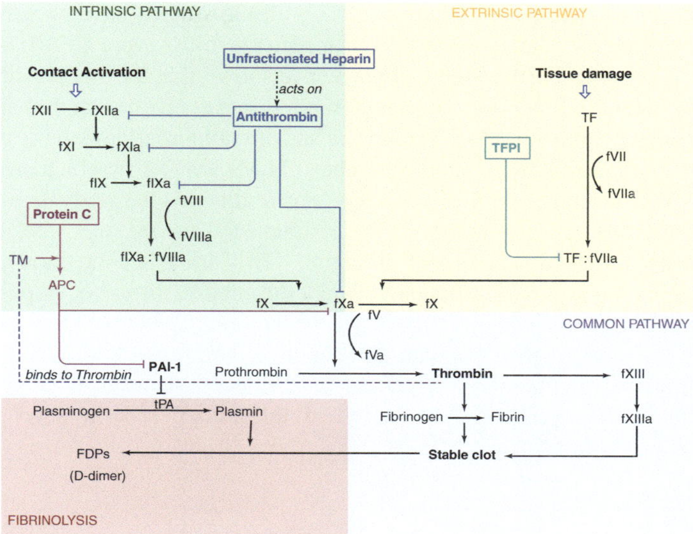

Fig. 19.1 Activation of coagulation pathways and the effects of common anticoagulants in acute respiratory distress syndrome. *F(number)a* factor, "a" indicates active, *TF* tissue factor, *TFPI* tissue factor pathway inhibitor, *FDP* fibrinogen degradation product, *tPA* tissue plasminogen activator, *PAI-1* plasminogen activator inhibitor 1, *TM* thrombomodulin, *APC* activated protein C. The activation of the extrinsic pathway (yellow) occurs due to tissue damage, while the activation of the intrinsic pathway (green) occurs with contact activation. Both of these lead to the common coagulation pathway (purple) and ultimately the fibrinolytic pathway (red). It can be seen that unfractionated heparin acts on antithrombin to inhibit coagulation factors XII, XI, IX, and X. Thrombomodulin is essential for the activation of protein C, and the subsequent inhibition of PAI-1. Finally TFPI inhibits the TF–fVIIa complex to halt coagulation

19.7 Role of VWF

VWF circulates in plasma and is stored in Weibel Palade bodies within endothelial cells. VWF can be thought of as the adhesive that helps platelets bind to exposed collagen at an injury site. During inflammatory states, including viral infection, stored VWF is released from endothelial cells. Multiple studies have shown elevated circulating VWF levels in patients with severe COVID-19 [26–29]. Further, these studies have shown that the amount of circulating VWF is associated with disease severity and that patients with reduced disintegrin and metalloproteinase with a thrombospondin like motif, member 13 (ADAMTS13), which is a VWF cleaving enzyme, have more severe illness. One study demonstrated that elevated VWF levels persisted for up to 3 weeks after initial SARS-CoV-2 infection [26]. In a second study, approximately 18% of patients had a thrombotic thrombocytopenic purpura (TTP) like disease where the ratio of ADAMTS13 to VWF antigen was less than 10 [28]. Together, these studies suggest that increased VWF release and reduced cleavage of large multimers contributes to increased thrombotic risk in severe COVID-19.

19.8 Increased Tissue Megakaryocytes and Increased Platelet Reactivity

Megakaryocytes are myeloid cells that reside primarily in the bone marrow. Each megakaryocyte is capable of producing thousands of individual platelets [30]. Autopsy studies of COVID-19 patients have shown increased numbers of pulmonary megakaryocytes, which suggests increased platelet production in patients with severe COVID-19 [31]. Platelets also appear to be more reactive in patients with severe COVID-19. Specifically, there is increased platelet degranulation and increased aggregation in response to thrombin and other agonists. Platelets from patients with severe COVID-19 also adhere to collagen more efficiently under shear, perhaps because of increased VWF levels [32–34].

19.9 Progressively Impaired Fibrinolysis

Activation of the fibrinolytic system occurs when tissue plasminogen activator (TPA) is released from endothelial cells. TPA converts fibrin bound plasminogen to plasmin. Plasmin cleaves fibrin in multiple locations (up to 34 distinct sites), which creates fibrin degradation products (FDPs) [35]. Urokinase converts plasminogen to plasmin, but has a smaller overall role in fibrinolysis. Patients with severe COVID-19 have elevated levels of TPA, PAI-1, and plasmin–antiplasmin complexes indicating that there is extensive activation of the fibrinolytic system, as SARS-CoV-2 infection progresses. Increased TPA and PAI-1 levels are associated with worse lung injury and mortality [14].

D-Dimer is formed when cross-linked fibrin is cleaved by plasmin. Multiple studies of patients with severe COVID-19 have shown that D-dimer elevation is associated with increased morbidity and mortality [36–39]. Interestingly, although D-dimer elevation is common in critically ill patients with COVID-19, significant fibrinolysis is not commonly observed on viscoelastic coagulation testing [40]. This suggests that fibrinolysis and D-dimer formation occurs mostly in the peripheral tissues and that systemic fibrinolysis is uncommon, even in patients with severe disease [41].

In the most severe cases of COVID-19, fibrinolysis becomes impaired. For example, in one study of 20 critically ill patients who had viscoelastic coagulation testing performed with the ClotPro device, patients had a prolonged lysis time on TPA test when compared to healthy controls [42]. In another study of 25 patients who had rotational thromboelastometry performed, 44% met criteria for fibrinolysis shutdown (maximum lysis <3.5%), with 73% of patients who had venous thromboembolism having fibrinolysis shutdown.

In summary, it appears that activation of the fibrinolytic system occurs early in COVID-19 and helps to compensate for excess thrombin generation and microthrombi formation. In patients who progress to severe disease, the fibrinolytic system becomes impaired and cannot keep pace with excess fibrin formation.

References

1. Newton AH, Cardani A, Braciale TJ. The host immune response in respiratory virus infection: balancing virus clearance and immunopathology. Semin Immunopathol. 2016;38:471–82.

2. Brandao SCS, Ramos JOX, Dompieri LT, et al. Is toll-like receptor 4 involved in the severity of COVID-19 pathology in patients with cardio-metabolic comorbidities? Cytokine Growth Factor Rev. 2020;58:102–10.
3. Oganesyan G, Saha SK, Guo B, et al. Critical role of TRAF3 in the toll-like receptor-dependent and -independent antiviral response. Nature. 2006;439:208–11.
4. Vinayagam S, Sattu K. SARS-CoV-2 and coagulation disorders in different organs. Life Sci. 2020;260:118431.
5. Petaja J. Inflammation and coagulation. An overview. Thromb Res. 2011;127(Suppl 2):S34–7.
6. Goeijenbier M, van Wissen M, van de Weg C, et al. Review: viral infections and mechanisms of thrombosis and bleeding. J Med Virol. 2012;84:1680–96.
7. Antoniak S, Mackman N. Multiple roles of the coagulation protease cascade during virus infection. Blood. 2014;123:2605–13.
8. Keller TT, van der Sluijs KF, de Kruif MD, et al. Effects on coagulation and fibrinolysis induced by influenza in mice with a reduced capacity to generate activated protein C and a deficiency in plasminogen activator inhibitor type 1. Circ Res. 2006;99:1261–9.
9. Key NS, Vercellotti GM, Winkelmann JC, et al. Infection of vascular endothelial cells with herpes simplex virus enhances tissue factor activity and reduces thrombomodulin expression. Proc Natl Acad Sci U S A. 1990;87:7095–9.
10. Shyu HW, Lin YY, Chen LC, et al. The dengue virus envelope protein induced PAI-1 gene expression via MEK/ERK pathways. Thromb Haemost. 2010;104:1219–27.
11. Ackermann M, Verleden SE, Kuehnel M, et al. Pulmonary vascular endothelialitis, thrombosis, and angiogenesis in Covid-19. N Engl J Med. 2020;383(2):120–8.
12. Varga Z, Flammer AJ, Steiger P, et al. Endothelial cell infection and endotheliitis in COVID-19. Lancet. 2020;395(10234):1417–8.
13. Libby P, Luscher T. COVID-19 is, in the end, an endothelial disease. Eur Heart J. 2020;41:3038–44.
14. Zuo Y, Warnock M, Harbaugh A, et al. Plasma tissue plasminogen activator and plasminogen activator inhibitor-1 in hospitalized COVID-19 patients. Sci Rep. 2021;11:1580.
15. Goshua G, Pine AB, Meizlish ML, et al. Endotheliopathy in COVID-19-associated coagulopathy: evidence from a single-centre, cross-sectional study. Lancet Haematol. 2020;7:e575–82.
16. Rosell A, Havervall S, von Meijenfeldt F, et al. Patients with COVID-19 have elevated levels of circulating extracellular vesicle tissue factor activity that is associated with severity and mortality. Arterioscler Thromb Vasc Biol. 2020;41(2):878–82.
17. Tabatabai A, Rabin J, Menaker J, et al. Factor VIII and functional protein C activity in critically ill patients with coronavirus disease 2019: a case series. A&A Pract. 2020;14:e01236.

18. Carty CL, Heagerty P, Heckbert SR, et al. Interaction between fibrinogen and IL-6 genetic variants and associations with cardiovascular disease risk in the cardiovascular health study. Ann Hum Genet. 2010;74:1–10.
19. Ranucci M, Sitzia C, Baryshnikova E, et al. Covid-19-associated coagulopathy: biomarkers of thrombin generation and fibrinolysis leading the outcome. J Clin Med. 2020;9:3487.
20. Bouck EG, Denorme F, Holle LA, et al. COVID-19 and sepsis are associated with different abnormalities in plasma procoagulant and fibrinolytic activity. Arterioscler Thromb Vasc Biol. 2021;41:401–14.
21. Gazzaruso C, Paolozzi E, Valenti C, et al. Association between antithrombin and mortality in patients with COVID-19. A possible link with obesity. Nutr Metab Cardiovasc Dis. 2020;30:1914–9.
22. von Meijenfeldt FA, Havervall S, Adelmeijer J, et al. Prothrombotic changes in patients with COVID-19 are associated with disease severity and mortality. Res Pract Thromb Haemost. 2021;5:132–41.
23. Anakli I, Ergin Ozcan P, Polat O, et al. Prognostic value of antithrombin levels in COVID-19 patients and impact of fresh frozen plasma treatment: a retrospective study. Turk J Haematol. 2021;38:15–21.
24. Lemke G, Silverman GJ. Blood clots and TAM receptor signalling in COVID-19 pathogenesis. Nat Rev Immunol. 2020;20:395–6.
25. Zhang Z. The efficacy of activated protein C for the treatment of sepsis: incorporating observational evidence with a Bayesian approach. BMJ Open. 2015;5:e006524.
26. Ward SE, Curley GF, Lavin M, et al. Von Willebrand factor propeptide in severe coronavirus disease 2019 (COVID-19): evidence of acute and sustained endothelial cell activation. Br J Haematol. 2020;192(4):714–9.
27. Mancini I, Baronciani L, Artoni A, et al. The ADAMTS13-von Willebrand factor axis in COVID-19 patients. J Thromb Haemost. 2020;19(2):513–21.
28. Doevelaar AAN, Bachmann M, Holzer B, et al. von Willebrand factor multimer formation contributes to immunothrombosis in coronavirus disease 2019. Crit Care Med. 2021;49(5):e512–20.
29. Philippe A, Chocron R, Gendron N, et al. Circulating Von Willebrand factor and high molecular weight multimers as markers of endothelial injury predict COVID-19 in-hospital mortality. Angiogenesis. 2021;24(3):505–17.
30. Patel SR, Hartwig JH, Italiano JE Jr. The biogenesis of platelets from megakaryocyte proplatelets. J Clin Investig. 2005;115:3348–54.
31. Valdivia-Mazeyra MF, Salas C, Nieves-Alonso JM, et al. Increased number of pulmonary megakaryocytes in COVID-19 patients with diffuse alveolar damage: an autopsy study with clinical correlation and review of the literature. Virchows Arch. 2020;478(3):487–96.
32. Zaid Y, Guessous F, Puhm F, et al. Platelet reactivity to thrombin differs between patients with COVID-19 and those with ARDS unrelated to COVID-19. Blood Adv. 2021;5:635–9.

33. Manne BK, Denorme F, Middleton EA, et al. Platelet gene expression and function in patients with COVID-19. Blood. 2020;136:1317–29.
34. Hottz ED, Azevedo-Quintanilha IG, Palhinha L, et al. Platelet activation and platelet-monocyte aggregate formation trigger tissue factor expression in patients with severe COVID-19. Blood. 2020;136:1330–41.
35. Hudson NE. Biophysical mechanisms mediating fibrin fiber lysis. Biomed Res Int. 2017;2017:2748340.
36. Zhang L, Yan X, Fan Q, et al. D-Dimer levels on admission to predict in-hospital mortality in patients with Covid-19. J Thromb Haemost. 2020;18:1324–9.
37. Artifoni M, Danic G, Gautier G, et al. Systematic assessment of venous thromboembolism in COVID-19 patients receiving thromboprophylaxis: incidence and role of D-dimer as predictive factors. J Thromb Thrombolysis. 2020;50:211–6.
38. Yao Y, Cao J, Wang Q, et al. D-Dimer as a biomarker for disease severity and mortality in COVID-19 patients: a case control study. J Intensive Care. 2020;8:49.
39. Berger JS, Kunichoff D, Adhikari S, et al. Prevalence and outcomes of D-dimer elevation in hospitalized patients with COVID-19. Arterioscler Thromb Vasc Biol. 2020;40:2539–47.
40. Madathil RJ, Tabatabai A, Rabin J, et al. Thromboelastometry and D-dimer elevation in Coronavirus-2019. J Cardiothorac Vasc Anesth. 2020;34(12):3495–6.
41. Panigada M, Meli A, Scotti E, et al. Viscoelastic coagulation monitor as a novel device to assess coagulation at the bedside. A single-center experience during the COVID-19 pandemic. ASAIO J. 2021;67:254–62.
42. Bachler M, Bosch J, Sturzel DP, et al. Impaired fibrinolysis in critically ill COVID-19 patients. Br J Anaesth. 2021;126:590–8.

20 Coagulation Disorders and Management

Mauro Panigada, Andrea Meli
and Heidi J. Dalton

20.1 Coagulation Disorders

Since the very first reports, SARS-COV2 has been associated with an increased concentration of inflammatory mediators [1]. High concentrations of blood D-dimer and fibrinogen has progressively become the hallmark of this syndrome, especially in severe presentations, and are associated with an overall increased risk of venous thrombosis and thromboembolism [2].

M. Panigada (✉)
Department of Anesthesia and Intensive Care, Fondazione IRCCS Ca' Granda Ospedale Maggiore Policlinico, Milan, Italy

A. Meli
Department of Anesthesiology, Intensive Care and Emergency, Fondazione IRCCS Ca' Granda Ospedale Maggiore Policlinico, Milan, Italy

H. J. Dalton
Department of Pediatrics INOVA Heart and Vascular Institute Falls Church, VA, USA

D. Battaglini, P. Pelosi (eds.), *COVID-19 Critical and Intensive Care Medicine Essentials*, https://doi.org/10.1007/978-3-030-94992-1_20

20.1.1 D-Dimer, Fibrinogen, and Standard Coagulation Tests

As mentioned, alteration of coagulation profiles in COVID-19 patients has been recognized since the very beginning of the pandemic; though, its pathophysiological substrate and clinical translation are still unclear [3]. The high incidence of venous thrombosis—both systemic and pulmonary—has been mainly ascribed to the increased inflammation triggered by SARS-COV2, which can result in the failure of macro- and microcirculation in affected regions (i.e., pulmonary circulation) [4]. The appraisal of laboratory test modifications has been the first step towards the understanding of this syndrome from a coagulative perspective.

In the seminal report by Guan et al. on 1099 patients diagnosticated with COVID-19, D-dimer >0.5 mg/mL was reported in 46.4% of studied patients, while the percentage increased to 59.6% in severe cases [1]. Of note, fibrinogen level was not described in this study, while platelets level seemed to show a mild decrease in severe patients, yet remaining within normal limits. More recently, Al-Samkari et al. retrospectively studied a cohort of 400 COVID-19 patients, of which 144 were critically ill, looking for risk factors associated with thrombosis and bleeding during the hospital stay [2]. In their study, a D-dimer level of >2500 ng/mL yielded a strong increase in the risk for venous thromboembolism, critical illness, and death (adjusted odds ratio [OR] 6.79 [95% CI 2.39–19.30]). Venous thromboembolism was radiographically detected in 4.8% of patients. In addition, the overall thrombotic complication rate was as high as 9.5%. Of note, the latter could be an underestimation of deep vein thrombosis and pulmonary embolism occurrence in this population as only patients with symptoms may get imaging. A report from Suh et al. detected an incidence of 14.8% for deep vein thrombosis and 16.5% for pulmonary embolism in a pooled population of 3342 COVID-19 hospitalized patients [5]. Again, platelet count did not seem to play a role in thrombotic risk; [2] on the other hand, a reduction in platelet count yielded increased risk for bleeding events. Finally, fibrinogen concentration was greatly increased in the subjects who developed thrombotic complications. Curiously, fibrinogen concentration was high (at least 486 [312–712] mg/dL) even in those subjects who showed bleeding events (2.3%).

The vast alteration of coagulation profiles was suspicious for a possible increase in the incidence of disseminated intravascular coagulation (DIC) [6], as diagnosed with shared criteria [7], due to the observed prolongation of prothrombin time (PT) and activated partial thromboplastin time (aPTT) coupled to the increase of D-dimer and fibrin degradation products in nonsurvivors. Yet, the increase in D-dimer results are disproportional with respect to the other markers of coagulation, and the DIC-score in most patient does not indicate overt DIC, despite D-dimer derangement [8]. Thus, DIC seems to be of lesser importance in the majority of COVID-19 population.

Finally, alteration of PT and aPTT has been described in COVID-19 patients. In a recent review by Xiang et al. [9], prolongation of PT was observed in severe cases, and this was associated with increased D-dimer and fibrinogen, while aPTT did not vary among severe and nonsevere COVID-19 subjects. Of note, this review reported that progressive prolongation of PT during hospital stay (together with gradual increase of D-dimers and fibrinogen, as markers of overall increased coagulation disfunction) accounted for augmented in-hospital mortality. On the other hand, prolongation of aPTT was associated with positive lupus anticoagulant test in 31/35 COVID-19 patients (91%) presenting with prolonged aPTT [10], once again propagating the risk for venous thromboembolism.

20.1.2 Viscoelastic Tests

Besides standard coagulation tests, viscoelastic monitoring was employed for a further understanding of the coagulation profile and its derangement during COVID-19. The viscoelastic reflection of increased blood fibrinogen is widely represented by a strong increase in maximum amplitude (MA) at TEG [11], maximum clot formation (MCF) at ROTEM (18), and clot strength (CS) with Quantra System [12] in COVID-19 subjects with respect of normal controls. C-reactive protein (CRP) and interleukin-6 elevation were linked to this viscoelastic pattern, as to underline the connection among inflammation and thrombogenic drift. While clot formation time (expressed as Reaction time at TEG or Clotting Time at ROTEM) was found to be normal or only slightly reduced in most samples—relegating a lesser role to coagulation factors in the prothrombotic picture of this syndrome, despite an increase in FVIII and von Willebrand factor concentration [11]—much of the attention is focused on fibrinolysis. Indeed, the simultaneous presence of elevated D-dimer and impaired fibrinolysis, or the so-called fibrinolysis shutdown (defined as a LY30 at TEG <0.8% or EXTEM maximum lysis of <3.5%) [13], has been reported recently, picturing a situation in which the endogenous inhibition of the fibrinolytic system is enhanced and conduces to poor clot lysis [14, 15]. This aspect is in contrast with the prevalence of high D-dimer concentration at admission and during the hospital stay of COVID-19 subjects, questioning the origin of the elevated D-dimer amount in the blood. Hypothetically, these D-dimers might be created in the lung from other sites than the peripheral circulation, such as in the alveoli, from a bronchoalveolar specific clot breakdown which might not be detected in the peripheral blood by viscoelastic tests [16]. Impaired fibrinolysis at viscoelastic tests in turn has been linked to an even more increased risk of venous thromboembolism, pulmonary embolism and need for renal replacement therapy in COVID-19 patients [17], thus playing a central role in patient prognosis.

The SARS-COV2 infection enhances the risk for venous thromboembolic events, especially in hospitalized and critically ill patients. Concerning the last two categories of subjects, prophylaxis for Venous Thromboembolism has been extensively applied in hospital wards to reduce thrombotic events. Yet endogenous inhibition of the fibrinolytic system may play a role in perpetuating the thrombotic tendency of COVID-19 patients. This complex picture concerning the coagulation profile of COVID-19 subjects has therefore deep implications in patient management and therapy.

20.2 Management

As discussed in the previous section, the clinical counterpart of COVID-19 coagulation disorders is thrombosis. When accounting for all thrombotic episodes (including also ischemic stroke, myocardial infarction, and systemic arterial embolism) the cumulative incidence raised up to 49% [18]. A later meta-analysis resized those data, estimating the pooled incidence of thrombotic events at 17.0% and at 7.1% for pulmonary embolism alone [19]. An important issue that emerged was that the rate of thrombosis appeared to be higher in more severe patients requiring critical care compared to those on the ward [20]. This propensity for thrombosis in COVID-19 alarmed the health care community, since it was much superior to what was previously described (e.g., 5–15% as in previous trials assessing the efficacy and safety of thromboprophylaxis) [21–23].

The pathogenic mechanism behind this hypercoagulable tendency is at present far from being elucidated. Yet it is supposed that inflammation and hypoxia following SARS-CoV-2 pneumonia favors microvascular thrombosis, which in turn causes the organ injury that we observe in clinical practice.

Heparin is the most commonly used anticoagulant drug in critical care and the available evidence [24] currently recommends thromboprophylaxis to all acutely ill patients requiring hospitalization. In COVID-19, high fibrinogen levels can lead to heparin resistance, thereby reducing the efficacy of standard thromboembolic prophylaxis [25]. Moreover, heparin may add further benefit because it shows antiviral and anti-inflammatory properties [26, 27]. Based on the pathophysiological rationale, clinical practice, and all the aforementioned reasons, many clinicians advocated the administration of higher doses of heparin (up to full anticoagulation) to counter COVID-19 thrombogenic tendency [28].

The benefits of heparin were soon reported in the pivotal study by Tang et al. [29] and later supported by many observational studies that suggested that anticoagulation beyond standard prophylactic doses was promising [30–32]. However, some of the first observational studies methodologically failed to deal with immortal time bias and were confounded by indication. Interestingly, in a retrospective analysis on more than 4000 patients, the hazards of in-hospital mortality or intubation was not different for therapeutic versus prophylactic heparin after restricting the analysis to those in whom anticoagulation was initiated within 48 h of admission [33], contradicting previous results.

Of note, increasing the dose of heparin in COVID-19 was generally reported to be safe [19, 33], with an occurrence of major bleeding similar to previous estimates of bleeding in non-COVID critically ill patients [34]. However, this is still debated. In fact, in a retrospective cohort study which compared COVID-19 patients with a matched cohort of patients with other respiratory viral illnesses, therapeutic anticoagulation on ICU admission was associated with a greater risk of major bleeding compared with standard thromboprophylaxis [35].

The uncertainty around optimal prophylactic anticoagulation regimen has translated into variability in expert recommendations, as reflected by several inconsistencies between international societies recommendations. Indeed, while thromboprophylaxis alone was often suggested, higher doses of heparin were indicated elsewhere; and last, heparin titration according to risk stratification (e.g., severity of the disease or D-dimer level) was also suggested [36–39].

We acknowledge that the evidence in this field is rapidly evolving and the latest evidence (at the time of writing of this text) is moving towards an absence of benefit of increased dose of heparin. In a recent large cohort study, the authors used a target trial framework emulation and inverse probability weighting to adjust for confounding and found that patients who received early therapeutic anticoagulation had a similar risk for death as those who did not [40]. The INSPIRATION trial was the first large multicenter open label randomized in this context. The authors compared intermediate-dose prophylactic anticoagulation with standard-dose prophylactic anticoagulation in critically ill patients. They did not find a difference in the primary outcome of a composite of venous or arterial thrombosis, treatment with ECMO or mortality within 30 days. Also, the prespecified safety outcome of major bleeding was noninferior in the standard-dose regimen, while overall incidence was limited (2.5% in the intermediate-dose group and 1.4% in the standard-dose prophylactic anticoagulation group) [41]. The latest evidence in this field is a prepublication of interim data—not peer reviewed—coming from a multiplatform open-label randomized controlled trial (ATTACC, REMAP-CAP, Activ-4a) [42]. The results showed that therapeutic anticoagulation did not improve survival or days free of organ support and had 89% probability of being inferior to usual care thromboprophylaxis. The explanation for the tendency for harm of the therapeutic regimen is difficult to interpret because bleeding complications were infrequent in both groups and therapeutic anticoagulation resulted in a numerical decrease in major thrombotic events.

Although increased dose of heparin has a strong rationale, the latest available evidence from trials shows that it does not seem to confer a protection. For this reason, standard prophylaxis in critically ill patients is probably the best option. However, COVID-19 shows a wide spectrum of illness severity; thus, the initiation of therapeutic anticoagulation once patients have already developed a severe form of illness might be too late to revert an established disease progression.

As previously mentioned, the use of viscoelastic assays provided an insight into the pathophysiology of COVID-19 acquired coagulopathy. They consistently showed hypercoagulability with a very high clot strength/firmness [11, 12, 43] and in some reports impaired fibrinolysis [15, 17, 44]. Although their utility in managing COVID-19 coagulopathy has not been demonstrated, it is at least thought-provoking: if impaired fibrinolysis is in part responsible for COVID-19 coagulation derangement, it raises the question whether a fibrinolytic drug can be of any benefit. Notwithstanding, it must be admitted that the fibrinolytic homeostasis in COVID-19 is very complex and still unclear. So far, there are only anecdotical reports on the use of rtPA in critically ill COVID-19, which resulted in a transient improvement of blood oxygenation that was lost by the end of the drug infusion [45].

Many other antithrombotic therapy trials are currently ongoing, evaluating drugs such as heparin derivatives, parenteral direct thrombin inhibitors, direct oral anticoagulants, aspirin and other antiplatelet agents, and also fibrinolytics [46]. All the listed trials target different aspects of the complex COVID-19 coagulation pathophysiology, recently labeled as "immunothrombosis" [47]. Besides the prophylaxis and/or anticoagulation with heparin and the thought-provoking use of rtPA, the administration of thrombomodulin (TM) might find its rationale in the enhanced shedding of TM from the endothelial cell surface of COVID-19 patients; this would result in low levels of activated protein C (APC), and thus reduced antithrombotic activity [48]. TM also activates thrombin activatable fibrinolysis inhibitor (TAFI), and exerts anti-inflammatory effects. The administration of rTM in non-COVID-19 ARDS patients seems to improve *P*/*F* ratio and ICU length of stay [49], thus representing a promising choice also in COVID-19 ARDS patients. On the other hand, direct administration of APC may constitute a feasible option, since its actions (degradation of fV and fVIII, anti-inflammatory effects via inhibition of the NF-kB pathway, profibrinolytic properties) [50] could be fostered by the hyper-inflammatory compound of COVID-19, as hypothesized in hyperinflamed ARDS subphenotypes. Although preliminary data on ARDS patients have been somewhat discouraging [51], APC administration in severe COVID-19 patients still needs to be tested. Tissue factor pathway inhibitor (TFPI) is known for its inactivation of the TF/fVIIa complex, thus limiting the extrinsic coagulation pathway. At the same time, low levels of functional TFPI have been found in ARDS patients, thus contributing to the prothrombotic environment of ARDS pulmonary microvasculature [52]. The administration of TFPI in small preclinical and clinical settings in ARDS has shown promising results [53], and so could result in COVID-19 subjects. Yet a rather simple and practical therapy would be represented by antithrombin (AT) administration. AT acts as thrombin, fIXa, fXa, fXIa, fXIIa, plasmin, trypsin, and kallikrein inhibitor. Moreover, AT is commonly supplemented as heparin cofactor to provide optimal anticoagulation during ECLS. Low levels of AT have been reported in ARDS subjects of both COVID-19 and non-COVID-19 etiology [54]. The administration of AT during ARDS—whether alone or in combination with rtPA and heparin—has led to improved shunt fraction and reduced neutrophil infiltration of the lungs [55, 56]. Its use in COVID-19 patients could therefore represent an accessible therapeutic/adjuvant option. At last, anectodical hypothesis of clinical immunothrombosis antagonism see the possible reduction of vWF activity via recombinant ADAMTS13 or caplacizumab, the use of statins and prostacyclin as actors against COVID-19 endotheliopathy and finally the administration of antiplatelet therapies to counteract COVID-19 derived thrombocytopathy [57].

However, at present, the evidence on the optimal management of COVID-19 acquired coagulopathy is still immature and the results of ongoing randomized controlled trials will help clarify whether an intervention might be effective. In the meanwhile, the old saying "first do no harm" is thus far the wisest choice.

References

1. Guan W, Ni Z, Hu Y, Liang W, Ou C, He J, et al. Clinical characteristics of coronavirus disease 2019 in China. N Engl J Med. 2020;382(18):1708–20.
2. Al-Samkari H, Karp Leaf RS, Dzik WH, Carlson JCT, Fogerty AE, Waheed A, et al. COVID-19 and coagulation: bleeding and thrombotic manifestations of SARS-CoV-2 infection. Blood. 2020;136(4):489–500.
3. Iba T, Levy JH, Connors JM, Warkentin TE, Thachil J, Levi M. The unique characteristics of COVID-19 coagulopathy. Crit Care. 2020;24(1):4–11.
4. Ackermann M, Verleden SE, Kuehnel M, Haverich A, Welte T, Laenger F, et al. Pulmonary vascular endothelialitis, thrombosis, and angiogenesis in Covid-19. N Engl J Med. 2020;383(2):120–8.
5. Suh Y, Hong H, Ohana M, Bompard F, Revel M-P, Valle C, et al. Pulmonary embolism and deep vein thrombosis in COVID-19: a systematic review and meta-analysis. Radiology. 2020;298:E70–80.
6. Tang N, Li D, Wang X, Sun Z. Abnormal coagulation parameters are associated with poor prognosis in patients with novel coronavirus pneumonia. J Thromb Haemost. 2020;18(4):844–7.
7. Taylor FB, Toh CH, Hoots WK, Wada H, Levi M, Scientific Subcommittee on Disseminated Intravascular Coagulation (DIC) of the International Society on Thrombosis and Haemostasis (ISTH). Towards definition, clinical and laboratory criteria, and a scoring system for disseminated intravascular coagulation. Thromb Haemost. 2001;86(5):1327–30.
8. Levi M, Hunt BJ. Thrombosis and coagulopathy in COVID-19: an illustrated review. Res Pract Thromb Haemost. 2020;4(5):744–51.

9. Xiang G, Hao S, Fu C, Hu W, Xie L, Wu Q, et al. The effect of coagulation factors in 2019 novel coronavirus patients: a systematic review and meta-analysis. Medicine (Baltimore). 2021;100(7):e24537.
10. Bowles L, Platton S, Yartey N, Dave M, Lee K, Hart DP, et al. Lupus anticoagulant and abnormal coagulation tests in patients with Covid-19. N Engl J Med. 2020;383(3):288–90.
11. Panigada M, Bottino N, Tagliabue P, Grasselli G, Novembrino C, Chantarangkul V, et al. Hypercoagulability of COVID-19 patients in intensive care unit: a report of thromboelastography findings and other parameters of hemostasis. J Thromb Haemost. 2020;18(7):1738–42.
12. Ranucci M, Ballotta A, Di Dedda U, Bayshnikova E, Dei Poli M, Resta M, et al. The procoagulant pattern of patients with COVID-19 acute respiratory distress syndrome. J Thromb Haemost. 2020;18(7):1747–51.
13. Gomez-Builes JC, Acuna SA, Nascimento B, Madotto F, Rizoli SB. Harmful or physiologic: diagnosing fibrinolysis shutdown in a trauma cohort with rotational thromboelastometry. Anesth Analg. 2018;127(4):840–9.
14. Creel-Bulos C, Auld SC, Caridi-Scheible M, Barker NA, Friend S, Gaddh M, et al. Fibrinolysis shutdown and thrombosis in a COVID-19 ICU. Shock. 2021;55(3):316–20.
15. Bachler M, Bösch J, Stürzel DP, Hell T, Giebl A, Ströhle M, et al. Impaired fibrinolysis in critically ill COVID-19 patients. Br J Anaesth. 2020;126(3):590–8.
16. Thachil J. Usefulness of combining D-dimers with thromboelastography. J Am Coll Surg. 2020;231(5):608.
17. Wright F, Vogler T, Moore E, Moore H, Wohlauer M, Urban S, et al. Fibrinolysis shutdown correlation with thromboembolic events in severe COVID-19 infection. J Am Coll Surg. 2020;231(2):193–203.
18. Klok FA, Kruip MJHA, van der Meer NJM, Arbous MS, Gommers D, Kant KM, et al. Confirmation of the high cumulative incidence of thrombotic complications in critically ill ICU patients with COVID-19: an updated analysis. Thromb Res. 2020;1(191):148–50.
19. Jiménez D, García-Sanchez A, Rali P, Muriel A, Bikdeli B, Ruiz-Artacho P, et al. Incidence of VTE and bleeding among hospitalized patients with coronavirus disease 2019: a systematic review and meta-analysis. Chest. 2021;159(3):1182–96.
20. Bilaloglu S, Aphinyanaphongs Y, Jones S, Iturrate E, Hochman J, Berger JS. Thrombosis in hospitalized patients with COVID-19 in a New York City health system. JAMA. 2020;324(8):799–801.
21. Samama MM, Cohen AT, Darmon JY, Desjardins L, Eldor A, Janbon C, Prophylaxis in Medical Patients with Enoxaparin Study Group, et al. A comparison of enoxaparin with placebo for the prevention of venous thromboembolism in acutely ill medical patients. N Engl J Med. 1999;341(11):793–800.

22. Leizorovicz A, Cohen AT, Turpie AGG, Olsson C-G, Vaitkus PT, Goldhaber SZ, et al. Randomized, placebo-controlled trial of dalteparin for the prevention of venous thromboembolism in acutely ill medical patients. Circulation. 2004;110(7):874–9.
23. Cohen AT, Davidson BL, Gallus AS, Lassen MR, Prins MH, Tomkowski W, et al. Efficacy and safety of fondaparinux for the prevention of venous thromboembolism in older acute medical patients: randomised placebo controlled trial. BMJ. 2006;332(7537):325–9.
24. Gerotziafas GT, Samama MM. Prophylaxis of venous thromboembolism in medical patients. Curr Opin Pulm Med. 2004;10(5):356–65.
25. Harr JN, Moore EE, Ghasabyan A, Chin TL, Sauaia A, Banerjee A, et al. Functional fibrinogen assay indicates that fibrinogen is critical in correcting abnormal clot strength following trauma. Shock. 2013;39:45–9.
26. Hippensteel JA, LaRiviere WB, Colbert JF, Langouët-Astrié CJ, Schmidt EP. Heparin as a therapy for COVID-19: current evidence and future possibilities. Am J Physiol Lung Cell Mol Physiol. 2020;319(2):L211–7.
27. Gozzo L, Viale P, Longo L, Vitale DC, Drago F. The potential role of heparin in patients with COVID-19: beyond the anticoagulant effect. A review. Front Pharmacol. 2020;11:1307.
28. de Montmollin E, Faille D, Andrieu V, Ajzenberg N, Timsit J-F. Intensified thromboprophylaxis in COVID-19 critically ill patients: is it enough? J Infect. 2021;82(5):e20–2.
29. Tang N, Bai H, Chen X, Gong J, Li D, Sun Z. Anticoagulant treatment is associated with decreased mortality in severe coronavirus disease 2019 patients with coagulopathy. J Thromb Haemost. 2020;18(5):1094–9. https://doi.org/10.1111/jth.14817.
30. Paranjpe I, Fuster V, Lala A, Russak A, Glicksberg BS, Levin MA, et al. Association of treatment dose anticoagulation with in-hospital survival among hospitalized patients with COVID-19. J Am Coll Cardiol. 2020;76(1):122–4.
31. Martinelli I, Ciavarella A, Abbattista M, Aliberti S, De Zan V, Folli C, et al. Increasing dosages of low-molecular-weight heparin in hospitalized patients with Covid-19. Intern Emerg Med. 2021;16(5):1223–9.
32. Tacquard C, Mansour A, Godon A, Godet J, Poissy J, Garrigue D, et al. Impact of high dose prophylactic anticoagulation in critically ill patients with COVID-19 pneumonia. Chest. 2021;159(6):2417–27.
33. Nadkarni GN, Lala A, Bagiella E, Chang HL, Moreno PR, Pujadas E, et al. Anticoagulation, bleeding, mortality, and pathology in hospitalized patients with COVID-19. J Am Coll Cardiol. 2020;76(16):1815–26.
34. PROTECT Investigators for the Canadian Critical Care Trials Group and the Australian and New Zealand Intensive Care Society Clinical Trials Group, Cook D, Meade M, Guyatt G, Walter S, Heels-Ansdell D, et al. Dalteparin versus unfractionated heparin in critically ill patients. N Engl J Med. 2011;364(14):1305–14.

35. Halaby R, Cuker A, Yui J, Matthews A, Ishaaya E, Traxler E, et al. Bleeding risk by intensity of anticoagulation in critically ill patients with COVID-19: a retrospective cohort study. J Thromb Haemost JTH. 2021;19(6):1533–45.
36. Thachil J, Tang N, Gando S, Falanga A, Cattaneo M, Levi M, et al. ISTH interim guidance on recognition and management of coagulopathy in COVID-19. J Thromb Haemost. 2020;18(5):1023–6. https://doi.org/10.1111/jth.14810.
37. Barnes GD, Burnett A, Allen A, Blumenstein M, Clark NP, Cuker A, et al. Thromboembolism and anticoagulant therapy during the COVID-19 pandemic: interim clinical guidance from the anticoagulation forum. J Thromb Thrombolysis. 2020;50(1):72–81. https://doi.org/10.1007/s11239-020-02138-z.
38. Moores LK, Tritschler T, Brosnahan S, Carrier M, Collen JF, Doerschug K, et al. Prevention, diagnosis, and treatment of VTE in patients with coronavirus disease 2019: CHEST guideline and expert panel report. Chest. 2020;158(3):1143–63.
39. Marietta M, Ageno W, Artoni A, De Candia E, Gresele P, Marchetti M, et al. COVID-19 and haemostasis: a position paper from Italian Society on Thrombosis and Haemostasis (SISET). Blood Transfus. 2020;18(3):167. https://doi.org/10.2450/2020.0083-20.
40. Al-Samkari H, Gupta S, Leaf RK, Wang W, Rosovsky RP, Brenner SK, et al. Thrombosis, bleeding, and the observational effect of early therapeutic anticoagulation on survival in critically ill patients with COVID-19. Ann Intern Med. 2021;26:M20–6739.
41. INSPIRATION Investigators, Sadeghipour P, Talasaz AH, Rashidi F, Sharif-Kashani B, Beigmohammadi MT, et al. Effect of intermediate-dose vs standard-dose prophylactic anticoagulation on thrombotic events, extracorporeal membrane oxygenation treatment, or mortality among patients with COVID-19 admitted to the intensive care unit: the INSPIRATION randomized clinical trial. JAMA. 2021;325(16):1620–30.
42. The REMAP-CAP, ACTIV-4a, ATTACC Investigators, Zarychanski R. Therapeutic anticoagulation in critically ill patients with Covid-19—preliminary report. Intensive Care Crit Care Med. 2021. Accessed 29 Mar 2021. https://doi.org/10.1101/2021.03.10.21252749
43. Yuriditsky E, Horowitz JM, Merchan C, Ahuja T, Brosnahan SB, McVoy L, et al. Thromboelastography profiles of critically ill patients with coronavirus disease 2019. Crit Care Med. 2020;48(9):1319–26.
44. Nougier C, Benoit R, Simon M, Desmurs-Clavel H, Marcotte G, Argaud L, et al. Hypofibrinolytic state and high thrombin generation may play a major role in SARS-COV2 associated thrombosis. J Thromb Haemost. 2020;18(9):2215–9.
45. Wang J, Hajizadeh N, Moore EE, McIntyre RC, Moore PK, Veress LA, et al. Tissue plasminogen activator (tPA) treatment for COVID-19 associated acute respiratory distress syndrome (ARDS): a case series. J Thromb Haemost. 2020;18(7):1752–5. https://doi.org/10.1111/jth.14828.

46. Talasaz AH, Sadeghipour P, Kakavand H, Aghakouchakzadeh M, Kordzadeh-Kermani E, Van Tassell BW, et al. Recent randomized trials of antithrombotic therapy for patients with COVID-19: JACC state-of-the-art review. J Am Coll Cardiol. 2021;77(15):1903–21.
47. O'Donnell JS, Peyvandi F, Martin-Loeches I. Pulmonary immuno-thrombosis in COVID-19 ARDS pathogenesis. Intensive Care Med. 2021;47(8):899–902.
48. Goshua G, Pine AB, Meizlish ML, Chang C-H, Zhang H, Bahel P, et al. Endotheliopathy in COVID-19-associated coagulopathy: evidence from a single-centre, cross-sectional study. Lancet Haematol. 2020;7(8):e575–82.
49. Uba T, Nishi K, Umegaki T, Ohashi N, Kusaka Y, Umegaki O, et al. The influence of human soluble recombinant thrombomodulin on in-hospital mortality in patients with acute respiratory distress syndrome and disseminated intravascular coagulation: a retrospective multicenter study. J Intensive Crit Care. 2017;3(3):40. http://criticalcare.imedpub.com/the-influence-of-human-soluble-recombinant-thrombomodulin-on-inhospital-mortality-in-patients-with-acute-respiratory-distress-synd.php?aid=21017.
50. Frantzeskaki F, Armaganidis A, Orfanos SE. Immunothrombosis in acute respiratory distress syndrome: cross talks between inflammation and coagulation. Respiration. 2017;93(3):212–25.
51. Ranieri VM, Thompson BT, Barie PS, Dhainaut J-F, Douglas IS, Finfer S, et al. Drotrecogin alfa (activated) in adults with septic shock. N Engl J Med. 2012;366(22):2055–64.
52. Bastarache JA, Wang L, Wang Z, Albertine KH, Matthay MA, Ware LB. Intra-alveolar tissue factor pathway inhibitor is not sufficient to block tissue factor procoagulant activity. Am J Physiol Lung Cell Mol Physiol. 2008;294(5):L874–81.
53. Camprubí-Rimblas M, Tantinyà N, Bringué J, Guillamat-Prats R, Artigas A. Anticoagulant therapy in acute respiratory distress syndrome. Ann Transl Med. 2018;6(2):36.
54. Koyama K, Katayama S, Tonai K, Shima J, Koinuma T, Nunomiya S. Biomarker profiles of coagulopathy and alveolar epithelial injury in acute respiratory distress syndrome with idiopathic/immune-related disease or common direct risk factors. Crit Care. 2019;23(1):283.
55. Rehberg S, Yamamoto Y, Sousse LE, Jonkam C, Zhu Y, Traber LD, et al. Antithrombin attenuates vascular leakage via inhibiting neutrophil activation in acute lung injury. Crit Care Med. 2013;41(12):e439–46.
56. Rehberg S, Yamamoto Y, Sousse LE, Jonkam C, Cox RA, Prough DS, et al. Advantages and pitfalls of combining intravenous antithrombin with nebulized heparin and tissue plasminogen activator in acute respiratory distress syndrome. J Trauma Acute Care Surg. 2014;76(1):126–33.
57. Lowenstein CJ, Solomon SD. Severe COVID-19 is a microvascular disease. Circulation. 2020;142(17):1609–11.

Part VII

Other Multiorgan Involvements

21 Gastrointestinal Manifestations of COVID-19

Matteo Bassetti, Antonio Vena, Daniele Roberto Giacobbe, Federica Briano, and Federica Portunato

21.1 Introduction

Although respiratory disease caused by SARS-CoV-2 accounts for most severe courses and hospital admissions, there has been emerging evidence on gastrointestinal manifestations of SARS-CoV-2 [1]. These manifestations are the most frequently reported extrapulmonary symptoms of COVID-19, affecting 10–50% of the patients. In most cases gastrointestinal manifestations include diarrhea, nausea and/or vomiting, and abdominal pain. Other common reported symptoms are anorexia, anosmia, and dysgeusia [2]. In a meta-analysis including 60 studies, Cheung et al. [3] found gastrointestinal symptoms in 17.6% of 4243 COVID-19 patients, with the most frequent manifestations being anorexia (26.8%), diarrhea (12.5%), nausea/vomiting (10.2%), and abdom-

M. Bassetti (✉) · A. Vena (✉) · D. R. Giacobbe · F. Briano
Infectious Diseases Unit, San Martino Policlinico Hospital—IRCCS for Oncology and Neurosciences, Genoa, Italy

Department of Health Sciences (DISSAL), University of Genoa, Genoa, Italy
e-mail: matteo.bassetti@hsanmartino.it

F. Portunato
Infectious Diseases Unit, San Martino Policlinico Hospital—IRCCS for Oncology and Neurosciences, Genoa, Italy

D. Battaglini, P. Pelosi (eds.), *COVID-19 Critical and Intensive Care Medicine Essentials*, https://doi.org/10.1007/978-3-030-94992-1_21

inal pain (9.2%). Similar data were also reported in two European cohorts in which gastrointestinal manifestations were observed in 16.9% at COVID-19 onset [4, 5] and at any time during the disease course in 29.9% [4, 5]. Higher age of gastrointestinal involvement were observed in studies from the USA, where the prevalence of gastrointestinal symptoms ranged between 35% and 61% [6, 7]. The differences in frequencies of gastrointestinal manifestations might be due to genetic factors including polymorphism in expression of the viral receptor angiotensin converting enzyme 2 (ACE-2) in the gastrointestinal tract, as well as SARS-CoV-2 strain variations [8].

Gastrointestinal manifestations are also of clinical relevance as they number among the first, and sometimes unique [9], symptoms of COVID-19. In a recent published report from Italy, out of total 411 consecutive patients, gastrointestinal symptoms were present at disease onset in 42 (10.2%) [10], with gastrointestinal features heralding COVID-19 on average 5–20 days before development of respiratory illness [10]. Therefore, that could potentially lead to delay in diagnosis with possible uncontrolled transmission of the infection.

21.2 Pathogenesis

The exact pathogenesis of gastrointestinal involvement in SARS-CoV-2 is not completed understood and four main factors have been hypothesized: (1) the direct ACE 2 mediated viral cytotoxicity, (2) cytokine-induced inflammation, (3) gut dysbiosis, and (4) vascular abnormalities.

SARS-CoV-2 use ACE-2 as an entry receptor to establish infection, which is expressed by various tissues, including epithelial cells of the tongue, small intestine, crypt cells, colon, hepatocytes, gallbladder epithelial cells and pancreatic ductal, acinar and islet cells [11, 12]. Evidence of gastrointestinal infection has also been provided by isolation of viral RNA from gastrointestinal epithelial cells and intracellular staining of viral nucleocapsid protein [13]. As a matter of fact, the presence of active viral replication in the intestinal tract of infected patients was demonstrated via both electronic microscopy and viral culture, suggesting the fecal–oral route as a possible mode of transmission [14, 15]. Moreover, it has been demonstrated that the alteration in gut microbiota in patients with COVID-19 may affect the patient's susceptibility and response to SARS-CoV-2 infection. A metagenomic sequencing analysis was performed on 15 COVID-19 cases, 6 pneumoniae controls and 15 healthy controls, showing that the first had significant alteration in fecal microbiome with an enrichment of opportunistic pathogens and depletion of beneficial commensals [16]. Gut dysbiosis persisted even after clearance of SARS-CoV-2 and inversely correlated with SARS-CoV-2 viral load in fecal samples. Finally, the use of antibiotic treatment was correlated with a more heterogeneous microbiome and a further shift away from a healthy one [16].

Between pathophysiological mechanisms of COVID-19 endothelial cell damage and thromboinflammation are fundamental during the first phase of the disease [17]. The infection causes endothelial injury and endotheliitis that can trigger excessive thrombin production, inhibit fibrinolysis, and activate complement pathways that finally lead to microthrombi deposition and microvascular dysfunction [18].

Finally, the overactivation of innate immunity in the setting of T cell lymphodepletion lead to dysregulated immune response and cytokine-release syndrome [19]. This imbalance is due to rapid viral replication that antagonize interferon signaling and activate neutrophils and monocyte-macrophages [20]. Markers of hyperinflammation such as C-reactive protein, ferritin, erythrocyte sedimentation rate, D-dimer, fibrinogen, and lactate dehydrogenase are predictive of mortality [21].

21.3 Clinical Manifestations

Diarrhea is the most common gastrointestinal symptom in patients affected by SARS-CoV-2 infection. Its role on prognosis of these patients is not clearly defined. Some studies showed a greater diarrhea age in patients with severe illness suggesting an association with disease severity [22]. However other studies did not confirm this correlation [23]. In this sense, it should be noted that these studies vary in their inclusion criteria, ascertainment of gastrointestinal symptoms, and definitions of severity of disease course. Therefore, further research is needed to better understand the correlation between diarrhea and COVID-19 outcome.

Abdominal pain has been reported most frequently in children, especially if they developed the multisystem inflammatory syndrome (MIS-C) [24]. In a systematic review, anosmia and dysgeusia were reported with a prevalence of 38.2% and 36.6%, respectively. These symptoms are prevalent in patients with COVID-19 compared to those with other respiratory infections [25].

21.4 Hepatic Manifestations

COVID-19 is commonly associated with hepatic dysfunction causing the elevation of alanine aminotransferase (ALT), aspartate aminotransferase (AST) and total bilirubin with a age that range between 14% and 53% depending on studies [26]. Due to the expression of ACE2 receptors in the cholangiocytes, it is not uncommon to see a mild elevation of alkaline phosphatase and gamma-glutamyl transferase (GGT) in patients with COVID-19 [27].

It has been demonstrated that liver damage is associated with severe COVID-19 illness and that elevation of liver biochemistries imply a higher risk of intensive care unit (ICU) admission and death [27, 28].

In an Italian cohort Taramasso et al., described 799 patients with COVID-19 and found that patients with liver enzyme elevation (AST and/or ALT between 2.5 and 5 upper limit of normal) had a higher hazard of death or ICU admission when compared with patients without liver enzyme elevation. In addition, the higher was the level of ALT and AST, the stronger was the association with mortality/ICU admission [29].

The pathogenesis of liver injury in COVID-19 patients is multifactorial and may include the following mechanism: ACE-2 viral replication mediated cytotoxicity, hypoxic or ischemic damage, hepatic congestion secondary to high positive end expiratory pressure during mechanical ventilation [30], immune-mediated inflammatory response and drug-induced liver injury (DILI) [31]. The systemic inflammatory response syndrome and multiorgan dysfunction contribute to the development to a cytokine storm and subsequently liver impairment.

21.5 Less Common Gastrointestinal Manifestations

Acute cholecystitis has been reported in patients with COVID-19, especially those who are critically ill [32, 33]. In most patients, the cholecystitis is acalculous, and the etiology remains largely unclear. While hypomotility of the gallbladder wall is expected in critical illness in general, a direct viral involvement in the pathophysiology in COVID-19 patients cannot be ruled out [34]. Other less common gastrointestinal manifestations of COVID-19 includes elevation of pancreatic enzymes, even if hyperlipasemia is not specific of pancreatitis and was not reflective of severe infection or poor clinical outcome [35].

As regards oral manifestations, mucosal lesions have been reported in COVID 19 confirmed and suspected individuals. These include ulcers, erosion, blisters, plaque-like lesions, reactivation of herpes simplex virus 1, and geographical tongue [36]. The lesions appear either before or along with systematic manifestations of COVID 19. It is hypothesized that taste impairment is the only oral symptom directly associated with viral damage and other oral lesion arise as a result of decreased immunity due to viral infection, opportunistic or secondary infection or medications used for treatment of COVID-19 [37].

21.6 Gastrointestinal Complications Associated with COVID-19

The gastrointestinal system is not only threatened by direct replication of SARS-CoV-2, but also from vascular and functional complications that are more commonly seen during long-term course of hospitalization or in ICU setting. In a retrospective review of 92 patients with severe COVID-19 admitted to the ICU, 44 patients (48%) had ileus, 4 (4%) had intestinal ischemia, and 2 (2%) had Ogilvie syndrome [38]. It also has been demonstrated that SARS-CoV-2 infection lead to a hypercoagulable state that ultimately can cause prothrombotic complications such as acute mesenteric ischemia and portal vein thrombosis [39]. Mesenteric ischemia represents the most serious gastrointestinal complication reported in patients with critical SARS-CoV-2 infection. In a cohort of critically ill COVID-19 patients admitted to a single institution, the reported incidence was between 3.8–4.0%, even if researchers found challenging to make definite diagnosis in this setting of patients, due to sedation and requirement of vasopressor that could lead to misdiagnosis [40]. The most common presenting symptoms are abdominal distension, increasing leukocytosis, increasing vasopressors requirements, and unexplained metabolic acidosis [41]. Computed tomography angiography is the modality of choice for the diagnosis of acute mesenteric ischemia along with clinical correlation.

Unfortunately, the mortality rate is extremely high, in fact, ages around 60–80% have been reported in non-COVID-19 patients [42].

Moreover, the virus can cause neuronal damage that alter colonic motility and could result in ileus or perforation. These complications could be also elicited by drugs used in critically ill patient like sedatives, opioids, steroids, and nonsteroidal anti-inflammatory drugs. In critical ill COVID-19 patients with rapidly deteriorating respiratory function, the use of tocilizumab, a monoclonal IL-6 receptor inhibitor, is indicated even if it can cause diverticulitis and perforation in susceptible patients [43].

Long-term hypoxia, preexisting or drug-induced coagulopathy and virus invasion of tissue cause gastrointestinal mucosal cell damage that could determine gastrointestinal bleeding. However, this complication may be also due to high doses of corticosteroid and heparin which are commonly used for treatment of COVID-19. In this setting the most common etiology for upper gastrointestinal bleeding are gastric or duodenal ulceration (80%) followed by rectal ulceration (50%) [44].

21.7 *Clostridioides difficile* Infection

During COVID-19 pandemic, most hospitals experienced overcrowding, emergency situations, and the need for strict isolation measures for infected patients, which in turn represented major factors for decreasing attention toward infection control measures. Paradoxically, in the management of SARS-CoV-2, despite the viral etiology of the disease, there has been an overuse of antibiotics with little concern for established antimicrobial stewardship programs [45, 46].

The inappropriate and excessive use of antibiotics has, therefore, led to an increase in *Clostridioides difficile* infection with consequent prolonged hospitalization and higher mortality. The clinicians should maintain a high clinical suspicion due to the common symptoms of COVID-19 GI manifestations and *Clostridioides difficile* infection [47].

21.8 Pediatric Population

In the pediatric population affected by SARS-CoV-2, the most common reported gastrointestinal symptoms are nausea, vomiting, diarrhea, abdominal pain and feeding difficulties. Like in the adult population, these manifestations may precede respiratory symptoms and in up 10% of children they could be the only presentation of the disease [48].

Children could present with rare manifestation such as terminal ileitis due to the significant mucosal inflammation in the acute phase of SARS-CoV-2 infection, mimicking an atypical appendicitis. Gastrointestinal symptoms are typical associated with SARS-CoV-2 related multisystem inflammatory syndrome in children (MIS-C), which is due to systemic hyperinflammation and could be confused with inflammatory bowel disease. In a retrospective chart review of 35 patients with MIS-C, gastrointestinal symptoms were present in 97% of children, requiring radiographic imaging in 54% of them and surgery in one child [49].

21.9 Conclusions

Gastrointestinal manifestations in patients infected with SARS-CoV-2 are extremely frequent and often could represent the only symptom of the disease. Clinicians should be aware of this in order not to delay diagnosis and hospitalization. It is still unclear if diarrhea is associated with worse prognosis. On the contrary, liver enzyme alterations are associated with worse outcomes and higher ICU admissions. Finally, it has to be underlined that SARS-CoV-2 could significantly alter gastrointestinal microbiome. This effect may be worsened by overuse of antibiotic therapy in COVID-19 patients.

References

1. Gupta A, Madhavan MV, Sehgal K, et al. Extrapulmonary manifestations of COVID-19. Nat Med. 2020;26(7):1017–32.
2. Han Cha M, Regueiro M, Sandhu DS, et al. Gastrointestinal and hepatic manifestations of COVID-19: a comprehensive review. World J Gastroenterol. 2020;26(19):2323–32.
3. Cheung KS, Hung IFN, Chan PPY, et al. Gastrointestinal manifestations of SARS-CoV-2 infection and virus load in fecal samples from a Hong Kong cohort: systematic review and meta-analysis. Gastroenterology. 2020;159(1):81–95.
4. Leal T, Costa E, Arroja B, et al. Gastrointestinal manifestations of COVID-19: results from a European Centre. Eur J Gastroenterol Hepatol. 2021;33(5):691–4.
5. Vena A, Giacobbe DR, Di Biagio A, et al. Clinical characteristics, management and in-hospital mortality of patients with coronavirus disease 2019 in Genoa, Italy. Clin Microbiol Infect. 2020;26(11):1537–154.
6. Nobel YR, Phipps M, Zucker J, et al. Gastrointestinal symptoms and COVID-19: case–control study from the United States. Gastroenterology. 2020;159:373–5.
7. Redd WD, Zhou JC, Hathorn KE, et al. Prevalence and characteristics of gastrointestinal symptoms in patients with severe acute respiratory syndrome coronavirus 2 infection in the United States: a multicenter cohort study. Gastroenterology. 2020;159:765–7.
8. Mao R, Qiu Y, He J-S, et al. Manifestations and prognosis of gastrointestinal and liver involvement in patients with COVID-19: a systematic review and meta-analysis. Lancet Gastroenterol Hepatol. 2020;5(7):667–78.

9. Sultan S, Altayar O, Siddique SM, et al. AGA institute rapid review of the gastrointestinal and liver manifestations of COVID-19, meta-analysis of international data, and recommendations for the consultative management of patients with COVID-19. Gastroenterology. 2020;159(1):320–34.
10. Buscarini E, Manfredi G, Brambilla G, et al. GI symptoms as early signs of COVID-19 in hospitalised Italian patients. Gut. 2020;69(8):1547–8.
11. Cao W, Li T. COVID-19: towards understanding of pathogenesis. Cell Res. 2020;30:367–9.
12. Devaux CA, Lagier J, Raoult D. New insights into the physiopathology of COVID-19: SARS-CoV-2 associated gastrointestinal illness. Front Med (Lausanne). 2021;8:640073.
13. Xiao F, Tang M, Zheung X, et al. Evidence for gastrointestinal infection of SARS-CoV-2. Gastroenterology. 2020;158(6):1831–3.
14. Parasa S, Desai M, Chandrasekar VT, et al. Prevalence of gastrointestinal symptoms and fecal viral shedding in patients with coronavirus disease 2019: a systematic review and meta-analysis. JAMA Netw Open. 2020;3(6):e2011335.
15. D'Amico F, Baumgart DC, Danese S, et al. Diarrhea during COVID-19 infection: pathogenesis, epidemiology, prevention, and management. Clin Gastroenterol Hepatol. 2020;18(8):1663–72.
16. Zuo T, Zhang F, Lui GC, et al. Alterations in gut microbiota of patients with COVID-19 during time of hospitalization. Gastroenterology. 2020;159(3):944–55.
17. Ackermann M, Verleden SE, Kuehnel M, et al. Pulmonary vascular endothelialitis, thrombosis and angiogenesis in COVID-19. N Engl J Med. 2020;383:120–8.
18. Varga Z, Flammer AJ, Steiger P, et al. Endothelial cell infection and endotheliitis in COVID-19. Lancet. 2020;395:1417–8.
19. Kim KD, Zhao J, Auh S, et al. Adaptive immune cells temper initial innate responses. Nat Med. 2007;13(10):1248–52.
20. Huang KJ, Su IJ, Theron M, et al. An interferon-gamma-related cytokine storm in SARS patients. J Med Virol. 2005;75(2):185–94.
21. Cummings MJ, Baldwin MR, Abrams D, et al. Epidemiology, clinical course, and outcomes of critically ill adults with COVID-19 in New York City: a prospective cohort study. Lancet. 2020;395:1763–70.
22. Wang D, Hu B, Hu C, et al. Clinical characteristics of 138 hospitalized patients with 2019 novel coronavirus-infected pneumonia in Wuhan, China. JAMA. 2020;323(11):1061–9.
23. Fang D, Ma J, Guan J, et al. Manifestations of digestive system in hospitalized patients with novel coronavirus pneumonia in Wuhan, China: a single-center, descriptive study. Chin J Dig. 2020;12:E005.
24. Rowley AH. Understanding SARS-CoV-2-related multisystem inflammatory syndrome in children. Nat Rev Immunol. 2020;20(8):453–4.
25. Mutiawati E, Fahriani M, Mamada SS, et al. Anosmia and dysgeusia in SARS-CoV-2 infection: incidence and effects on COVID-19 severity and

mortality, and the possible pathobiology mechanisms—a systematic review and meta-analysis. F1000Res. 2021;10:40.
26. Xu L, Liu J, Lu M, et al. Liver injury during highly pathogenic human coronavirus infections. Liver Int. 2020;40(5):998–1004.
27. Zhang C, Shi L, Wang FS. Liver injury in COVID-19: management and challenges. Lancet Gastroenterol Hepatol. 2020;5(5):428–30.
28. Hajifathalian K, Krisko T, Mehta A, et al. Gastrointestinal and hepatic manifestations of 2019 novel coronavirus disease in a large cohort of infected patients from New York: clinical implications. Gastroenterology. 2020;159(3):1137–40.
29. Taramasso L, Vena A, Bovis F, et al. Higher mortality and intensive care unit admissions in COVID-19 patients with liver enzyme elevations. Microorganisms. 2020;8(12):2010.
30. Bangash MN. COVID-19 and the liver: little cause concern. Lancet Gastroenterol Hepatol. 2020;5:529–30.
31. Li J, Fan JG. Characteristics and mechanism of liver injury in 2019 coronavirus disease. J Clin Transl Hepatol. 2020;8(1):13–7.
32. Sun JK, Liu Y, Zou L, et al. Acute gastrointestinal injury in critically ill patients with COVID-19 in Wuhan, China. World J Gastroenterol. 2020;26(39):6087–97.
33. Scutari R, Piermatteo L, Ciancio Manuelli M, et al. Long-term SARS-CoV-2 infection associated with viral dissemination in different body fluids including bile in two patients with acute cholecystitis. Life (Basel). 2020;10(11):302.
34. Mattone E, Sofia M, Schembari E, et al. Acute acalculous cholecystitis on a COVID-19 patient: a case report. Ann Med Surg (Lond). 2020;58:73–5.
35. McNabb-Baltar J, Jin DX, Grover AS, et al. Lipase elevation in patients with COVID-19. Am J Gastroenterol. 2020;115(8):1286–8.
36. Farid H, Khan M, Jamal S, et al. Oral manifestations of Covid-19—a literature review. Rev Med Virol. 2021;32:e2248.
37. Brandão TB, Gueiros LA, Melo TS, et al. Oral lesions in patients with SARS-CoV-2 infection: could the oral cavity be a target organ? Oral Surg Oral Med Oral Pathol Oral Radiol. 2021;131(2):e45–51.
38. El Moheb M, Naar L, Christensen MA, et al. Gastrointestinal complications in critically ill patients with and without COVID-19. JAMA. 2020;324(18):1899–901.
39. Parry AH, Wani AH, Yaseen M. Acute mesenteric ischemia in severe Coronavirus-19 (COVID-19): possible mechanisms and diagnostic pathway. Acad Radiol. 2020;27(8):1190.
40. Kaafarani HMA, El Moheb M, Hwabejire JO, et al. Gastrointestinal complications in critically ill patients with COVID-19. Ann Surg. 2020;272(2):e61–2.
41. Gartland RM, Velmahos GC. Bowel necrosis in the setting of COVID-19. J Gastrointest Surg. 2020;24(12):2888–9.

42. Kerawala AA, Das B, Solangi A. Mesenteric ischemia in COVID-19 patients: a review of current literature. World J Clin Cases. 2021;9(18):4700–8.
43. Vikse J, Henry BM. Tocilizumab in COVID-19: beware the risk of intestinal perforation. Int J Antimicrob Agents. 2020;56(1):106009.
44. Martin TA, Wan DW, Hajifathalian K, et al. Gastrointestinal bleeding in patients with coronavirus disease 2019: a matched case-control study. Am J Gastroenterol. 2020;115(10):1609–16.
45. Rawson TM, Moore LS, Castro-Sánchez E, et al. COVID-19 and the potential long-term impact on antimicrobial resistance. J Antimicrob Chemother. 2020;75:1681–4.
46. Magnasco L, Mikulska M, Giacobbe DR, et al. Spread of carbapenem-resistant Gram-Negatives and *Candida auris* during the COVID-19 pandemic in critically ill patients: one step back in antimicrobial stewardship? Microorganisms. 2021;9(1):95.
47. Khanna S, Kraft CS. The interplay of SARS-CoV-2 and *Clostridioides difficile* infection. Future Microbiol. 2021;16:439–43. https://doi.org/10.2217/fmb-2020-0275.
48. Puoti MG, Rybak A, Kiparissi F, et al. SARS-CoV-2 and the gastrointestinal tract in children. Front Pediatr. 2021;9:617980.
49. Sahn B, Eze OP, Edelman MC, et al. Features of intestinal disease associated with COVID-related multisystem inflammatory syndrome in children. J Pediatr Gastroenterol Nutr. 2021;72(3):384–7.

Nutritional Therapy

22

Samir Giuseppe Sukkar, Stefano Kayali,
Arianna Prister, Livia Pisciotta,
and Manuele Furnari

22.1 Introduction

Nutritional status is a major player in the complex management of patients affected by Covid-19 requiring intensive care unit (ICU) treatment. These represent the 20% of the hospitalized population infected by SARS-CoV2 [1].

Comorbidities are strongly associated with disease severity and mortality risk [2]. Moreover, multiple chronic diseases like diabetes and cardiovascular disease affect the majority of Covid-19 hospitalized patients ad are associated with malnutrition and severe outcomes [3, 4]. Their nutritional risk depends on the course of the infection itself, its treatments (e.g., ventilation, sedation) and pathophysiologic changes such as hyperpyrexia and hypermetabolism [5]. Malnutrition involves 38–78% of patients admitted to intensive care units and is independently associated with poorer clinical outcomes [6]. Moreover, it is the first cause of immunodeficiency indirectly affecting physiological routes of

S. G. Sukkar (✉) · A. Prister · L. Pisciotta
Dietetics and Clinical Nutrition Unit, IRCCS-Policlinic Hospital San Martino, Genoa, Italy
e-mail: samir.sukkar@hsanmartino.it

S. Kayali · M. Furnari
Gastroenterology Unit, Department of Internal Medicine, IRCCS-Policlinic Hospital San Martino, Genoa University, Genoa, Italy
e-mail: stefano.romagnoli@unifi.it

D. Battaglini, P. Pelosi (eds.), *COVID-19 Critical and Intensive Care Medicine Essentials*, https://doi.org/10.1007/978-3-030-94992-1_22

response to viral infections. Thus, nutritional risk assessment embodies a pivotal role in stratifying patients and optimizing their management. Nutritional status and infection outcomes are strictly linked and their important relationship has been studied since the initial spread of the pandemic. At least 10 international guidelines have been developed based on clinician experiences, expert consensus and evidences extrapolated from previous guidelines about nutrition in critically ill patients without Covid-19 [7]. Nevertheless, to date, there is no international consensus on the gold standard nutritional support practice for critically ill patients affected by Covid-19.

22.2 Nutritional Assessment

In order to identify the patients who are at greatest nutritional risk and to integrate nutritional interventions into the overall medical therapy, carrying out a nutrition screening once the patient has been admitted to ICU is crucial [8]. Several screening tools have been developed by different workgroups. In a recent systematic review of nutritional screening tools in adults affected by COVID-19, the European NRS-2002, the Mini Nutritional Assessment (MNA), the Malnutrition Universal Screening Tool (MUST), the Nutrition Risk Index (NRI), the Geriatric NRI (GNRI), and the modified nutrition risk in critically ill (mNUTRIC) were compared [9, 10]. Nutritional risk was prevalent regardless of the tool used, ranging from 27.5 (MNA) to 100% (GNRI). The MNA demonstrated higher predicting validity for weight loss and poor appetite, prolonged hospitalization was better predicted by NRS-2002 while complications and mortality at 28 days were better associated with the results of mNUTRIC score. Moreover, malnourished patients in nonintensive medical units accounted for 23% of the total, malnutrition was higher in patients transferred to ICU involving 39% of patients [11].

Albumin is historically known as biochemical marker of malnutrition and indicator of nutritional status. Thus, its role in the management of critically ill COVID-19 patients has been inda-gated. A recent study by Evans et al., approved by the American Society for parenteral and enteral nutrition (ASPEN), proposes albumin as marker of inflammation rather than nutrition status alone [12]. These results are in line with Bedock et al. and Liu e al. who reported how hypoalbuminemia is independently associated with the risk of patients transfer to ICU, to twofold higher risk of mortality and to fivefold increase in acute respiratory distress syndrome (ARDS) [11, 13]. Therefore, as stated by Thomas et al., albumin should be used and analysed in the context of COVID-19 related inflammation to stratify and identify patients who are at major risk of severe outcomes if adequate and timely nutrition support is not provided [9].

The correct type of nutritional support for each patient in a delicate and fragile context such as that of COVID-intensive care unit is as important as the correct timing with which this is carried out.

22.3 Timing and Route of Nutrition Delivery

The correct nutritional assessment has to be followed by an early and patient-tailored nutrition delivery. COVID-19 is more likely to affect severely old patients and to be associated with comorbidities thus leading to long ICU stay. Despite placing a nasogastric tube exposes healthcare personnel at higher risk of SARS-CoV2 transmission, EN is preferable to PN if no contraindications are present. As several studies reported that early EN reduces infections and mortality compared to delayed or withheld EN provision, EN should be started within 24–36 h of the admission to the ICU or within 12 h of the placement on mechanical ventilation [14, 15].

If intolerance to gastric EN is encountered, prokinetic agents are recommended as first approach, followed by post-pyloric EN in case of therapeutic failure. Once an enteral feeding tube is placed, continuous rather than bolus EN is then recommended because of the lower risk to develop diarrhea and to expose the healthcare personnel to SARS-CoV-2 [16].

In case of refractory enteral feeding intolerance, high risk patients should be switched to PN. Early PN is also recommended in case of rising lactate levels and hemodynamic instability with high dose of vasopressors, while it could be postponed up to 7 days in patients with lower risk [14].

However, Patel et al. demonstrated that EN at trophic rate is well tolerated in patients with circulatory shock or sepsis when escalation of vasopressors is not required [17]. Moreover, in patients with severe COVID-19 PN might be preferred to EN due to the development of GI manifestations and the higher risk of bowel ischemia [18].

In case of hypoxemia refractory to mechanical ventilation, prone position could be necessary in order to ameliorate both oxygenation and bronchial clearance [19].

Several studies demonstrated EN in prone position is safe and therefore it should be started early [20, 21].

22.4 Dose and Formula Selection

Feeding should be started with trophic EN and slowly increased to reach about 75% of the caloric goal that is about 15–20 kcal/kg Adjust Body Weight (ABW)/day and protein 1.2–2.0 g/kg ABW/day. The caloric threshold should be further adjusted for BMI > 30 [22].

Glucose and propofol administration should be also taken into account as uncalculated nonnutrient calories.

It is important to assess the risk of refeeding syndrome, which is high in ICU patients with severe COVID-19. In these patients is suggested to start cautiously with about 25% of the caloric goal and to assess the potassium, magnesium and phosphate serum level particularly within the first 72 h.

Triglycerides levels should be monitored in patients receiving PN and propofol, keeping in mind that severe increase of TGs might be due to secondary hemophagolymphocytic histiocytosis (HLH).

An isosmotic enteral formulation with high energy density (>1.25 kcal/mL) and high protein content (>20% protein) is generally recommended in the early phase, with a more concentrated formulation recommended for restrictive fluid management. Moreover, withholding soybean lipids from PN is recommended, whereas preliminary data from animal studies showed benefit in immune modulation helping clearance of viral infection for fish oil containing formulations [23]. Similarly, based on results from animal studies about the role of ketogenic diet on antiviral resistance against influenza A virus, a recent retrospective study by Sukkar et al. shows how a ketogenic nutrition is able to support drug therapy in improving prognosis in COVID-19 patients [24]. However, there are no strong evidence to support their routinely use, yet.

Fibers could be added in a later phase if no GI manifestations are present. In addition, nutritional supplements, such as niacin and folic acid, are suggested in postacute patients with Covid-19 in order to intervene and improve the muscle and the cardiovascular functions that are often impaired in the so-called "post-Covid-19 chronic illness" [25].

Among nonintubated critically ill patients who suffer from dyspnea, tachypnea, fatigue, poor appetite, and dysphagia several guidelines recommend that a high energy and protein diet with oral nutrition supplements should be provided [7, 26, 27]. Moving to enteral nutrition should be considered when energy and protein targets are not met after 5 days of oral nutrition.

In conclusion, as showed above, ICU COVID-19 patients are at higher nutritional risk. This is strictly linked to worse prognosis and poorer outcomes. Thus, rapid assessment, correct timing, route, and type of nutrition are crucial, even if probably underestimated, in the management of severely and critically ill COVID-19 patients.

References

1. Wiersinga WJ, Rhodes A, Cheng AC, Peacock SJ, Prescott HC. Pathophysiology, transmission, diagnosis, and treatment of coronavirus disease 2019 (COVID-19): a review. JAMA. 2020;324(8):782–93.
2. Wu C, Chen X, Cai Y, Xia J, Zhou X, Xu S, et al. Risk factors associated with acute respiratory distress syndrome and death in patients with coro-

navirus disease 2019 pneumonia in Wuhan, China. JAMA Intern Med. 2020;180(7):934–43.
3. Barazzoni R, Bischoff SC, Breda J, Wickramasinghe K, Krznaric Z, Nitzan D, et al. ESPEN expert statements and practical guidance for nutritional management of individuals with SARS-CoV-2 infection. Clin Nutr. 2020;39(6):1631–8.
4. Gomes F, Schuetz P, Bounoure L, Austin P, Ballesteros-Pomar M, Cederholm T, et al. ESPEN guidelines on nutritional support for polymorbid internal medicine patients. Clin Nutr. 2018;37(1):336–53.
5. Eden T, McAuliffe S. Critical care nutrition and COVID-19: a cause of malnutrition not to be underestimated. BMJ Nutr Prev Health. 2021;4(1):342.
6. Lew CCH, Yandell R, Fraser RJL, Chua AP, Chong MFF, Miller M. Association between malnutrition and clinical outcomes in the intensive care unit: a systematic review [formula: see text]. JPEN J Parenter Enteral Nutr. 2017;41(5):744–58.
7. Chapple LAS, Tatucu-Babet OA, Lambell KJ, Fetterplace K, Ridley EJ. Nutrition guidelines for critically ill adults admitted with COVID-19: is there consensus? Clin Nutr Espen. 2021;44:69–77.
8. Thibault R, Seguin P, Tamion F, Pichard C, Singer P. Nutrition of the COVID-19 patient in the intensive care unit (ICU): a practical guidance. Crit Care. 2020;24(1):447.
9. Thomas S, Alexander C, Cassady BA. Nutrition risk prevalence and nutrition care recommendations for hospitalized and critically-ill patients with COVID-19. Clin Nutr Espen. 2021;44:38–49.
10. Silva DFO, Lima S, Sena-Evangelista KCM, Marchioni DM. Nutritional risk screening tools for older adults with COVID-19: a systematic review. Nutrients. 2020;12(10):2956.
11. Bedock D, Bel Lassen P, Mathian A, Moreau P, Couffignal J, Ciangura C, et al. Prevalence and severity of malnutrition in hospitalized COVID-19 patients. Clin Nutr Espen. 2020;40:214–9.
12. Evans DC, Corkins MR, Malone A. The use of visceral proteins as nutrition markers: an ASPEN position paper. Nutr Clin Pract. 2021;36(1):22–8.
13. Liu W, Tao ZW, Wang L, Yuan ML, Liu K, Zhou L, et al. Analysis of factors associated with disease outcomes in hospitalized patients with 2019 novel coronavirus disease. Chin Med J (Engl). 2020;133(9):1032–8.
14. McClave SA, Taylor BE, Martindale RG, Warren MM, Johnson DR, Braunschweig C, et al. Guidelines for the provision and assessment of nutrition support therapy in the adult critically ill patient: Society of Critical Care Medicine (SCCM) and American Society for Parenteral and Enteral Nutrition (A.S.P.E.N.). JPEN J Parenter Enteral Nutr. 2016;40(2):159–211.
15. Taylor BE, McClave SA, Martindale RG, Warren MM, Johnson DR, Braunschweig C, et al. Guidelines for the provision and assessment of

nutrition support therapy in the adult critically ill patient: Society of Critical Care Medicine (SCCM) and American Society for Parenteral and Enteral Nutrition (A.S.P.E.N.). Crit Care Med. 2016;44(2):390–438.
16. Singer P, Blaser AR, Berger MM, Alhazzani W, Calder PC, Casaer MP, et al. ESPEN guideline on clinical nutrition in the intensive care unit. Clin Nutr. 2019;38(1):48–79.
17. Patel JJ, Rice T, Heyland DK. Safety and outcomes of early enteral nutrition in circulatory shock. JPEN J Parenter Enteral Nutr. 2020;44(5):779–84.
18. Pan L, Mu M, Yang P, Sun Y, Wang R, Yan J, et al. Clinical characteristics of COVID-19 patients with digestive symptoms in Hubei, China: a descriptive, cross-sectional, multicenter study. Am J Gastroenterol. 2020;115(5):766–73.
19. Guérin C, Reignier J, Richard JC, Beuret P, Gacouin A, Boulain T, et al. Prone positioning in severe acute respiratory distress syndrome. N Engl J Med. 2013;368(23):2159–68.
20. Saez de la Fuente I, Saez de la Fuente J, Quintana Estelles MD, Garcia Gigorro R, Terceros Almanza LJ, Sanchez Izquierdo JA, et al. Enteral nutrition in patients receiving mechanical ventilation in a prone position. JPEN J Parenter Enteral Nutr. 2016;40(2):250–5.
21. van der Voort PH, Zandstra DF. Enteral feeding in the critically ill: comparison between the supine and prone positions: a prospective crossover study in mechanically ventilated patients. Crit Care. 2001;5(4):216–20.
22. Martindale R, Patel JJ, Taylor B, Arabi YM. Nutrition therapy in critically ill patients with Coronavirus Disease 2019. J Parenter Enteral Nutr. 2020;44(7):1174–84.
23. Baillie JK, Digard P. Influenza—time to target the host? N Engl J Med. 2013;369(2):191–3.
24. Sukkar SG, Cogorno L, Pisciotta L, Pasta A, Vena A, Gradaschi R, et al. Clinical efficacy of eucaloric ketogenic nutrition in the COVID-19 cytokine storm: a retrospective analysis of mortality and intensive care unit admission. Nutrition. 2021;89:111236.
25. Mohammadpour H, MacDonald CR, Qiao G, Chen M, Dong B, Hylander BL, et al. β2 Adrenergic receptor-mediated signaling regulates the immunosuppressive potential of myeloid-derived suppressor cells. J Clin Investig. 2019;129(12):5537–52.
26. Chapple LS, Fetterplace K, Asrani V, Burrell A, Cheng AC, Collins P, et al. Nutrition management for critically and acutely unwell hospitalised patients with coronavirus disease 2019 (COVID-19) in Australia and New Zealand. Nutr Diet. 2020;77(4):426–36.
27. Cena H, Maffoni S, Braschi V, Brazzo S, Pallavicini C, Vietti I, et al. Position paper of the Italian association of medical specialists in dietetics and clinical nutrition (ANSISA) on nutritional management of patients with COVID-19 disease. Mediterr J Nutr Metab. 2020;13:113–7.

Part VIII

Principles of Therapy

Sedation, Analgesia, and Myorelaxants

23

Giselle Carvalho de Sousa,
Pedro Leme Silva,
and Patricia Rieken Macedo Rocco

Patients with severe acute respiratory distress syndrome due to coronavirus (SARS-CoV-2) who need sedation represent a challenge in the intensive care unit (ICU). Although improvement in overall gas exchange is an important goal, there is also the need to adapt the patient during mechanical ventilation (MV). Therefore, it is important to obtain deep sedation to promote comfort during MV and minimize ventilator-induced lung injury. However, a deeper anesthesia plan can be harmful, favoring delirium, hemodynamic instability, difficulty in weaning from MV, abstinence syndrome, propofol infusion syndrome (PRIS), and increasing the consumption of anesthetics in a pandemic situation when there may be a shortage of sedatives [1, 2].

G. C. de Sousa (✉)
Laboratory of Pulmonary Investigation, Carlos Chagas Filho Biophysics Institute, Federal University of Rio de Janeiro, Centro de Ciências da Saúde, Rio de Janeiro, RJ, Brazil

Department of Anesthesiology, Federal University of Rio de Janeiro, Rio de Janeiro, RJ, Brazil

P. L. Silva · P. R. M. Rocco
Laboratory of Pulmonary Investigation, Carlos Chagas Filho Biophysics Institute, Federal University of Rio de Janeiro, Centro de Ciências da Saúde, Rio de Janeiro, RJ, Brazil

D. Battaglini, P. Pelosi (eds.), *COVID-19 Critical and Intensive Care Medicine Essentials*, https://doi.org/10.1007/978-3-030-94992-1_23

Patients with SARS-CoV-2 seem to need higher doses to achieve analgesia and sedation compared with classic acute respiratory distress syndrome due to younger age and good health, high respiratory drive, and intense inflammatory responses (linked to tolerance mechanisms) [3, 4].

Deep sedation associated with or without myorelaxants suppresses the ventilatory drive, which favors adaptation to MV and promotes hypercapnia tolerance due to low tidal volume in patients with SARS-CoV-2 [5]. It can also reduce the risk of patient self-extubation, mainly in the prone position, and avoid environmental exposure to new coronavirus [4]. On the other hand, because lung compliance is normal initially, and the ventilatory drive may not be altered (even when hypoxemic most of the time, patients do not have tachypnea), it may not be necessary to use deep sedation in all cases. In addition, it is well know that pain assessment and control in mechanically ventilated patients is independently associated with a reduction in the duration of ventilatory support and ICU stay, in addition to reduced risk of delirium [6, 7]. This may be related to a restricted use of hypnotics when pain is assessed [6]. Therefore, recent guidelines recommend the need for individualization of sedation and analgesia, adjustable over time, reaching the lightest level of sedation (i.e., a Richmond Agitation Sedation Scale [RASS] score between 2 and +1) and prioritizing pain control, which means obtaining a Behavioral Pain Scale score <5 at rest and during nociceptive procedures [1, 6, 8, 9]. This sedation plan can be achieved with propofol or continuous infusion of dexmedetomidine (0.5–1.4 μg/kg/h, without bolus), in combination with opioid and nonopioid analgesics (acetaminophen, nefopam) [1, 5].

For patients with SARS-CoV-2 on MV, Payen et al. [5] suggested a flowchart for the choice of anesthetic as shown in Fig. 23.1, depending on the ventilatory mode and patient's clinical condition. For instance, during pressure-support ventilation, deep sedation is not needed; opioids in association with other drugs are used in cases of severe pain or persistent dyspnea despite adjusting the ventilator settings. In patients with SARS-CoV-2 with low lung compliance, ventilator asynchrony, incoercible cough, or agitation (RASS +2 to +4) despite optimization of ven-

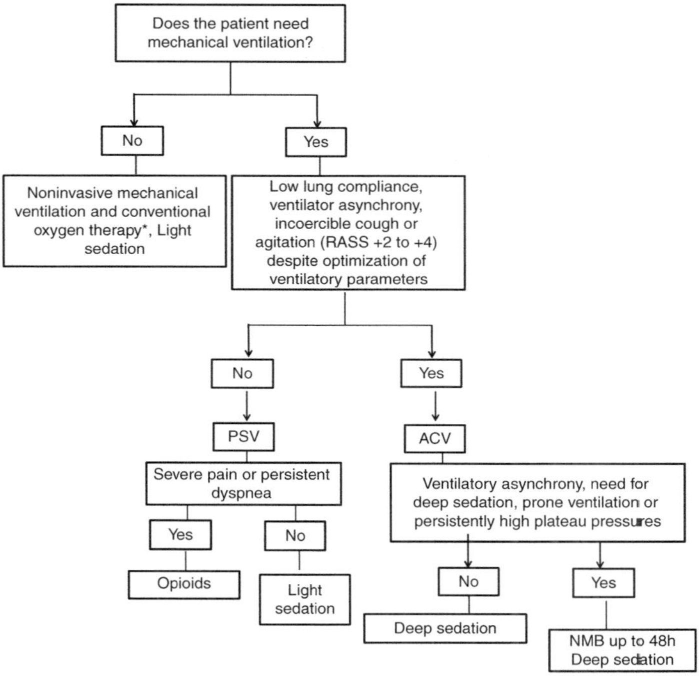

Fig. 23.1 Flowchart for the choice of anesthetic. *ACV* assisted controlled ventilation, *NMB* neuromuscular blocking, *PSV* pressure support ventilation, *RASS* Richmond Agitation Sedation Scale. (Adapted from Payen et al. [5])

tilatory parameters, it is necessary to offer a higher level of analgesia, sedation, and anxiolysis.

Propofol, a short-acting and titratable drug with a good pharmacokinetic profile, can be used as a sedative, allowing for easy management and less time to wake up compared with benzodiazepines, in addition to deeper sedation than dexmedetomidine. A disadvantage of using propofol is the risk of PRIS, a rare complication with high mortality. PRIS may occur after a prolonged period under MV (more than 48 h), as well as with the use of doses >5 mg/kg/h [10]. It can also cause hypotension secondary to a reduction in vascular sympathetic tone [11]. Benzodiazepines are an alternative for patients with SARS-CoV-2 who need prolonged sedation to avoid hypotension. The potential disadvantage is accumulation due to its pharmacokinetic profile, as well as withdrawal syndrome after sudden interruption, characterized by anxiety and panic, usually accompanied by tachycardia, arterial hypertension, and hyperthermia [12]. Gradual withdrawal of benzodiazepines can prevent such symptoms [12]. There is also a risk of delirium and psychomotor agitation, especially in the elderly [13, 14]. The use of halogenates, such as sevoflurane and isoflurane, in ICU is a good option, mainly due to the ease of use, and because they do not cause tachyphylaxis [5]. An effective concentration in the brain is achieved quickly, and dosage adjustment is simple based on clinical manifestations. They are also bronchodilators, with a good profile in patients with SARS-CoV-2 who have a background history of asthma or chronic obstructive pulmonary disease [15]. Compared with propofol or midazolam, sevoflurane did not show adverse hepatic or renal events, in addition to decreased awakening and extubation times, less morphine consumption after extubation, and even increased the quality of awakening [16]. In contrast, they are cardiovascular depressants and sensitize the myocardium to the effects of catecholamines, which can cause arrhythmias [17, 18]. Moreover, team training is required on the use of sevoflurane, and the delivery method involves a scavenging device [5]. Fentanyl and morphine are the first-line opioids for analgesia [5]. The ultrashort-acting opioids, sufentanil and alfentanil, are not commonly used in ICUs, but they can become options in situations of drug shortages [19]. They are 5–10 times more potent than fentanyl and can provide the necessary analgesia as well as an acceptable infusion volume, preserving the volume of patients who need high doses of opioids [19, 20]. Remifentanil can also be administered as a continuous infusion; the advantage is its context-sensitive half-life due to its metabolism by plasma esterase [21]. Nonetheless, progressive dose reduction is necessary to avoid withdrawal syndrome and pain due to the short half-life of remifentanil [22]. Apnea, bradycardia, and hypotension can also occur and, in patients without muscle relaxation, there is a risk of chest stiffness especially at the start of drug infusion and with high doses [23, 24]. Nonopioid analgesics, such as a low dose of ketamine (1–2 μg/kg/min) are also used, with the aim of sparing opioid use and improving analgesic effectiveness [1]. Intravenous lidocaine (1 mg/kg/h) can be used as a co-analgesic and to reduce incoercible coughing [1, 5].

In situations of persistent ventilatory asynchrony, the need for deep sedation, prone ventilation, or persistently high plateau pressures, continuous infusion of a neuromuscular blocker is necessary [5]. This should be used for a short period of up to 48 h [5]. It should be administered intermittently whenever possible for economic reasons and preferably with monitoring of neuromuscular block obtaining a train-of-four scan of 0–2, followed by reassessment of the need for muscle relaxation [5]. When placing the patient in the prone position, a muscle relaxant may be necessary.

Patients with severe SARS-CoV-2 can require prolonged sedation (often >2 weeks), which can lead to many side effects, such as drug accumulation and delirium (benzodiazepines), tolerance and tachyphylaxis (dexmedetomidine), hypertriglyceridemia and PRIS (propofol), QT interval prolongation (haloperidol), psychomimetic effects (ketamine), and hyperalgesia or opioid dependence (fentanyl, hydromorphone, remifentanil) [4]. The weaning process may be difficulty for several reasons, such as alteration of the ventilatory drive, asynchrony of the ventilator, frequent coughing, tolerance, and withdrawal syndrome [4, 5]. To limit excessive use of these drugs with prolonged MV, and even in the context of scarcity of resources, other drugs such as antipsychotics and alpha-2 agonists (clonidine, dexmedetomidine) are associated with these sedatives.

References

1. Devlin JW, Skrobik Y, Gelinas C, Needham DM, Slooter AJC, Pandharipande PP, et al. Clinical practice guidelines for the prevention and management of pain, agitation/sedation, delirium, immobility, and sleep disruption in adult patients in the ICU. Crit Care Med. 2018;46:e825–73.
2. Chanques G, Drouot X, Payen JF. 2008–2018: Ten years of gradual changes in the sedation guidelines for critically ill patients. Anaesth Crit Care Pain Med. 2018;37:509–11.

3. Kapp CM, Zaeh S, Niedermeyer S, Punjabi NM, Siddharthan T, Damarla M. The use of analgesia and sedation in mechanically ventilated patients with COVID-19 acute respiratory distress syndrome. Anesth Analg. 2020;131:e198–200.
4. Hanidziar D, Bittner EA. Sedation of mechanically ventilated COVID-19 patients: challenges and special considerations. Anesth Analg. 2020;131:e40–1.
5. Payen JF, Chanques G, Futier E, Velly L, Jaber S, Constantin JM. Sedation for critically ill patients with COVID-19: which specificities? One size does not fit all. Anaesth Crit Care Pain Med. 2020;39:341–3.
6. Payen JF, Bosson JL, Chanques G, Mantz J, Labarere J, Investigators D. Pain assessment is associated with decreased duration of mechanical ventilation in the intensive care unit: a post hoc analysis of the DOLOREA study. Anesthesiology. 2009;111:1308–16.
7. Shehabi Y, Bellomo R, Kadiman S, Ti LK, Howe B, Reade MC, et al. Sedation intensity in the first 48 hours of mechanical ventilation and 180-day mortality: a multinational prospective longitudinal cohort study. Crit Care Med. 2018;46:850–9.
8. Sessler CN, Gosnell MS, Grap MJ, Brophy GM, O'Neal PV, Keane KA, et al. The Richmond Agitation-Sedation Scale: validity and reliability in adult intensive care unit patients. Am J Respir Crit Care Med. 2002;166:1338–44.
9. Payen JF, Bru O, Bosson JL, Lagrasta A, Novel E, Deschaux I, et al. Assessing pain in critically ill sedated patients by using a behavioral pain scale. Crit Care Med. 2001;29:2258–63.
10. Hemphill S, McMenamin L, Bellamy MC, Hopkins PM. Propofol infusion syndrome: a structured literature review and analysis of published case reports. Br J Anaesth. 2019;122:448–59.
11. Devlin JW, Roberts RJ. Pharmacology of commonly used analgesics and sedatives in the ICU: benzodiazepines, propofol, and opioids. Crit Care Clin. 2009;25:431–49.
12. Arroyo-Novoa CM, Figueroa-Ramos MI, Puntillo KA. Opioid and benzodiazepine iatrogenic withdrawal syndrome in patients in the intensive care unit. AACN Adv Crit Care. 2019;30:353–64.
13. Dell'osso B, Lader M. Do benzodiazepines still deserve a major role in the treatment of psychiatric disorders? A critical reappraisal. Eur Psychiatry. 2013;28:7–20.
14. Cavallazzi R, Saad M, Marik PE. Delirium in the ICU: an overview. Ann Intensive Care. 2012;2:49.
15. Woods BD, Sladen RN. Perioperative considerations for the patient with asthma and bronchospasm. Br J Anaesth. 2009;103(Suppl 1):157–65.
16. Mesnil M, Capdevila X, Bringuier S, Trine PO, Falquet Y, Charbit J, et al. Long-term sedation in intensive care unit: a randomized comparison between inhaled sevoflurane and intravenous propofol or midazolam. Intensive Care Med. 2011;37:933–41.

17. Himmel HM. Mechanisms involved in cardiac sensitization by volatile anesthetics: general applicability to halogenated hydrocarbons? Crit Rev Toxicol. 2008;38:773–803.
18. De Hert SG. Volatile anesthetics and cardiac function. Semin Cardiothorac Vasc Anesth. 2006;10:33–42.
19. Ammar MA, Sacha GL, Welch SC, Bass SN, Kane-Gill SL, Duggal A, et al. Sedation, analgesia, and paralysis in COVID-19 patients in the setting of drug shortages. J Intensive Care Med. 2021;36:157–74.
20. Monk JP, Beresford R, Ward AS. A review of its pharmacological properties and therapeutic use. Drugs. 1988;36:286–313.
21. Michelsen LG, Hug CC Jr. The pharmacokinetics of remifentanil. J Clin Anesth. 1996;8:679–82.
22. Delvaux B, Ryckwaert Y, Van Boven M, De Kock M, Capdevila X. Remifentanil in the intensive care unit: tolerance and acute withdrawal syndrome after prolonged sedation. Anesthesiology. 2005;102:1281–2.
23. Videira RL, Cruz JR. Remifentanil in the clinical practice. Rev Bras Anestesiol. 2004;54:114–28.
24. Joshi GP, Warner DS, Twersky RS, Fleisher LA. A comparison of the remifentanil and fentanyl adverse effect profile in a multicenter phase IV study. J Clin Anesth. 2002;14:494–9.

24 Antibiotics, Antiretroviral, Corticosteroids, Other Therapies Against SARS-CoV-2

Dayene de Assis Fernandes Caldeira, Patricia Rieken Macedo Rocco, and Fernanda Ferreira Cruz

Pharmacological treatment for COVID-19 is still exclusively supportive [1]. Drugs have been tested based on the pathogenesis events, particularly considering the potential impact on? (1) the viral infection and replication cycle (early phase); and (2) the inflammatory response phase marked by a cytokine storm that leads to tissue damage [2, 3].

24.1 Antibiotics

Empirical therapy or prophylaxis with antibiotics is not effective for the treatment of COVID-19 and is associated with antimicrobial resistance (AMR) [4]. Bacterial coinfection is relatively

D. de Assis Fernandes Caldeira · P. R. M. Rocco · F. F. Cruz (✉)
Laboratory of Pulmonary Investigation, Carlos Chagas Filho Institute of Biophysics, Federal University of Rio de Janeiro, Centro de Ciências da Saúde, Ilha do Fundão, Rio de Janeiro, RJ, Brazil
e-mail: dayenecaldeira@biof.ufrj.br; ffcruz@biof.ufrj.br

D. Battaglini, P. Pelosi (eds.), *COVID-19 Critical and Intensive Care Medicine Essentials*, https://doi.org/10.1007/978-3-030-94992-1_24

infrequent in patients hospitalized with COVID-19 (6–9%) and is more common in critically ill patients [5]. Despite that, around 72% of patients with COVID-19 have received antibiotics even when not clinically indicated [5].

The use of antibiotics should be recommended for patients with suspected or confirmed severe COVID-19 only when clinical suspicion of bacterial infection exists based on clinical judgement, radiological findings and/or compatible laboratory markers [6]. The strategy is to follow the guidelines for antibacterial treatment of community-acquired pneumonia (CAP) [7, 8]. Guidelines also recommend assessing the presence of ventilator-associated pneumonia or hospital-acquired pneumonia (HAP) by running semiquantitative cultures on respiratory samples: spontaneous expectoration, sputum induction, nasotracheal suctioning in a patient who is unable to cooperate to produce a sputum sample, and endotracheal aspiration in a patient with HAP who subsequently requires mechanical ventilation [7]. Urinary pneumococcal antigen testing has been recommended for all patients and a positive result might support the diagnosis of bacterial coinfection to initiate the antibiotic therapy [8]. Antibiotic treatment in adults with clinically suspected and radiographically confirmed CAP should be initiated regardless of the initial serum procalcitonin level [9]. None of the diagnostic modalities (procalcitonin level, C-reactive protein level, or the Modified Clinical Pulmonary Infection Score) were of additional value compared with clinical criteria alone [7, 8]. The guidelines suggest that antibiotic treatment should be as short as possible (5–7 days) and should be followed by improvement in signs, symptoms, and inflammatory markers. Regimens depend on the severity of disease and epidemiological data. Amoxicillin is recommended as the first choice (oral, 750 mg every 8 h) for mild and moderate CAP and a second- or third-generation cephalosporin is recommended for patients with severe CAP [8, 10].

24.2 Antiviral Therapy

Several antiviral drugs have been proposed with potential to inhibit viral entry, viral membrane fusion and endocytosis, activity on 3-chymotrypsin-like protease (3CLpro), pivotal for the replication of SARS-CoV-2, and RNA-dependent RNA polymerase [11, 12]. Remdesivir is a nucleoside analogue that targets RNA-dependent polymerase and blocks viral RNA synthesis in a broad spectrum of viruses, including human coronaviruses [11, 13–15].

Clinical trials were conducted to evaluate the efficacy and safety of this therapeutic agent in patients hospitalized with COVID-19 [16, 17]. The multicentric, randomized, double-blind, placebo-controlled trial (ACTT-1) shed light on the effectiveness of remdesivir for patients hospitalized with moderate COVID-19 who required low-flow supplemental oxygen. Compared with supportive care, patients in the remdesivir group (intravenous, 200 mg loading dose on day 1, 100 mg maintenance dose on days 2–10 or until hospital discharge or death) presented a shorter time to recovery than those in the placebo group (median, 10 days vs. 15 days), length of initial hospital stay (median, 12 days vs. 17 days), and all-cause mortality (11.4% with remdesivir and 15.2% with placebo), with a low rate of adverse events similar to the placebo group [18].

However, the Interim WHO Solidary Trial, a multicentre and randomized mortality trial of four repurposed antiviral drugs—remdesivir (intravenous, 200 mg on day 0, 100 mg on days 1–9), hydroxychloroquine, lopinavir, and interferon beta-1a—demonstrated that no drug reduced mortality or reduced initiation of ventilation or hospitalization duration in patients hospitalized with COVID-19. It refuted early hopes, based on smaller or non-randomized studies, that this regimen would be efficient to treat SARS-CoV-2 infection [19]. The World Health Organization (WHO) has a conditional recommendation against the use of remdesivir for patients hospitalized with COVID-19 [6].

24.3 Anti-Inflammatory Therapy

24.3.1 Corticosteroids

A subgroup of patients with COVID-19 can develop a dysfunctional immune response with a massive cytokine release and increased levels of inflammatory markers, including C-reactive protein, ferritin, interleukin-1, and interleukin-6, leading to severe COVID-19 and organ failure [20, 21]. Thus, the use of glucocorticoids has been debated because they suppress gene expression of pro-inflammatory cytokines, linked to the severity of COVID-19 [22, 23]. They were initially recommended to be used in patients with COVID-19 with acute respiratory distress syndrome and refractory shock to mitigate the cytokine storm and reduce peripheral vasodilation [24–26].

The recommendation of dexamethasone for the treatment of patients with COVID-19 who needed supplemental oxygen to keep their oxygen saturation above 94% or those on mechanical ventilation was largely based on the RECOVERY trial (2104 patients), demonstrating lower mortality at 28 days, shorter duration of hospitalization, and greater probability of discharge alive within 28 days in the dexamethasone group (6 mg once daily, orally or intravenously for 10 days) compared with the standard care group [20]. Patients with COVID-19 who do not require oxygen support should not use steroids because a risk of worse outcomes has been implicated. If dexamethasone is not available, equivalent doses of other corticosteroids such as prednisone, methylprednisolone, or hydrocortisone may be used.

24.3.2 Tocilizumab

The positive correlation between higher levels of interleukin-6 in cases of severe COVID-19 and prediction of mechanical ventilation led to studies to understand possible outcomes after treatment with tocilizumab, an anti-interleukin-6 receptor monoclonal antibody approved for the treatment of multiple inflammatory diseases

[27–29]. Favourable results were found in observational studies and suggested that early treatment with tocilizumab is associated with a lower mortality rate and improved clinical outcome in patients critically ill with COVID-19 [30, 31].

A global, randomized, double-blind, placebo-controlled, phase 3 clinical trial, EMPACTA (Evaluating Minority Patients with Actemra, NCT04372186), treated non-mechanically ventilated patients with COVID-19 pneumonia with tocilizumab (8 mg/kg/body weight, to a maximum of 800 mg per dose) and observed a reduction in the likelihood of mechanical ventilation and death (from 19.3 to 12.0% on the cumulative proportion of patients at day 28) [32]. However, before or during the trial, (1) patients treated with tocilizumab received concomitant systemic glucocorticoids (80.3%) or antiviral therapy (78.7%); and (2) patients also received dexamethasone (55.4%) or remdesivir (52.6%) [32]. Thus, even though not yet recommended, these results suggest that tocilizumab may add to the potential benefit of antiviral treatment and glucocorticoids.

24.3.3 Other Immunomodulatory Therapies

Despite having the potential to reduce the inflammatory storm associated with COVID-19, other classes of target immune modulators, such as interleukin (IL)-1 inhibitors (e.g. anakinra), anti-IL-6 monoclonal antibodies (e.g. siltuximab), interferons (alfa or beta), and kinase inhibitors (e.g. acalabrutinib, ibrutinib, tofacitinib), have no reported findings or outcomes compared with placebo or standard care and cannot be recommended for the treatment of COVID-19, except in a clinical trial [6, 33].

24.4 Combined Therapy

Despite the use of remdesivir, there was a high rate of mortality demonstrating that treatment with an antiviral drug alone is not likely to be sufficient for all patients [8]. A double-blind, placebo-controlled trial (ATCC-2) involving eight countries demonstrated that the combination of the baricitinib with remdesivir was more effective in patients with moderate COVID-19 pneumonia compared with a combination of remdesivir and placebo. Treatment with baricitinib (4 mg daily dose, orally, for 14 days or until hospital discharge) plus remdesivir (in accordance with ATCC-1) reduced the median time to recovery and improved the clinical status [12]. Baricitinib is a Janus kinase (JAK) inhibitor with a powerful anti-inflammatory function, as a JAK-STAT signalling inhibitor, and is likely to be effective against the consequences of the increased levels of cytokines observed in people with COVID-19 [13].

The ACTT-2 and RECOVERY trials cannot be compared directly because of their different trial designs, and baricitinib and dexamethasone have important biological differences. Despite the fact that these two therapies have not been evaluated in clinical trials to define the better approach, dexamethasone demonstrates a reduction in mortality in the subgroup of patients receiving supplemental oxygen [20].

24.5 Other Therapies

24.5.1 COVID-19 Convalescent Plasma

Results suggest that high antibody titres may be more beneficial than low-titre plasma in non-intubated patients. The US Food and Drug Administration has issued an Emergency Use Authorization for the use of convalescent plasma for patients hospitalized with COVID-19. However, the lack of larger randomized trials, untreated control groups and studies with other large limitations do not permit a recommendation for or against the use of convalescent plasma, or establish its safety and efficacy [33].

24.5.2 Stem Cell Therapy

Mesenchymal stromal cells (MSCs) have been tested to reduce the inflammatory response and lung injury in SARS-CoV-2 infection, especially for their immunomodulatory properties [34]. Furthermore, the lack of angiotensin-converting enzyme 2 (ACE2) in MSCs, a receptor that SARS-CoV-2 uses for viral entry into cells, provided more resistance to infection [34, 35]. However, because of the lack of data to support the use of MSCs in patients who have viral infections, their use is not recommended for the treatment of COVID-19, except in a clinical trial [33].

24.6 Final Comments

The following speculative agents have not shown efficacy and are not recommended for treatment of COVID-19, except when administered in a clinical trial [6, 33]:

- Angiotensin-converting enzyme inhibitors or angiotensin II receptor blockers.
- Chloroquine or hydroxychloroquine with or without azithromycin.
- Ivermectin.
- Lopinavir/ritonavir.
- Nitazoxanide.
- Oseltamivir.
- Ribavirin.
- Vitamin C and D, and zinc.

There is no evidence that these agents are harmful when prescribed for the treatment of other conditions in patients with COVID-19. COVID-19 clinical trials conducted to date with antivirals are in shown in Table 24.1.

Table 24.1 Complete COVID-19 clinical trials conducted with antivirals

Antiviral drug	Mechanism of action	Clinical trial ID
Remdesivir	A nucleoside analogue blocks viral RNA synthesis in a broad spectrum of viruses [13, 14, 36], including in vitro activity against severe acute respiratory syndrome coronavirus 2 (SARS-CoV-2) [33]	NCT04292899, NCT04292730, NCT04280705, NCT04315948, NCT04257656, NCT04492501, NCT04409262, NCT04401579, NCT04492475, NCT04349410
Lopinavir/ritonavir	Acts by inhibiting coronavirus proteases, 3-chymotrypsin-like protease (3CLpro) and papain-like protease (PLpro), producing immature viruses [36]. Lopinavir has low bioavailability when administered alone. For this reason, ritonavir is widely co-formulated with lopinavir to increase its plasma half-life by strongly inhibiting cytochrome P450 3A4 (CYP3A4) and discreetly inhibiting CYP2D6 [36]	NCT04376814, NCT04343768, NCT04276688, NCT04386876
Oseltamivir	Inhibitor of neuraminidase enzymes, known to cleave sialic acid groups from glycoproteins and required for virus replication [37, 38]	NCT04338698
Favipiravir	Intracellularly, converts to its metabolite ribofuranosyl 5′-triphosphate (favipiravir-RTP), which can then be recognized as a pseudopurine by viral RNA-dependent RNA polymerase (RdRp) and incorporated in the viral RNA chain or act by binding to their polymerase domains, preventing viral RNA replication [39, 40]	NCT04542694, NCT04376814, NCT04349241

Table 24.1 (continued)

Antiviral drug	Mechanism of action	Clinical trial ID
Chloroquine or hydroxychloroquine with or without azithromycin	In vitro studies have suggested that chloroquine gathers in the endosomes and lysosomes and leads to pH neutralization, which hinders the effects of proteases, thus preventing S protein cleavage and, ultimately, the process of viral access into a host organism [41]. In vitro studies have suggested that both chloroquine and hydroxychloroquine may block the transport of SARS-CoV-2 from early endosomes to endolysosomes, possibly preventing the release of the viral genome [42]	NCT04332991, NCT04381936, NCT04322123, NCT04323527, NCT04308668, NCT04420247, NCT04338698, NCT04491994, NCT04331600, NCT04384380, NCT04391127, NCT04321278, NCT04788355, NCT04334148, NCT04358081, NCT04420247, NCT04342650, NCT04331834, NCT04333225, NCT04391127, NCT04261517, NCT04328961, NCT04652648, NCT04358068, NCT04334148, NCT04349592, NCT04408456, NCT04370782, NCT04321278, NCT04350281, NCT04322396, NCT04376814, NCT04746365, NCT04423991, NCT04446104, NCT04668469, NCT04354870, NCT04441424, NCT04347031, NCT04497519, NCT04461353, NCT04343768, NCT04349410

(continued)

Table 24.1 (continued)

Antiviral drug	Mechanism of action	Clinical trial ID
Ivermectin	In vitro studies suggest that ivermectin acts by inhibiting the host importin alpha/beta-1 nuclear transport proteins, which are part of a key intracellular transport process that viruses hijack to enhance infection by suppressing the host's antiviral response [43]. It may also interfere with attachment of the SARS-CoV-2 spike protein to the human cell membrane [44]	NCT04390022, NCT04391127, NCT04523831, NCT04646109, NCT04343092, NCT04422561, NCT04746365, NCT04668469, NCT04381884, NCT04405843, NCT04591600, NCT04391127, NCT04739410, NCT04407130, NCT04784481, NCT04701710, NCT04446104

References

1. Robba C, Battaglini D, Ball L, Patroniti N, Loconte M, Brunetti I, et al. Distinct phenotypes require distinct respiratory management strategies in severe COVID-19. Respir Physiol Neurobiol. 2020;279:103455.
2. Battaglini D, Robba C, Ball L, Cruz FF, Silva PL, Pelosi P, et al. Emerging therapies for COVID-19 pneumonia. Expert Opin Investig Drugs. 2020;29:633–7.
3. Tay MZ, Poh CM, Rénia L, MacAry PA, Ng LFP. The trinity of COVID-19: immunity, inflammation and intervention. Nat Rev Immunol. 2020;20:363–74.
4. Strathdee SA, Davies SC, Marcelin JR. Confronting antimicrobial resistance beyond the COVID-19 pandemic and the 2020 US election. Lancet. 2020;396:1050–3.
5. Langford BJ, So M, Raybardhan S, Leung V, Westwood D, MacFadden DR, et al. Bacterial co-infection and secondary infection in patients with COVID-19: a living rapid review and meta-analysis. Clin Microbiol Infect. 2020;26:1622–9.
6. World Health Organization. Clinical management of COVID-19: interim guidance, 27 May 2020. Geneva: World Health Organization; 2020.

7. Kalil AC, Metersky ML, Klompas M, Muscedere J, Sweeney DA, Palmer LB, et al. Management of adults with hospital-acquired and ventilator-associated pneumonia: 2016 clinical practice guidelines by the Infectious Diseases Society of America and the American Thoracic Society. Clin Infect Dis. 2016;63:e61–111.
8. Sieswerda E, de Boer MGJ, Bonten MMJ, Boersma WG, Jonkers RE, Aleva RM, et al. Recommendations for antibacterial therapy in adults with COVID-19—an evidence based guideline. Clin Microbiol Infect. 2021;27:61–6.
9. Metlay JP, Waterer GW, Long AC, Anzueto A, Brozek J, Crothers K, et al. Diagnosis and treatment of adults with community-acquired pneumonia. An official clinical practice guideline of the American Thoracic Society and Infectious Diseases Society of America. Am J Respir Crit Care Med. 2019;200:e45–67.
10. Wiersinga WJ, Bonten MJ, Boersma WG, Jonkers RE, Aleva RM, Kullberg BJ, et al. Management of community-acquired pneumonia in adults: 2016 guideline update from the Dutch Working Party on Antibiotic Policy (SWAB) and Dutch Association of Chest Physicians (NVALT). Neth J Med. 2018;76:4–13.
11. Sanders JM, Monogue ML, Jodlowski TZ, Cutrell JB. Pharmacologic treatments for coronavirus disease 2019 (COVID-19): a review. JAMA. 2020;323:1824–36.
12. Mody V, Ho J, Wills S, Mawri A, Lawson L, Ebert MCCJC, et al. Identification of 3-chymotrypsin like protease (3CLPro) inhibitors as potential anti-SARS-CoV-2 agents. Commun Biol. 2021;4:93.
13. Li G, De Clercq E. Therapeutic options for the 2019 novel coronavirus (2019-nCoV). Nat Rev Drug Discov. 2020;19:149–50.
14. Agostini ML, Andres EL, Sims AC, Graham RL, Sheahan TP, Lu X, et al. Coronavirus susceptibility to the antiviral remdesivir (GS-5734) is mediated by the viral polymerase and the proofreading exoribonuclease. MBio. 2018;9:e00221–18.
15. Sheahan TP, Sims AC, Graham RL, Menachery VD, Gralinski LE, Case JB, et al. Broad-spectrum antiviral GS-5734 inhibits both epidemic and zoonotic coronaviruses. Sci Transl Med. 2017;9:eaal3653.
16. Spinner CD, Gottlieb RL, Criner GJ, Arribas López JR, Cattelan AM, Soriano Viladomiu A, et al. Effect of remdesivir vs standard care on clinical status at 11 days in patients with moderate COVID-19: a randomized clinical trial. JAMA. 2020;324:1048–57.
17. Goldman JD, Lye DCB, Hui DS, Marks KM, Bruno R, Montejano R, et al. Remdesivir for 5 or 10 days in patients with severe Covid-19. N Engl J Med. 2020;383:1827–37.
18. Beigel JH, Tomashek KM, Dodd LE, Mehta AK, Zingman BS, Kalil AC, et al. Remdesivir for the treatment of Covid-19—final report. N Engl J Med. 2020;383:1813–26.

19. WHO Solidarity Trial Consortium, Pan H, Peto R, Henao-Restrepo A-M, Preziosi M-P, Sathiyamoorthy V, et al. Repurposed antiviral drugs for Covid-19—Interim WHO Solidarity Trial results. N Engl J Med. 2021;384:497–511.
20. RECOVERY Collaborative Group, Horby P, Lim WS, Emberson JR, Mafham M, Bell JL, et al. Dexamethasone in hospitalized patients with Covid-19—preliminary report. N Engl J Med. 2021;384:693–704.
21. Moore JB, June CH. Cytokine release syndrome in severe COVID-19. Science. 2020;368:473–4.
22. Zhong J, Tang J, Ye C, Dong L. The immunology of COVID-19: is immune modulation an option for treatment? Lancet Rheumatol. 2020;2:e428–36.
23. Ahmed MH, Hassan A. Dexamethasone for the treatment of coronavirus disease (COVID-19): a review. SN Compr Clin Med. 2020;2(12): 2637–46.
24. Alhazzani W, Møller MH, Arabi YM, Loeb M, Gong MN, Fan E, et al. Surviving sepsis campaign: guidelines on the management of critically ill adults with coronavirus disease 2019 (COVID-19). Crit Care Med. 2020;48:e440–69.
25. Mattos-Silva P, Felix NS, Silva PL, Robba C, Battaglini D, Pelosi P, et al. Pros and cons of corticosteroid therapy for COVID-19 patients. Respir Physiol Neurobiol. 2020;280:103492.
26. Wang Y, Jiang W, He Q, Wang C, Wang B, Zhou P, et al. A retrospective cohort study of methylprednisolone therapy in severe patients with COVID-19 pneumonia. Signal Transduct Target Ther. 2020;5:57.
27. Zhu J, Pang J, Ji P, Zhong Z, Li H, Li B, et al. Elevated interleukin-6 is associated with severity of COVID-19: a meta-analysis. J Med Virol. 2021;93:35–7.
28. Herold T, Jurinovic V, Arnreich C, Lipworth BJ, Hellmuth JC, von Bergwelt-Baildon M, et al. Elevated levels of IL-6 and CRP predict the need for mechanical ventilation in COVID-19. J Allergy Clin Immunol. 2020;146:128–36.
29. Aziz M, Fatima R, Assaly R. Elevated interleukin-6 and severe COVID-19: a meta-analysis. J Med Virol. 2020;92:2283–5.
30. Gupta S, Wang W, Hayek SS, Chan L, Mathews KS, Melamed ML, et al. Association between early treatment with tocilizumab and mortality among critically ill patients with COVID-19. JAMA Intern Med. 2021;181:41–51.
31. Xu X, Han M, Li T, Sun W, Wang D, Fu B, et al. Effective treatment of severe COVID-19 patients with tocilizumab. Proc Natl Acad Sci U S A. 2020;117:10970–5.
32. Salama C, Han J, Yau L, Reiss WG, Kramer B, Neidhart JD, et al. Tocilizumab in patients hospitalized with Covid-19 pneumonia. N Engl J Med. 2021;384:20–30.

33. COVID-19 Treatment Guidelines Panel. Coronavirus Disease 2019 (COVID-19) treatment guidelines. National Institutes of Health. https://www.covid19treatmentguidelines.nih.gov/. Accessed 23 Feb 2021.
34. Li N, Hua J. Interactions between mesenchymal stem cells and the immune system. Cell Mol Life Sci. 2017;74:2345–60.
35. Shetty AK. Mesenchymal stem cell infusion shows promise for combating coronavirus (COVID-19)-induced pneumonia. Aging Dis. 2020;11:462–4.
36. Uzunova K, Filipova E, Pavlova V, Vekov T. Insights into antiviral mechanisms of remdesivir, lopinavir/ritonavir and chloroquine/hydroxychloroquine affecting the new SARS-CoV-2. Biomed Pharmacother. 2020;131:110668.
37. Moscona A. Oseltamivir resistance—disabling our influenza defenses. N Engl J Med. 2005;353:2633–6.
38. Chow EJ, Doyle JD, Uyeki TM. Influenza virus-related critical illness: prevention, diagnosis, treatment. Crit Care. 2019;23:214.
39. Furuta Y, Komeno T, Nakamura T. Favipiravir (T-705), a broad spectrum inhibitor of viral RNA polymerase. Proc Jpn Acad Ser B Phys Biol. 2017;93:449–63.
40. Delang L, Abdelnabi R, Neyts J. Favipiravir as a potential countermeasure against neglected and emerging RNA viruses. Antiviral Res. 2018;153:85–94.
41. Satarker S, Ahuja T, Banerjee M, Dogra S, Agarwal T, Nampoothiri M. Hydroxychloroquine in COVID-19: potential mechanism of action against SARS-CoV-2. Curr Pharmacol Rep. 2020;6(5):203–11. https://doi.org/10.1007/s40495-020-00231-8.
42. Liu J, Cao R, Xu M, Wang X, Zhang H, Hu H, et al. Hydroxychloroquine, a less toxic derivative of chloroquine, is effective in inhibiting SARS-CoV-2 infection in vitro. Cell Discov. 2020;6:16.
43. Yang SN, Atkinson SC, Wang C, Lee A, Bogoyevitch MA, Borg NA, et al. The broad spectrum antiviral ivermectin targets the host nuclear transport importin $\alpha/\beta1$ heterodimer. Antiviral Res. 2020;177:104760.
44. Lehrer S, Rheinstein PH. Ivermectin docks to the SARS-CoV-2 spike receptor-binding domain attached to ACE2. In Vivo. 2020;34:3023–6.

Coagulation and Haemostasis

25

Nathane Santanna Felix,
Hugo C. Castro Faria Neto,
and Fernanda Ferreira Cruz

25.1 Introduction

A notable feature of coronavirus disease 2019 (COVID-19), caused by severe acute respiratory syndrome coronavirus (SARS-CoV-2), is the high emergence of pulmonary and extrapulmonary thrombosis observed in patients with severe disease. The incidence of venous thromboembolism (VTE) varies between 6 and 86% depending on the investigations performed, follow-up time documented, and thromboprophylactic regimens used; the prevalence ranges between 15 and 40%. These are important numbers, especially compared with the prevalence of VTE associated with non-COVID-19 diseases (5–30%) [1]. Thus, VTE is an important consideration in the management of patients hospitalized with COVID-19 [2].

N. S. Felix (✉) · F. F. Cruz
Laboratory of Pulmonary Investigation, Institute of Biophysics Carlos Chagas Filho, Federal University of Rio de Janeiro, Rio de Janeiro, Brazil

Hugo C. Castro Faria Neto
Laboratory of Immunopharmacology, Oswaldo Cruz Institute, Fiocruz, Rio de Janeiro, Brazil

D. Battaglini, P. Pelosi (eds.), *COVID-19 Critical and Intensive Care Medicine Essentials*, https://doi.org/10.1007/978-3-030-94992-1_25

SARS-CoV-2 infects monocytes and endothelial cells, leading to a complex downstream cascade, cytokine storm, and eventual intravascular thrombosis [3]. Extensive crosstalk exists between the coagulation and immune systems, with both working together to provide effective host defence. This, activation of the coagulation system is an integral part of the immune response to infection; a dysregulated immune response leads to overactivation of the coagulation system, which can progress to disseminated intravascular coagulation and multi-organ failure [1]. Under physiological conditions, the body's fibrinolytic components are kept in a state of balance between the profibrinolytic and the antifibrinolytic factors. In COVID-19, an abnormal fibrinolytic balance is one of the players in its coagulopathy [4].

Aiming at better management of COVID-19 coagulopathy, the prompt recognition of haemostasis and coagulation disorders is essential. During hospitalization, treatment should be individualized according to laboratory test results and clinical status [5].

COVID-19-associated coagulopathy is characterized by features of coagulation that mimic disseminated intravascular coagulation (DIC) but differs from sepsis-related DIC by less prominent thrombocytopaenia and lower consumption of coagulation factors; clinical and pathological signs of thrombotic microangiopathy; and increased D-dimer levels that are predictive of unfavourable prognosis [6].

Increased D-dimer levels are associated with the need for hospitalization and admission to the intensive care unit (ICU), reflecting the severity of disease and predicting outcomes. Prothrombin time (PT) was found to be modestly prolonged at admission in non-survivors and in patients requiring ICU admission, but not in those not requiring ICU admission [7]. Given the associations between coagulation test results and patient outcomes, routine measurement of D-dimer, PT and platelet count are highly recommended in all patients with SARS-CoV-2 infection to identify those at higher risk of adverse outcome, including a worsening coagulopathy [1].

Conventional tests to diagnose VTE and pulmonary embolism (PE), such as Doppler ultrasonography and angiotomography, became difficult to perform in patients with COVID-19 due to the risk of infection, the need to minimize contact with health care workers, and the instability of critically ill patients hospitalized with COVID-19, especially in the ICU [2].

Prophylactic anticoagulation is vital in patients hospitalized with COVID-19. The disease can cause both arterial and venous thromboses, especially PE and pulmonary microthrombi. A high index of suspicion is indispensable in recognizing these complications, and timely institution of therapeutic anticoagulation is vital in pursuit of a better outcome [3]. The risks/benefits of anticoagulation should be reassessed at each step of treatment, especially after discharge, considering the risk of haemorrhage and the patient's clinical status and clinical events (such as PE, venous thrombosis, local bleeding, and haemorrhagic shock) [5].

Currently, clinical trials are ongoing to fully elucidate the pathways associated with COVID-19 hypercoagulable state, determine optimal doses of anticoagulation therapies, and study other treatment modalities. In the meantime, general guidelines for anticoagulation have been put in place by societies such as the American Society of Hematology (ASH) and the International Society of Thrombosis and Haemostasis (ISTH), with room for modifications to suit the needs of specific institutions [8].

25.2 Thromboprophylaxis

Critically ill hospitalized patients, including those with viral infections such as COVID-19 pneumonia, are at increased risk for VTE due to a combination of risk factors, including immobilization, indwelling catheters, mechanical ventilation and inflammation [1]. Given the relatively high rates of VTE found in early reports, the use of a "universal" thromboprophylactic strategy for all patients hospitalized with COVID-19 appears more appropriate than an individualized VTE risk assessment approach at present. Antithrombotic practice guidelines recommend thromboprophylaxis with twice or thrice daily subcutaneous unfractionated heparin (UFH), once daily subcutaneous low-molecular-weight heparin (LMWH) or fondaparinux to reduce this risk [2].

All patients hospitalized with COVID-19 should be considered for thromboprophylaxis with either UFH or LMWH unless there are absolute contraindications. Advantages of LMWH over UFH include once daily versus twice or thrice daily injections and less heparin-induced thrombocytopenia. In patients who show renal impairment, UFH is preferred over LMWH. Routine thromboprophylaxis with a prophylactic dose of UFH or LMWH should be used after careful assessment of bleed risk. An intermediate dose of LMWH (50% of respondents) can also be considered in high-risk patients [2]. For patients with active bleeding, or in whom anticoagulant therapy is contraindicated for other reasons, mechanical thromboprophylaxis, preferably with intermittent pneumatic compression devices, should be utilized, although there is limited evidence of efficacy in hospitalized medically ill patients [2, 5]. In cases of suspicion of heparin-induced thrombocytopenia, oral anticoagulants should be used. Danaparoid, argatroban, or bivalirudin may be preferred over rivaroxaban or fondaparinux [5].

One other possibility that is currently under investigation is the use of novel oral anticoagulants (NOACs; e.g. edoxaban, betrixaban, and apixaban), which are direct factor Xa inhibitors. In addition, these drugs may have direct antiviral effects providing an additional benefit in the case of patients with COVID-19. Apixaban presented higher theoretical affinity for SARS-CoV-2 main protease (Mpro; 7.0 kcal/mol) than for factor Xa (5.1 kcal/mol) [9]. Mpro activity is of vital importance for viral replication, and its inhibition is being target as an antiviral strategy. This finding highlights the potential of NOACs as a weapon against widespread hypercoagulability syndrome, but also as antiviral therapies preventing viral replication by inhibiting Mpro within the host cells or when it is released from infected damaged cells.

The risk of hospital-associated VTE extends for up to 6 weeks after hospital discharge in medically ill patients at high risk of VTE, including those with pneumonia, sepsis, and any condition requiring management in an ICU setting. It is reasonable to consider extended-duration thromboprophylaxis with LMWH or a direct oral anticoagulant (DOAC) for at least 2 weeks and up to 6 weeks after hospital discharge in selected patients with COVID-19 who are at low risk for bleeding and with key VTE risk factors such as advanced age, stay in the ICU, cancer, a previous history of VTE, thrombophilia, severe immobility or high D-dimer levels [2].

Although the ISTH guidance recommends LMWH prophylaxis, it is important to take the use of UFH into consideration in patients with risk of renal failure, and the existence of the UFH protamine sulphate antidote [10]. Some institutional protocols provide more aggressive anticoagulation with an intermediate or even therapeutic dose of anticoagulation for all patients with COVID-19 admitted to the ICU [11].

25.3 Treatment of COVID-19-Associated Coagulation

Hospitalized patients with confirmed VTE or PE should be given a therapeutic dose of anticoagulation, unless contraindicated [11]. It is important to note the advantages of LMWH in the inpatient setting and DOACs after hospital discharge, and the need to make the transition from parenteral to oral medication during hospitalization, especially for patients in critical care settings or with relevant concomitant medications, and dependent on renal function and platelet counts. Anticoagulant regimens should not change based solely on D-dimer levels [2].

Due to the difficulty with diagnostic tests, a change in anticoagulant regimen (i.e. from a prophylactic or intermediate dose to a therapeutic regimen) can be considered in patients without established VTE but with deteriorating pulmonary status or acute respiratory distress syndrome.

Preliminary reports have suggested that treatment with LMWH reduces mortality in patients with COVID-19 with an increased D-dimer level or increased sepsis-induced coagulopathy score [12].

25.4 Haemostasis

The main risk factors for bleeding are the use of antiplatelet drugs, anticoagulation, and underlying vascular lesions. A recent report of major bleeding in anticoagulated patients with macrothrombosis prompted caution in using therapeutic doses of heparin and recommended close monitoring [4].

Bleeding does not appear to be a major manifestation of COVID-19, but patients may have bleeding for other reasons, including trauma and/or treatment with anticoagulation drugs. If it occurs, treatment is similar to that for non-COVID-19 patients and may include transfusions, anticoagulant reversal or discontinuation, or haemoderivates for underlying bleeding disorders [11]. Importantly, all anticoagulants have associated risks of bleeding, which should be weighed against the clinical antithrombotic benefit. This risk should be considered on a patient-by-patient basis, taking into account potential coagulopathies and renal insufficiency [10].

25.5 Conclusion

Patients with COVID-19 present increased incidence of coagulopathy, but at the same time, there are difficulties in diagnosing VTE or PE. Thus, it is necessary to establish routine thromboprophylaxis and treatment, as well as identification of bleeding and haemostasis. In this context, biomarkers such as D-dimer, PT, and platelet count are used to predict the risk of thrombus formation.

All patients hospitalized with COVID-19 require thromboprophylaxis, preferably with LMWH. UFH should be used in cases of renal disfunction. Pharmacological prophylaxis should only be avoided when contraindicated. In this case, intermittent pneumatic compression should be adopted.

Treatment should be started immediately VTE or PE is diagnosed. In cases of sudden deterioration of lung function, PE should be suspected and the prophylactic dose increased to a therapeutic dose. Finally, the risk of haemorrhage should be evaluated before its use to avoid this complication.

References

1. Waite AAC, Hamilton DO, Pizzi R, Ageno W, Welters ID. Hypercoagulopathy in severe COVID-19: implications for acute care. Thromb Haemost. 2020;120:1654–67.

2. Spyropoulos AC, Levy JH, Ageno W, Connors JM, Hunt BJ, Iba T, et al. Scientific and Standardization Committee Communication: clinical guidance on the diagnosis, prevention, and treatment of venous thromboembolism in hospitalized patients with COVID-19. J Thromb Haemost. 2020;18:1859–65.
3. Rahi MS, Jindal V, Reyes SP, Gunasekaran K, Gupta R, Jaiyesimi I. Hematologic disorders associated with COVID-19: a review. Ann Hematol. 2021;100:309–20.
4. Robba C, Battaglini D, Ball L, Valbusa A, Porto I, Della Bona R, et al. Coagulative disorders in critically ill COVID-19 patients with acute distress respiratory syndrome: a critical review. J Clin Med. 2021;10:140.
5. Kwaan HC. The central role of fibrinolytic response in trauma-induced coagulopathy: a hematologist's perspective. Semin Thromb Hemost. 2020;46:116–24.
6. Mazilu L, Katsiki N, Nikolouzakis TK, Aslanidis MI, Lazopoulos G, Kouretas D, et al. Thrombosis and haemostasis challenges in COVID-19—therapeutic perspectives of heparin and tissue-type plasminogen activator and potential toxicological reactions—a mini review. Food Chem Toxicol. 2021;148:111974.
7. Tang N, Li D, Wang X, Sun Z. Abnormal coagulation parameters are associated with poor prognosis in patients with novel coronavirus pneumonia. J Thromb Haemost. 2020;18:844–7.
8. Salabei JK, Fishman TJ, Asnake ZT, Ali A, Iyer UG. COVID-19 coagulopathy: current knowledge and guidelines on anticoagulation. Heart Lung. 2021;50:357–60.
9. Biembengut ÍV, de Souza TACB. Coagulation modifiers targeting SARS-CoV-2 main protease Mpro for COVID-19 treatment: an in silico approach. Mem Inst Oswaldo Cruz. 2020;115:e200179.
10. Page EM, Ariëns RAS. Mechanisms of thrombosis and cardiovascular complications in COVID-19. Thromb Res. 2021;200:1–8.
11. Zanza C, Racca F, Longhitano Y, Piccioni A, Franceschi F, Artico M, et al. Risk management and treatment of coagulation disorders related to COVID-19 infection. Int J Environ Res Public Health. 2021;18:1268.
12. Lachant DJ, Lachant NA, Kouides P, Rappaport S, Prasad P, White RJ. Chronic therapeutic anticoagulation is associated with decreased thrombotic complications in SARS-CoV-2 infection. J Thromb Haemost. 2020;18:2640–5.

26 Rescue Therapies

Renata Mendes, Felipe Saddy, and Pedro Leme Silva

This chapter will discuss four rescue therapies—prone positioning, extracorporeal membrane oxygenation (ECMO) and CO_2 removal ($ECCO_2R$), inhaled nitric oxide (INO), and renal replacement therapy (RRT)—and their role in the management of critically ill patients with COVID-19.

R. Mendes (✉)
Laboratório de Produtos Naturais Bioativos (LPNB), Departamento de Bioquímica, Instituto de Ciências Biológicas, Universidade Federal de Juiz de Fora, Juiz de Fora, MG, Brazil

Nephrology Department, Rio de Janeiro State University, Rio de Janeiro, Brazil

Nephrology Department, Federal University of Rio de Janeiro, Rio de Janeiro, Brazil

F. Saddy
Ventilatory Intensive Care Unit, Hospital Copa D'Or, Rio de Janeiro, Brazil

General Intensive Care Unit, Hospital Pró-Cardiaco, Rio de Janeiro, Brazil

P. L. Silva
Laboratory of Pulmonary Investigation, Carlos Chagas Filho Institute of Biophysics, Federal University of Rio de Janeiro, Rio de Janeiro, Brazil

D. Battaglini, P. Pelosi (eds.), *COVID-19 Critical and Intensive Care Medicine Essentials*, https://doi.org/10.1007/978-3-030-94992-1_26

26.1 Prone Positioning

The first rationale to use prone position in COVID-19 patients is the dramatic improvement observed in oxygenation [1, 2]. Based on the relationship between hypoxemia and SARS-CoV-2 infection outcomes found in observational studies, prone positioning is very attractive for widespread use. The second rationale relies on the mechanisms by which oxygenation improves, which are attributable to a reduction in intrapulmonary shunt in the dorsal lung regions, which become nondependent in prone position. This phenomenon results from the increase in alveolar ventilation in the previously dorsal regions and maintenance of pulmonary blood flow [3], which promotes a more homogeneous distribution of lung aeration along a ventral-to-dorsal gradient. The third rationale is the ability of prone position to reduce or prevent ventilator-induced lung injury (VILI) [4]. Prone positioning in classical ARDS has been shown to reduce global lung stress and strain [5], expression of pro-inflammatory cytokines [6], the amount of overdistended lung areas [7], and the magnitude of the opening and closing phenomenon. The likely mechanism may again rely on homogeneous lung aeration [7]. The *P*ROSEVA trial [8] included 26 ICUs in France and Spain. In patients receiving protective ventilation (V_T 6 mL/kg PBW, $Pplat_{RS} < 31$ cmH_2O) and sedation holidays in preparation for weaning, prone positioning (for at least 16 h) reduced the relative risk of mortality by 50%.

Case Study

A 60-year-old female, RT-PCR positive for COVID-19, presented with an initial CT scan showing 50% compromised lung area with interstitial and alveolar infiltrates. Despite anticoagulation and corticosteroids, 13 days after symptom onset, she required endotracheal intubation. After 1 h on mechanical ventilation, the PaO_2/FiO_2 was 210 and the C_{RS} was 27 ml/cmH_2O. Protective mechanical ventilation settings were applied. After 7 days, gas exchange had deteriorated, with PaO_2/FiO_2 decreasing to 130 and a $PaCO_2$ of 67 mmHg. CT angiography of the chest showed no evidence of pulmonary thrombosis, but revealed extensive lung parenchymal injury (Fig. 26.1).

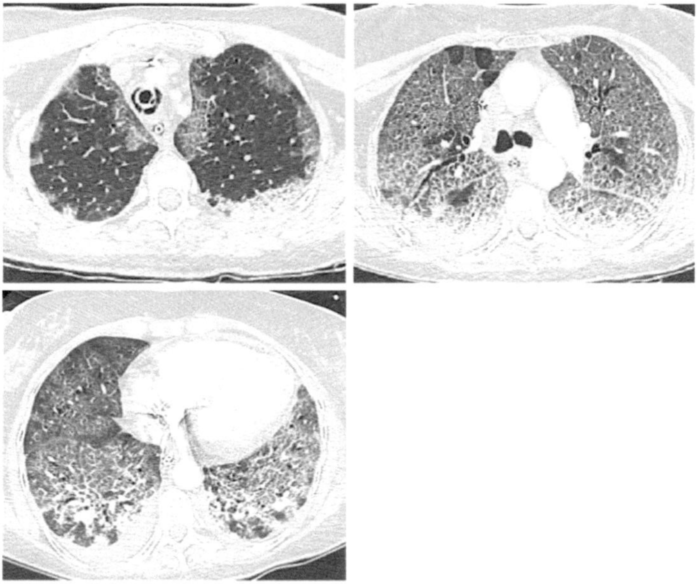

Fig. 26.1 Chest CT scan showing extensive bilateral ground-glass opacities and alveolar infiltrates

Since the PaO_2/FiO_2 was less than 150 and mechanical ventilation has been used for 7 days, prone positioning was indicated and implemented as a rescue therapy. After PEEP titration, V_T and ΔP_{RS} were adjusted and PaO_2/FiO_2 increased up to 350, followed by a decrease in $PaCO_2$ to 42 mmHg. The chest X-ray is shown in Fig. 26.2.

26.2 Extracorporeal Membrane Oxygenation (ECMO) and Extracorporeal CO_2 Removal ($ECCO_2R$)

During the COVID-19 pandemic, several cases of refractory hypoxemia and/or hypercapnia requiring extracorporeal lung support (ECLS) have been observed. Venovenous (VV) ECMO is the

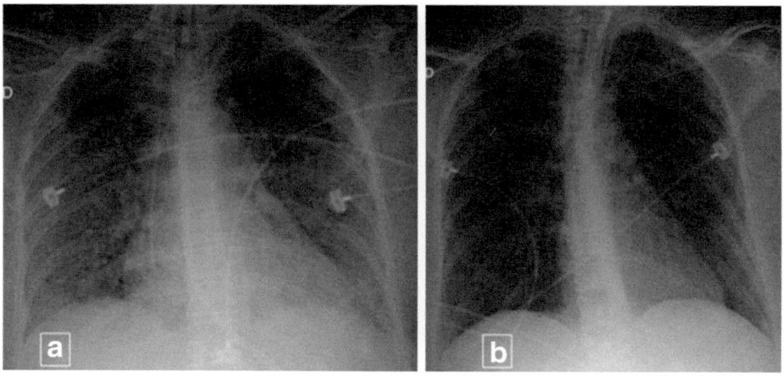

Fig. 26.2 Chest X-ray prior to prone positioning (**a**) and after 16 h in prone position (**b**). Prone positioning was done after PEEP titration and V_T and ΔP_{RS} adjustments. *V*/*Q* was adjusted and gas exchange improved. *PEEP* positive end-expiratory pressure, V_T tidal volume, *V*/*Q* ventilation–perfusion ratio

configuration of choice for patients with refractory hypoxemia. However, none of the four RCTs conducted to date demonstrated efficacy of routine application of ECLS in patients with classical ARDS as compared to conventional therapy [9, 10]. The Extracorporeal Life Support Organization (ELSO) guidelines (www.elso.org) suggest ECLS for patients with a predicted risk of mortality > 80%, identified by a $PaO_2/FIO_2 < 80$ mmHg when the FiO_2 is > 90% and a Murray score of 3–4. However, ECLS could also be considered in less severely ill hypoxemic patients, with a mortality risk > 50%, identified by $PaO_2/FIO_2 < 150$ mmHg when the FiO_2 is > 90% and a Murray score of 2–3.

$ECCO_2R$ represents a therapeutic approach for critical hypercapnia, which may precede the progression to refractory hypoxemia associated with critical respiratory acidosis. By reducing V_T and RR, $ECCO_2R$ may interrupt this vicious cycle related to dynamic hyperinflation and/or increased dead space, and reestablish appropriate oxygen delivery. Current indications suggested by the ELSO guidelines include CO_2 retention due to asthma or extreme hypercapnia associated with inability to achieve safe inflation pressures ($Pplat_{RS} \leq 30$ cmH_2O, as well as V_T and ΔP_{RS}) (www.elso.org). Table 26.1 lists typical characteristics for initiat-

Table 26.1 Triggers for initiation of ultraprotective ventilation in ARDS and of $ECCO_2R$ as rescue therapy [11]

Parameters	Trigger for ultraprotective ventilation	Trigger for $ECCO_2R$
ΔP_{RS} (cmH_2O)	>13–15	>15–20
P_{PLAT} (cmH_2O)	≥25	>30–35
$PaCO_2$ (mmHg)	≥60	≥60
pH	<7.25–7.30	<7.25–7.30
RR (bpm)	>20	>20–30
PaO_2/FiO_2 (mmHg)	<150	<150
PEEP (cmH_2O)	≥8	>8–15

ing $ECCO_2R$ as rescue therapy and to facilitate ultraprotective ventilation in ARDS, as discussed in a recently published consensus [11].

26.3 Inhaled Nitric Oxide (INO)

Nitric oxide (NO) is produced from arginine in a limited range of mammalian cells: neuronal (nNOS), endothelial (eNOS), and other cells expressing inducible nitric oxide synthase (iNOS) [12]. In endothelial cells, NO production is maintained by biophysical stimuli such as pulsatile flow and shear stress [13]. NO diffuses into adjacent vascular smooth muscle and decreases vascular tone in the systemic and pulmonary circulations. When administered exogenously by inhalation, it selectively dilates the pulmonary vasculature [14], improving the V/Q ratio.

Although there is no evidence to support the use of INO in COVID-19 patients, NO donation to SARS-CoV2 infected cells had an inhibitory effect on the virus protease, reducing viral replication [15]. NO-depleted vasculature exhibits persistent inflammation and impaired oxygen delivery and removal of toxic products, due to stagnation of blood flow into and out of hypoxic tissue [16]. Interestingly, NO generation by eNOS decreases with aging and in patients with important comorbidities, such as type 2 diabetes mellitus, the metabolic syndrome, chronic obstructive pulmonary disease, obesity, and hemoglobinopathies [17, 18]. This may explain at least in part why patients with these conditions have the highest risk of developing more severe COVID-19 and experiencing adverse outcomes.

As a therapy during the SARS epidemic of 2003, iNO at 30 ppm improved oxygenation in hypoxemic patients. In addition, a small randomized clinical study showed that iNO treatment improved oxygenation and allowed noninvasive pressure support to be discontinued in patients with severe classical ARDS [19]. Additional research in the specific context of COVID-19 is required.

26.4 Renal Replacement Therapy (RRT)

The incidence of acute kidney injury (AKI) in critically ill patients with COVID-19 [20] ranges from 4 to 32%. Several pathways are likely to be involved [21, 22]. Reported rates of RRT also vary widely, from 2 to 73% overall [23–25].

There is no specific treatment guideline for AKI related to COVID-19. Thus, general management should follow current recommendations for AKI of any etiology [26, 27]: (1) optimization of fluid balance, for example, fluid replacement in hypovolemic patients and diuretics/fluid restriction in fluid nonresponders; (2) prevention and treatment of acid–base disorders; (3) control of electrolytes, particularly potassium; (4) dosage adjustment of renally excreted drugs; (5) avoidance of nephrotoxic drugs; and (6) hemodynamic adjustments to avoid secondary kidney damage. When conservative management cannot maintain fluid, electrolyte, and acid–base homeostasis, RRT should be considered.

The decision to initiate RRT is also controversial in severely ill patients, since most studies exclude them [28–30]. It would not be different in severe COVID-19; the more critical a patient's illness, the lower the threshold for RRT initiation. Peritoneal dialysis (PD) is rarely used to manage patients with AKI in high-resource settings, but in developing countries, it is widely used in intensive-care settings as an alternative to continuous RRT [31, 32]. In severe COVID-19 patients requiring ventilatory support in the ICU, PD has been considered a safe and effective form of RRT. This represents another therapeutic option for COVID-19-related AKI, with the potential to stabilize hyperkalemia, acidosis, and fluid balance [33].

References

1. Nakos G, et al. Effect of the prone position on patients with hydrostatic pulmonary edema compared with patients with acute respiratory distress syndrome and pulmonary fibrosis. Am J Respir Crit Care Med. 2000;161(2 Pt 1):360–8.
2. Gattinoni L, et al. Effect of prone positioning on the survival of patients with acute respiratory failure. N Engl J Med. 2001;345(8):568–73.
3. Richard JC, et al. Effects of prone position and positive end-expiratory pressure on lung perfusion and ventilation. Crit Care Med. 2008;36(8):2373–80.
4. Broccard A, et al. Prone positioning attenuates and redistributes ventilator-induced lung injury in dogs. Crit Care Med. 2000;28(2):295–303.
5. Mentzelopoulos SD, et al. Prone position reduces lung stress and strain in severe acute respiratory distress syndrome. Eur Respir J. 2005;25(3):534–44.
6. Papazian L, et al. Comparison of prone positioning and high-frequency oscillatory ventilation in patients with acute respiratory distress syndrome. Crit Care Med. 2005;33(10):2162–71.
7. Galiatsou E, et al. Prone position augments recruitment and prevents alveolar overinflation in acute lung injury. Am J Respir Crit Care Med. 2006;174(2):187–97.
8. Guerin C, et al. Prone positioning in severe acute respiratory distress syndrome. N Engl J Med. 2013;368(23):2159–68.
9. Peek GJ, et al. Efficacy and economic assessment of conventional ventilatory support versus extracorporeal membrane oxygenation for severe adult respiratory failure (CESAR): a multicentre randomised controlled trial. Lancet. 2009;374(9698):1351–63.
10. Combes A, et al. Extracorporeal membrane oxygenation for severe acute respiratory distress syndrome. N Engl J Med. 2018;378(21):1965–75.
11. Combes A, et al. ECCO$_2$R therapy in the ICU: consensus of a European round table meeting. Crit Care. 2020;24(1):490.
12. Askenazi DJ, et al. Renal replacement therapy in critically ill patients receiving extracorporeal membrane oxygenation. Clin J Am Soc Nephrol. 2012;7(8):1328–36.

13. Moncada S. The 1991 Ulf von Euler lecture. The L-arginine: nitric oxide pathway. Acta Physiol Scand. 1992;145(3):201–27.
14. Ichinose F, et al. Inhaled nitric oxide: a selective pulmonary vasodilator: current uses and therapeutic potential. Circulation. 2004;109(25):3106–11.
15. Akaberi D, et al. Mitigation of the replication of SARS-CoV-2 by nitric oxide in vitro. Redox Biol. 2020;37:101734.
16. Uchimido R, et al. The glycocalyx: a novel diagnostic and therapeutic target in sepsis. Crit Care. 2019;23(1):16.
17. Lee HY, et al. Nox4 regulates the eNOS uncoupling process in aging endothelial cells. Free Radic Biol Med. 2017;113:26–35.
18. Csoma B, et al. Dysregulation of the endothelial nitric oxide pathway is associated with airway inflammation in COPD. Respir Res. 2019;20(1):156.
19. Chen L, et al. Inhalation of nitric oxide in the treatment of severe acute respiratory syndrome: a rescue trial in Beijing. Clin Infect Dis. 2004;39(10):1531–5.
20. Gabarre P, et al. Acute kidney injury in critically ill patients with COVID-19. Intensive Care Med. 2020;46(7):1339–48.
21. Sharkey RA, et al. The acute effects of oxygen and carbon dioxide on renal vascular resistance in patients with an acute exacerbation of COPD. Chest. 1999;115(6):1588–92.
22. Su H, et al. Renal histopathological analysis of 26 postmortem findings of patients with COVID-19 in China. Kidney Int. 2020;98(1):219–27.
23. Chan L, et al. Acute kidney injury in hospitalized patients with COVID-19. medRxiv. 2020;51:786.
24. Wang D, et al. Clinical characteristics of 138 hospitalized patients with 2019 novel coronavirus-infected pneumonia in Wuhan, China. JAMA. 2020;323(11):1061–9.
25. Rubin S, et al. Characterization of acute kidney injury in critically ill patients with severe coronavirus disease 2019. Clin Kidney J. 2020;13(3):354–61.
26. Palevsky PM, et al. KDOQI US commentary on the 2012 KDIGO clinical practice guideline for acute kidney injury. Am J Kidney Dis. 2013;61(5):649–72.
27. Ronco C, et al. Management of acute kidney injury in patients with COVID-19. Lancet Respir Med. 2020;8(7):738–42.
28. Gaudry S, et al. Initiation strategies for renal-replacement therapy in the intensive care unit. N Engl J Med. 2016;375(2):122–33.
29. Barbar SD, et al. Timing of renal-replacement therapy in patients with acute kidney injury and sepsis. N Engl J Med. 2018;379(15):1431–42.
30. Zarbock A, et al. Effect of early vs delayed initiation of renal replacement therapy on mortality in critically ill patients with acute kidney injury: the ELAIN randomized clinical trial. JAMA. 2016;315(20):2190–9.

31. Almeida CP, et al. Effect of peritoneal dialysis vs. haemodialysis on respiratory mechanics in acute kidney injury patients. Clin Exp Nephrol. 2018;22(6):1420–6.
32. Li PK, et al. Changes in the worldwide epidemiology of peritoneal dialysis. Nat Rev Nephrol. 2017;13(2):90–103.
33. Bowes E, et al. Acute peritoneal dialysis with percutaneous catheter insertion for COVID-19-associated acute kidney injury in intensive care: experience from a UK tertiary center. Kidney Int Rep. 2021;6(2):265–71.

MIX
Papier aus verantwortungsvollen Quellen
Paper from responsible sources
FSC® C105338

If you have any concerns about our products, you can contact us on
ProductSafety@springernature.com

In case Publisher is established outside the EU, the EU authorized representative is:
Springer Nature Customer Service Center GmbH
Europaplatz 3, 69115 Heidelberg, Germany

Printed by Libri Plureos GmbH
in Hamburg, Germany